Register Now for Online Access to Your Book!

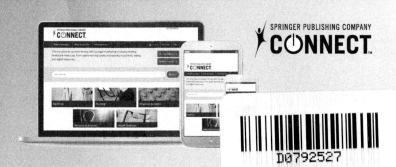

Your print purchase of *Handbook of Sup...
Palliative Care,* **includes online access to the contents of your
book**—increasing accessibility, portability, and searchability!

Access today at:

**http://connect.springerpub.com/content/book/978-0-8261-2828-7
or scan the QR code at the right with your smartphone
and enter the access code below.**

H937DP3Y

*Scan here for
quick access.*

If you are experiencing problems accessing the digital component of this product, please contact our
customer service department at cs@springerpub.com

The online access with your print purchase is available at the publisher's discretion and may be
removed at any time without notice.

Publisher's Note: New and used products purchased from third-party sellers are not guaranteed for
quality, authenticity, or access to any included digital components.

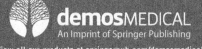

demosMEDICAL
An Imprint of Springer Publishing

View all our products at springerpub.com/demosmedical

Handbook of Supportive Oncology and Palliative Care

Whole-Person Adult and Pediatric Care

Editors

Ann M. Berger, MSN, MD
Pain and Palliative Care
Bethesda, Maryland

Pamela S. Hinds, PhD, RN, FAAN
Executive Director
Department of Nursing Science, Professional Practice & Quality
The William and Joanne Conway Chair of Nursing Research
The Research Integrity Officer
Children's National Health System
Professor of Pediatrics
The George Washington University School of Medicine and
*   Health Sciences*
Washington, DC

Christina M. Puchalski, MD, MS, FACP, FAAHPM
Professor of Medicine and Health Sciences
Director
The George Washington Institute for Spirituality and Health
*   (GWish)*
The George Washington University School of Medicine and
*   Health Sciences*
Washington, DC

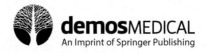

demosMEDICAL
An Imprint of Springer Publishing

Visit our website at www.Springerpub.com

ISBN: 9780826128249
ebook ISBN: 9780826128287
DOI: 10.1891/9780826128287

Acquisitions Editor: David D'Addona
Compositor: Exeter Premedia Services Pvt Ltd.

Library of Congress Cataloging-in-Publication Data

Names: Berger, Ann (Ann M.), editor. | Hinds, Pamela S., editor. | Puchalski, Christina M., editor.
Title: Handbook of supportive oncology and palliative care : whole-person adult and pediatric care / editors, Ann Berger, Pamela S. Hinds, Christina Puchalski.
Description: New York : Springer Publishing Company, [2019] | Includes bibliographical references and index.
Identifiers: LCCN 2018040265| ISBN 9780826128249 | ISBN 9780826128287 (ebook)
Subjects: | MESH: Neoplasms—therapy | Palliative Care—methods | Neoplasms—complications | Pain Management | Evidence-Based Medicine | Child | Adult
Classification: LCC RC271.P33 | NLM QZ 266 | DDC 616.99/4029—dc23
LC record available at https://lccn.loc.gov/2018040265

Printed in the United States of America.
18 19 20 21 22 / 5 4 3 2 1

To our spouses and children,
whose love and support make our work possible.
Carl, Stephen, Rebecca.
Ann M. Berger

With deep and lasting gratitude, I thank each patient, each family,
each student, and each colleague for patiently teaching me about
the needs of the human spirit while experiencing suffering.
Pamela S. Hinds

To all my patients who have inspired me through their strength
and courage in the midst of their suffering; they have taught me the
meaning of compassionate presence and love. To my students who
continually inspire me with their hopes and determination to bring
compassionate, whole-person care to all their patients.
Christina M. Puchalski

Contents

I. The Whole-Person Approach to Supportive Oncology and Palliative Care

II. Symptom Management of Advanced Cancer and Cancer Treatment

III. Supportive Oncology and Quality of Life Considerations for Patients, Families, and Caregivers

Contributors

Kevin Adams, MDiv, PhD, Staff Chaplain, Department of Chaplaincy Services and Pastoral Education, University of Virginia Health System, Charlottesville, Virginia

Rezvan Ameli, PhD, Clinical Psychologist, Clinical Center, National Institute of Mental Health, National Institutes of Health, Bethesda, Maryland

Ashley Anderson, BS, Student, Special Volunteer Pediatric Oncology Branch, National Cancer Institute, National Institutes of Health, Bethesda, Maryland

Allison J. Applebaum, PhD, Assistant Attending Psychologist, Director, Caregivers Clinic, Memorial Sloan Kettering Cancer Center, New York, New York

Karen Baker, MSN, CRNP, Clinician in Pain and Palliative Care, Faculty Member for Hospice and Palliative Care Medicine Fellowship, Clinical Center Pain and Palliative Care, National Institutes of Health, Bethesda, Maryland

Jill Bechaz, PharmD, Clinical Pharmacist, Department of Pediatrics, Children's Hospital and Medical Center, Omaha, Nebraska

Ann M. Berger, MSN, MD, Pain and Palliative Care, Bethesda, Maryland

Rebecca Berger, MSN, CPNP-AC, Nurse Practitioner, Johns Hopkins All Children's Hospital, Cancer and Blood Disorders Institute, St. Petersburg, Florida

Tara Berman, MD, Oncologist/Medical Officer, Gynecologic Malignancies, Food and Drug Administration, Silver Spring, Maryland

Margaret Bevans, PhD, RN, AOCN®, FAAN, Associate Director, Clinical Research, Office of Research on Women's Health, National Institutes of Health, Bethesda, Maryland

M. Jennifer Cheng, MD, Associate Program Director, Hospice and Palliative Medicine Fellowship Program, Senior Attending Physician, Pain and Palliative Care Service, Clinical Center, National Institutes of Health, Bethesda, Maryland

Julia Cheringal, MD, Fellow, Department of Pain and Palliative Care, Clinical Center, National Institutes of Health, Bethesda, Maryland

Jaydira Del Rivero, MD, Medical Oncology and Clinical Endocrinology, Director CCR Rare Tumor Clinic, Rare Tumor Initiative, Medical Oncology Service/Pediatric Oncology Branch, National Cancer Institute/ National Institutes of Health, Bethesda, Maryland

Brian Detwiler, BS, JD, Chief Legal Officer, Cobro Ventures, Inc., Arlington, Virginia

Kathryn Detwiler, BS, Parent and Program Lead for the Complex Care Program Within the Goldberg Center for Primary Care, Children's National Health System, Washington, DC

Deborah Fisher, PhD, RN, PPCNP-BC, CHPPN, Pediatric Nurse Practitioner / PANDA Palliative Care Team, Division of Hospitalist Medicine, Children's National Health System, Washington, DC

Amy M. Garee, PhD(c), RN, PNP, Pediatric Palliative Care Nurse Practitioner, Pain and Palliative Medicine, Nationwide Children's Hospital, Columbus, Ohio

Monika Gasiorek, BSc, Medical Student, Georgetown University School of Medicine, Washington, DC

Gleynora J. GilBhrighde, DO, Attending and Consulting Physician, Internal Medicine / Palliative Medicine, Summers County Appalachian Regional Hospital, Hinton, West Virginia

Laura Hofmann, MD, Fellow, Hospice and Palliative Medicine, Department of Geriatrics and Palliative Medicine, The George Washington University School of Medicine and Health Sciences, Washington, DC

Michael H. Hsieh, MD, PhD, Associate Professor, Urology and Pediatrics, Children's National Health System, Washington, DC

Shana S. Jacobs, MD, Associate Professor of Pediatrics, The George Washington University School of Medicine and Health Sciences; Attending Physician, Children's National Health System, Washington, DC

Najmeh Jafari, MD, Research Program Director, The George Washington Institute for Spirituality and Health (GWish), The George Washington School of Medicine and Health Sciences, Washington, DC

Anna B. Jolliffe, DO, FAAP, Clinical Instructor, Department of Psychiatry, University of Pittsburgh Medical Center, Pittsburgh, Pennsylvania

Robert M. Kaiser, MD, MHSc, Attending Physician, Geriatrics and Extended Care, Veterans Affairs Medical Center; Associate Professor of Medicine, Division of Geriatrics and Palliative Medicine, The George Washington University School of Medicine and Health Sciences, Washington, DC

Jessica Keim-Malpass, PhD, RN, Assistant Professor, School of Nursing, University of Virginia, Charlottesville, Virginia

Katherine Patterson Kelly, PhD, RN, Nurse Scientist, Department of Nursing Science, Professional Practice, and Quality; Associate Professor, The George Washington University School of Medicine and Health Sciences, Children's National Health System, Washington, DC

Ann H. Lichtenstein, DO, Associate Medical Director, Montgomery Hospice, Rockville, Maryland

Lisa C. Lindley, PhD, RN, FPCN, Associate Professor, College of Nursing, University of Tennessee, Knoxville, Tennessee

Maureen E. Lyon, PhD, ABPP, Professor of Pediatrics, The George Washington University School of Medicine and Health Sciences, Children's National Health System, Center for Translational Science/ Children's Research Institute, Washington, DC

Margaret M. Mahon, PhD, CRNP, FAAN, FPCN, Nurse Practitioner, Pain and Palliative Care, National Institutes of Health, Bethesda, Maryland

Rita A. Manfredi, MD, FACEP, Associate Professor of Clinical Emergency Medicine; Fellow, Hospice and Palliative Medicine, Department of Geriatrics and Palliative Medicine, The George Washington University School of Medicine and Health Sciences, Washington, DC

Ambereen K. Mehta, MD, MPH, Assistant Professor, Palliative Medicine, Department of Medicine, University of California Los Angeles, Los Angeles, California

Kim Mooney-Doyle, PhD, CPNP-AC, RN, Assistant Professor, Department of Family and Community Health, University of Maryland, School of Nursing, Baltimore, Maryland

Catriona Mowbray, PhD, BSN, RN, Research Nurse Coordinator for Supportive Care Studies, Division of Oncology, Children's National Medical Center, Washington, DC

Rachel Ombres, MD, Geriatric Medicine Fellow, Division of General, Geriatric, Palliative and Hospital Medicine, University of Virginia School of Medicine, Charlottesville, Virginia

Victoria D. Powell, MD, Hospice and Palliative Medicine Fellow, Pain and Palliative Care, National Institutes of Health, Bethesda, Maryland

Christina M. Puchalski, MD, MS, FACP, FAAHPM, Professor of Medicine and Health Sciences, Director, The George Washington Institute for Spirituality and Health (GWish), The George Washington University School of Medicine and Health Sciences, Washington, DC

Katalin Eve Roth, JD, MD, Professor of Medicine, Director, Division of Geriatrics and Palliative Medicine, The George Washington University School of Medicine and Health Sciences, Washington, DC

Juanita L. Smith, MD, Assistant Professor of Medicine, The Glennan Center for Geriatrics and Gerontology, Eastern Virginia Medical School, Norfolk, Virginia

David M. Steinhorn, MD, Professor of Pediatrics – Palliative Care and Critical Care, Children's National Medical Center, Washington, DC

Sarah M. Verga, DO, Hospice and Palliative Medicine Fellow, Department of Internal Medicine, Division of General Medicine, Geriatrics, Palliative and Hospital Medicine, University of Virginia Health System, Charlottesville, Virginia

Jeffrey Villanueva, MD, Chief Resident, Department of Urology, Medstar Georgetown Hospital, Washington, DC

Anne Watson, MSc, PhD, BSN, RN, Case Manager II, Clinical Resource Management, Children's National Health System, Washington, DC

Meaghann Weaver, MD, MPH, FAAP, Chief, Pediatric Palliative Care, Children's Hospital and Medical Center, Omaha, Nebraska

Andrew Whitman, PharmD, Clinical Pharmacist – Oncology/Palliative Care, University of Virginia Health System, Charlottesville, Virginia

Lori Wiener, PhD, DCSW, Co-Director, Behavioral Health Core, Head, Psychosocial Support and Research Program, Pediatric Oncology Program, National Cancer Institute, National Institutes of Health, Bethesda, Maryland

Preface

Palliative care begins at the time of diagnosis of any chronic and/or life-threatening disorder. As part of quality patient care, this care must focus on physical, psychological, social, and spiritual dimensions for the patient, caregiver, and family to achieve the best quality of life possible for any patient going through any phase of the oncological journey from diagnosis to cure or to end of life.

Palliative care is healthcare which focuses care on all aspects of the patient—emotional, social, and spiritual as well as physical issues. Thus, palliative care focuses on preventing, assessing, and treating all dimensions of pain and suffering. Palliative care additionally concentrates on accompanying patients and families during their illness journey to help them find healing and peace whether cure of the disease is possible or not. This care focus is done concurrently with the work of the oncologist, who primarily focuses on treatments given to an oncology patient that includes chemotherapy, immunotherapy, surgery, and radiation, all of which are focused on treating the cancer. The primary care doctor, nurse practitioner, and/or physician assistants, who are collaborating to treat the cancer, need to understand the principles of palliative care and, in particular, of primary palliative care. Treating the disease is important, but to achieve health and well-being to the extent possible for the patient and family, clinicians need to treat the whole person, including addressing psychosocial and spiritual suffering with a goal of helping patients find acceptance and healing as they define both. This can be done through the practice of primary palliative care (or basic palliative care) and, oftentimes, in collaboration with specialty palliative care providers.

Palliative care focuses on value-based care. Care is provided by a large interdisciplinary team, essentially an entire community of providers who treat the whole person and family. Doctors and nurses work with a larger interdisciplinary team with staff from multiple departments, including social work, chaplaincy, psychiatry, nutrition, recreation therapy, and pharmacy. The services offered are anything that needs to be done to relieve total pain and suffering and help quality of life. This includes pharmacologic management, emotional and spiritual counseling, and complementary modalities, such as acupuncture, massage therapy, art therapy, reiki, hypnosis, biofeedback, labyrinth, mandala, and pet therapy.

To achieve whole-person care, the oncologist, oncology nurse practitioner, and physician assistant must understand how to support an integrated care team. The provider needs to start by getting a patient story that includes all physical–medical, psychological, social, and spiritual dimensions. The provider needs to learn how to coordinate a single longitudinal care plan that is fluid and changes throughout the disease process but can also be delivered by all members of the interdisciplinary team. In addition, the provider needs to learn humanistic integrative care and how to communicate with a community of healthcare providers.

This book is meant to be a practical handbook for oncologists, residents, fellows, nurse practitioners, nurses, psychosocial providers, and physician assistants so that they understand and will be able to provide primary palliative care to patients and families who live with cancer. What is additionally emphasized is how to support an integrated team. Because medical care and oncologic care can be fragmented, we felt an urgent need to put this resource together for anyone entering oncology, nursing, primary care, or palliative care specialties. With this book, we hope to help the reader understand practical ways of integrating curing and healing and improve the quality of life for all patients and their families enduring disease-related and treatment-related symptoms.

Ann M. Berger, MSN, MD
Pamela S. Hinds, PhD, RN, FAAN
Christina M. Puchalski, MD, MS, FACP, FAAHPM

The Whole-Person Approach to Supportive Oncology and Palliative Care

Understanding the Adult Cancer Patient and Caregiver Perspective—The Illness Experience

1

Kim Mooney-Doyle

Recent estimates from the American Cancer Society indicate that nearly 610,000 people died from cancer in 2018, that is nearly 1,700 people each day. In most cases, these individuals are cared for by a family member or friend. Indeed, 7% of the general population is a caregiver to someone with cancer (1,2). This translates to approximately 4 million caregivers for adults with cancer in the United States. While most of these caregivers are women caring for their spouses and partners, nearly 20% are adult children of the individuals with cancer. In this role, caregivers often coordinate care and appointments, advise on treatment decision making, manage finances, and provide emotional support to the person with cancer. In fact, recent estimates indicate that even 1 year after diagnosis, caregivers still provided, on average, 8 hours of care each day (1). The number of hours likely increases in advanced cancer given that as the severity of disease increases, symptoms and their management become more intense, and care moves into the home. Taken together, we see that many individuals in the United States are providing increasingly intense supportive and instrumental care to family members and potentially feel overwhelmed and underprepared (1).

"Daddy, I love you, but you drive me crazy."

These were the last words I spoke to my father before he died approximately 6 months after being diagnosed with renal cell carcinoma. At this point, he had been receiving home hospice care for several weeks. My family and I cared for him throughout this time with the support of hospice nursing and social work services. It was a privilege to care for him at the end of his life and I strove to be the best daughter I could be in this heartbreaking context, yet it was hard. I can smile about the above quote now, 15 years later. But it still reminds me of the bittersweet and complex dynamics families experience as they lose a loved one. Caring for my father was both transformational and stifling, complete with times of laughter and frustration, and it prompted me to become both other-focused and withdrawn. My perspective on this experience was, and continues to be, informed by the fact that I am both an oncology nurse and a child affected by a parent's cancer. Being the person in two worlds can be confusing. One world is where I can understand the systems of oncology, palliative, and end-of-life (EOL) care that surrounded my father and family and the experiences of the healthcare providers. There is a bittersweet world where the image of my father lives on in the sweet faces of grandchildren he never met. This duality informs and inspires my work as a pediatric oncology nurse and palliative care researcher. This chapter offers theoretically and experientially based approaches to help oncology clinicians in their interactions with family caregivers of adult patients approaching their EOL.

- A theoretical framework for use by clinicians to interpret and gain understanding of interactions with family caregivers of the dying adult oncology patient:
  - The family ecological framework illuminates the multiple actors and their intersecting relationships when a loved one nears the end of life and will guide the chapter.
  - This framework is rooted in systems theory and has four underlying tenets:
    - "Individual behavior can only be understood within its social context" (3).
    - "Individuals exist within a number of interdependent systems and contexts" (3).
    - "The reciprocal relationship between individual and social systems with which they interact are vital for understanding development" (3).
    - "Variables beyond the level of individual attributes (social and cultural), especially those that address the interaction between individual and system, must be included to understand adaptation processes" (3).
  - This framework maintains that:
    - Individuals, in considering their development, are nested within families or other groups of loved ones; within communities, schools, neighborhoods, workplaces; within healthcare systems; within the sociopolitical context of their immediate area and beyond (healthcare and social policy that influences coverage of care, family leave, work protections; science policy that directs funding for particular areas of research).
    - Individual actors and systems change over time, as do their interactions.
    - The patient is at the center of this model.
    - Patients affected by life-threatening conditions experience a range of emotions, are often afraid, and may have had an extensive "diagnostic odyssey" (4) by the time they reach oncology.
    - They are exhausted, yet often have to initiate marathon-like treatment that involves travel, role adjustments, employment changes, and fears of burdening their families or friends.
  - Immediately surrounding the patient is the family and family caregivers or care partners, a close group of intimately involved individuals with a history and a past (5).
    - The group has also traveled along the "diagnostic odyssey" of monitoring symptoms; suggesting the patient get a symptom

checked out; accompanying the patient to initial primary care and specialist appointments; providing frontline emotional, psychological, and possibly financial support; scheduling second opinions and treatment centers; consulting Dr. Google for information about the disease that is disrupting their lives; and living with uncertainty.

- ○ As the AARP policy statement reports, caregivers are a precious, but limited resource (2).
- ○ Considering the toll this can take on an individual, standardized, accessible support for family caregivers' mental health has been recommended (6).
- ▪ These two groups are surrounded by the wider community that includes places of employment, neighborhoods, places of worship, and healthcare systems and providers.
  - ○ These sites can be both sources of support or sources of stress.
  - ○ Family caregivers and patients traverse their surrounding environments; thus, not only is each person affected by his or her own interactions with agencies and institutions, but also by how similar interactions affect family members. For example, I was not only affected by my own interactions with my father's healthcare providers, but also by his interactions with those same providers.
  - ○ These interactions have implications for the patient and the caregiver.
- • Understanding adults within the context of a family system:
  - ▪ It is vitally important for healthcare providers to broaden their understanding of the patient with cancer to the context in which the person lives as a parent, grandparent, spouse/partner, friend, employee, and community member.
  - ▪ Going through this experience, as both a caregiving daughter and an oncology nurse, it became increasingly clear to me that this broader thinking was missing in the care of adults with cancer.
  - ▪ I recognized that the clinicians were trying to get by (and, probably, often felt overwhelmed and distressed as I often did in my own work) and I hated to bother them.
  - ▪ Yes, they were overwhelmed and distressed from a night shift load of 13 patients per nurse or from caring for an entire unit as a resident where multiple patients experience cardiac and respiratory arrest in one shift. I don't want to minimize the pain and distress of multiple losses we experience as clinicians. It is incredibly painful to bear witness to suffering, to feel powerless, and to work daily in a context in which one's own suffering is not recognized (7).
  - ▪ Yet, there were limits to their understanding of our family or that, I as a family caregiver, was overwhelmed and distressed, too. This was our suffering; our family did not get a second chance to do this the right way. Our beloved family member was dying. We did not get to leave (8).

- Caregivers and support:
  - There has been a long-standing debate about whether providing support for bereaved care partners or family caregivers should fall within the scope of palliative care (9).
  - Yet, recent research demonstrates that caregiver health is an important component of cancer care and should be routinely assessed.
  - There are several compelling reasons to assess and support care partners or family caregivers:
    - Supporting the family caregiver can improve the patient's symptom and emotional outcomes.
    - Assessing distress and providing meaningful support to the family caregivers may improve their health outcomes.
    - The healthcare system that cares for aging adults with chronic life-threatening illnesses is built on the backs of family caregivers and care partners; quite often, the treatment plans we make as healthcare providers would not be achievable without care partner and family caregiver support (18).
    - Family caregivers and care partners have identified positive elements of this role. Targeted interventions for them based in the palliative care setting can help to elucidate these potential sources of posttraumatic growth (20).
    - Supporting the family caregiver is the right thing to do. No matter how much one prepares for the death of a family member and no matter how old the dying person is, the losing and the loss are still difficult.
  - Family caregivers perform medical and nursing tasks that lessen the ill person's pain and symptoms, allow for greater independence, and avoid out-of-home placement (2).
    - These effects were especially magnified for those patients with five or more chronic conditions (19).
      - The presence and support of family caregivers influenced patient quality of life by performing medical/nursing tasks that decreased pain, promoted involvement in the family, and avoided institutionalization for the patient (19).
      - This report (2) reminds healthcare professionals and policymakers that family caregivers are often invisible in the adult healthcare system, that nearly half perform medical/nursing tasks in addition to personal care of the patient and household management, with minimal support and training (2,19).
      - "A healthcare system that relies on untrained and unpaid family members to perform skilled medical/nursing tasks, but does not train and support them, has lost sight of its primary mission of providing humane and compassionate care to sick people and their families" (2, p. 34).
        - While the creation of caregiver-friendly healthcare environments requires collective effort, "…such action will not be effective without individual commitment" (2, p. 34).

- Healthcare providers across disciplines can encourage questions, assess learning needs, and provide information regarding additional supports.
- Organizations must create environments that facilitate transitions of patients and caregivers across settings, from acute care to community settings, and within community settings as people live with their life-limiting illnesses.

- Family caregivers of adults can experience greater distress and anxiety than the patient (9):
  - Over 40% of care partners and family caregivers report at least 10 unmet needs (9), including gaps in illness management information and lack of emotional support.
  - It is difficult to predict which family caregivers or care partners will have issues, thus systematic assessment is required that directs interventions and services.
  - This is especially true as the population ages and care partners and family caregivers face increased duties and responsibilities of illness management, emotional support, care coordination, and information seeking.
  - Caregivers of older adults experience nearly twice as much psychological distress versus controls (10).
    - "Family caregiving for older adults with cancer is the result of both demographic and healthcare delivery changes...Cancer leads to change in family and identity roles, daily functioning, and the effects of such change can be profound and long-lasting" (10, p. 269).
  - Brief interventions that assess caregiver emotional/social health in late-stage cancer diagnoses have demonstrated a positive influence on the caregiver's perception of EOL care (18);
  - Caregivers who perceive that their loved one is receiving high-quality EOL care may experience better social health than those who did not receive the intervention (11).
  - Family caregivers report positive effects of providing care to the patient, such as perception of inner growth and strength, meaning appreciation of humor, love, resilience, and feeling a sense of reward (12).
    - Perceived benefits include increased sensitivity and empathy, greater appreciation for life, development of meaningful interpersonal relationships, potentially increased self-efficacy, motivation to reconnect family relationships.
    - In adult children of people with cancer, posttraumatic growth moderated the relationship between the stress of the illness situation of their parent and posttraumatic stress disorder (PTSD) (20).
      - The meaning ascribed to the experience or the perceived growth that results from the experience of caring for a parent with cancer can minimize the effect of psychological distress for daughters who are caregivers to their parents with cancer.

        □ Targeted interventions that support meaning-making or social connection may help decrease psychological distress in family caregivers as they live with and survive cancer in their loved one.

- Five points to guide family-focused care for the adult family caregiver:
  - The relationship between healthcare professionals and family members is vitally important. Similar to the concept of "being a good parent to a seriously ill child" (13), adults caring for their family members near the EOL may also strive to fulfill their internal definition of being a good spouse, partner, child, sibling, parent, cousin, or friend. Thoughtful words can help to reframe negative beliefs and limit feelings of guilt.
  - As vitally important as healthcare professionals are, they are but one part of a system that orbits loved ones with cancer at EOL (14). Adult caregivers have feet in multiple worlds; sometimes these worlds coexist peacefully and sometimes they collide.
  - Language matters across all sectors of healthcare, EOL care, and bereavement services. Communication across all sectors of the healthcare system, from the daily, mundane communication to the intense, life-altering communication, makes a difference and influences a caregiver's perception of the system and those who work in it.
    - Communication may be considered part of the "microethics: the ethics of every day clinical practice" (15, p.11).
      - The conversations between clinicians and nonclinicians within a clinical setting contribute to constructing the narrative of the family member's experiences as the patient and the experiences of the caregivers.
      - "Microethics are created in the relational space between participants. . .at a particular moment in time...through verbal and nonverbal communication" (15, p.12).
      - The following scenarios I experienced walking the line between oncology nurse and caregiver daughter illustrate gaps in communication. These were likely unintentional microethics infractions; a clinician or nonclinician representative of the healthcare system (both the one I personally encountered and the system communicated through research) entered that relational space between us and I was left confused and disappointed in both systems.
        - Although comical now, it was infuriating when the billing representative at the hospital asked when my father expired (I responded, "Uh, he wasn't a carton of milk.").
        - Or when the insurance representative told me that they simply could not share billing information with me, that they had to talk to my father, after he had already died (I responded, "Um, I wish you could, however, as I mentioned earlier, he died.").

- Or when the nurse caring for him states, "You know he's going to die, right?," when I ask when the team is going on the round, after I have waited at his bedside all day (I responded, "Yes, I know, but that doesn't mean they give up on him.").
- Or when research studies and papers call us "informal caregivers" (I still don't laugh at this; it still feels pejorative and classist). I am confident that other terms can be created by this erudite group, including care partners or caregivers. Researchers and authors should consider using a term that is more descriptive of our role.
  - While "informal" versus "professional" denotes the difference between those paid for their caregiving and those who are not paid, the truth is that we, as "informal caregivers," can pay dearly for our role in strained relationships, lost wages, lapses in career development, diminished physical and mental health, diminished quality of life, and strong emotions and negative thoughts that follow us into bereavement and beyond.
  - There is growth and transformation that comes from the experience of caring for a loved one at the EOL. You live daily with the humbling recognition that life is so very short. This growth carries heft with it.
- Even though adults with cancer are the model on which so much of our hospice system is built, the American health care system is still built on the backs of family caregivers (2). This takes a toll, yet many of the caregivers perceive it to be their duty. Health professionals must help them fulfill this duty in a way that does not harm them. The experiences of parents caring for children with life-threatening and life-limiting illnesses may illuminate the drive and strategies that healthcare providers can utilize (16,17).
- Healthcare has got to and can do better. Healthcare providers in any given field may have limited knowledge of what it is like to live with the illnesses of their specialty or to be involved as a family caregiver. Healthcare professionals may also have limited insights into the role and function if they do not occupy a similar role themselves. For example, it may be hard to empathize with a hovering parent if one does not have children.

In pediatrics, family is a recognized system and integral part of development. I think there is a place for it in adult palliative care and oncology, too, to benefit patients, caregivers, and healthcare providers. It is not enough to have "next of kin" or a spouse/child's phone number recorded in the chart or a healthcare proxy/decision maker. The envelope of care needs to be broadened since family members suffer, as do the involved healthcare providers. An earlier inclusion of palliative care could potentially address that, but the oncology team has to adopt the mindset that family matters. Family is not just something within the purview of the palliative care team.

Some might say, "Pediatrics is a different beast." Parents care for a vulnerable child, who has limited decision-making capacity and make decisions in the child's best interest. Or, in the case of adolescents/young adults, they serve as surrogate decision makers and incorporate the young person's values and goals into the process. Yet, not extending family-centered care to ill adults erects a false dichotomy. Adult patients may have reached the age of majority and may have demonstrated capacity, yet the shock and grief that accompanies diagnosis and life threat, as well as the cognitive and physical side effects of treatment, amplify the uncertainty and isolation of the situation. A healthcare system, which cares for ill adults, yet does not incorporate the family, sets the patient up for failure and the caregivers up for increasing burden, poor quality of life, diminished health, and potentially complex grief and bereavement. Adult-focused healthcare providers may like to rely on the four traditional bioethical principles: autonomy, beneficence, nonmaleficence, and justice. However, this concept has limitations in that it does not take relationships into account. In the context of oncology and palliative care, relationships are everything.

REFERENCES

1. American Cancer Society. *Cancer Facts and Figures 2018*. Atlanta: American Cancer Society; 2018.
2. American Association of Retired Persons (AARP). *Caregiving in the U.S. Executive Summary*. Washington, DC: AARP Public Policy Institute and National Institute for Caregiving; 2015.
3. Pedersen S, Revenson TA. Parental Illness, Family Functioning, and Adolescent Well-Being. *J Fam Psychol*. 2005;19(3):404–409. doi:10.1037/0893-3200.19.3.404
4. Basel D, McCarrier J. Ending a diagnostic odyssey: Family education, counseling, and response to eventual diagnosis. *Pediatr Clin N Am*. 2017;64(1):265–272. doi:10.1016/j.pcl.2016.08.017
5. Rolland JS. Chronic illness and the life cycle: a conceptual framework. *Family Process*. 1987; 26(2):203–221. doi:10.1111/j.1545-5300.1987.00203.x
6. Cadovius N. Who cares for the caregivers? We all do." Health Affairs Blog". 2017. https://www.healthaffairs.org/do/10.1377/hblog20171022.320285/full/
7. Campbell SM, Ulrich CM, Grady C. A broader understanding of moral distress. *Am J Bioeth*. 2016;16(12):2–9. doi:10.1080/15265161.2016.1239782
8. Janvier A. I would never want this for my baby. *Pediatr Crit Care Med*. 2009;10(1):113–114. doi:10.1097/pcc.0b013e3181937adf
9. Sklenarova H, Krumpelmann A, Haun MW, et al. When do we need to care about the caregiver? Supportive care needs, anxiety, and depression among informal caregivers of patients with cancer and cancer survivors. *Cancer*. 2015;121(9):1513–1519. doi:10.1002/cncr.29223
10. Weitzner MA, Haley WE, Chen H. The family caregiver of the older cancer patient. *Hematol Oncol Clin North Am*. 2000;14(1):269–281. doi:10.1016/S0889-8588(05)70288-4
11. Douglas SL, Daly BJ. Effect of an integrated cancer support team on caregiver satisfaction with end-of-life care. *Oncol Nurs Forum*. 2014;41(4):E248–E255. doi:10.1188/14.ONF.E248-E255
12. Weisser FB, Bristowe K, Jackson D. Experiences of burden, needs, rewards and resilience in family caregivers of people living with motor neuron disease, amyotrophic lateral sclerosis: a secondary thematic analysis of qualitative interviews. *Palliat Med*. 2015;29(8):737–745. doi:10.1177/0269216315575851
13. Hinds PS, Oakes LL, Hicks J, et al. "Trying to be a good parent" as defined by interviews with parents who made phase I, terminal care, and resuscitation decisions for their children. *J Clin Oncol*. 2009;27(35):5979–5985. doi:10.1200/jco.2008.20.0204

14. Palacio RJ. *Wonder*. New York, NY: Knopf; 2012.
15. Truog RD, Brown SD, Browning D, et al. Microethics: the ethics of everyday clinical practice. *Hastings Cent Rep*. 2015;45(1):11–17. doi:10.1002/hast.413
16. Mooney-Doyle K, dos Santos MR, Szylit R, Deatrick JA. Parental expectations of support from healthcare providers during pediatric life-threatening illnesses: a secondary qualitative analysis. *J Pediatr Nurs*. 2017;36:163–172. doi:10.1016/j.pedn.2017.05.008
17. Janvier A, Lantos J, Aschner J, et al. Stronger and more vulnerable: a balanced view of the impacts of the NICU experience on parents. *Pediatrics*. 2016;138(3):e201606655. doi:10.1542/peds.2016-0655
18. National Academies of Sciences, Engineering, and Medicine. *Families caring for an aging America*. Washington, DC: National Academies Press; 2016.
19. Reinhard SC, Levine C, Samis S. *Home Alone: Family Caregivers Providing Complex Chronic Care*. Washington, DC: AARP Public Policy Institute; 2012.
20. Teixeira RJ, Pereira MG. Factors contributing to posttraumatic growth and its buffering effect in adult children of cancer patients undergoing treatment. *J Psychosoc Oncol*. 2013;31(3):235–265. doi:10.1080/07347332.2013.778932

Understanding the Pediatric Cancer Patient and Caregiver Perspective — The Illness Experience

2

Kathryn Detwiler, Brian Detwiler, Deborah Fisher, and Katherine Patterson Kelly

INTRODUCTION AND BACKGROUND

In the United States, over 500,000 children and their families cope with potentially life-threatening, complex chronic conditions (1). Childhood cancer accounts for less than 20% of children under the care of a pediatric palliative care (PPC) program. Children with chronic progressive conditions including genetic/congenital and neuromuscular conditions, among others, account for the vast majority of children in palliative care programs (2). While cancer continues to be the most common diagnosis for adult palliative care patients, it is less common in PPC. As such we illustrate common issues in PPC using a case representative of other complex chronic conditions that are more commonplace within PPC. Case illustrations are italicized throughout the chapter.

A FAMILY'S VIEW

Nolan's Story

Most parents want to be good parents (3), which is why there are thousands of books, blogs, and Pinterest boards dedicated to this topic. My husband and I are no exception; we too strive to be good parents to our 2-year-old son, Nolan (Figure 2.1). However, our definition of "good" might be a little different from the norm because we are the adoptive parents of a seriously ill, medically fragile child. Our son was born full-term with complex gastroschisis (Box 2.1). He is now an intestinal rehabilitation patient with short-gut syndrome. He is dependent on a central line for total parenteral nutrition (TPN) and a g-tube for enteral feeds, and he is likely to have multiple surgeries in the future to lengthen his bowel.

In Nolan's first year of life, he spent over 3 months in the hospital and another 45 days in the outpatient setting. As parents, we struggle to find the right balance between providing care and letting him grow up like any other healthy kid. We want to focus on his health but also give him the opportunities to become a young man who is not defined by his condition. He has such a warm personality and an inquisitive mind that is just waiting to explore the world. We believe that palliative care can help us achieve the right balance.

From the moment Nolan became a member of our family, we knew that we wanted the good moments to outnumber the bad. And they have. On his first birthday, after months of physical therapy, Nolan crawled for the very first

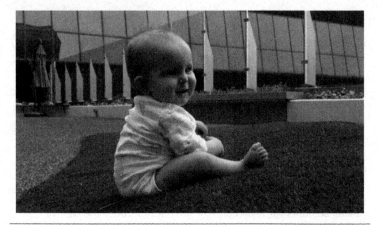

Figure 2.1 Nolan at age 2 playing in the children's hospital healing garden.

time across his grandparents' living room to get his bottle, which he craved so dearly. During one of his countless admissions, Nolan met with six members of Congress to share his story and the valuable role of Medicaid. Nolan is an ambassador—literally a poster child—for one of our hospital's annual fundraisers. Every good moment has been the direct result of the village that works so hard every day to support our family. Our biggest advocates have provided primary palliative care and include our primary pediatrician and advance practice registered nurse, as well as our providers on the consultative complex care team.

Many said we were the ideal parents for Nolan, well-resourced and informed about palliative medicine and its benefits. We know that . . .

- PPC is an organized system of holistic care for children with life-threatening conditions and their families, which focuses on relief of symptoms, pain, and stress caused by a serious illness or its treatment, combining aggressive symptom control with provision of timely, accurate information and support in decision making to help families live as normally as possible (4).
- Palliative medicine is **not** another word for hospice or euthanasia.

Box 2.1 Definition of Gastroschisis

Gastroschisis is one of the most common fetal abdominal wall defects. It is characterized by the absence of a covering membrane surrounding the protrusion of fetal bowel. Although the survival rate is relatively high at 90%, surviving children may suffer lifelong complex health problems including short bowel syndrome necessitating multiple specialty providers and leading to technology dependence and increased risk of mortality.

- Palliative medicine **does not** mean giving up treatment, hope, or curative options; but using them concurrently.
- Palliative medicine is a fellowship-trained and boarded subspecialty.
- Some primary providers may resist incorporating palliative medicine into their patients' care teams because disparity exists between the physician and nonphysician pediatric providers in terms of their perceptions of palliative care.
- Physicians may be concerned that palliative care could affect their role with their own patients, that palliative care is inconsistent with cure-directed therapy, or that their emotions could bias recommendations for different treatment modalities (5).
- Other concerns include caring for children with uncertain prognoses, role overlap among teams, perceptions that the family is not ready to acknowledge a potentially incurable disease, cultural barriers, time constraints, and lack of knowledge regarding novel pain management strategies used in palliative care (6).

COMMUNICATION

In addition to worrying about Nolan's symptoms, our family bears a heavy burden of anticipatory grief. Anticipatory grief is the emotional and physical manifestation of knowing that you will lose a child, leaving you haunted by a lifetime of wondering. While not all-consuming, we carry this grief every day, knowing that we may outlive our child. We fret about milestones that Nolan may never attain. We hope that medical science makes great leaps and saves him just in time. Palliative medicine teams help families cope with anticipatory grief. They provide the tools necessary to actualize Rose Kennedy's sentiment that "life isn't a matter of milestones, but of moments" (7).

Decision Making

Medical information can be overwhelming and difficult to understand. As a family navigates a new diagnosis or approaches a decision-making juncture, they seek clear and honest verbal and written information from their providers to help them understand and accept the diagnosis or problem (8). Families will be tasked with numerous medical decisions. Families prefer shared decision making, which is the cornerstone of patient and family-centered care. In shared decision making:

- Parents want support both during and after the decision-making process (8).
- They want to hear their providers' recommendations, but retain the option to pursue a different path.
- Incongruent messages from providers contribute to the stress of decision making.
- Other factors that may impact decision making include (9):
  - Prognostic uncertainty
  - Perception of child's quality of life
  - Staff acknowledgment of parents' role as experts on their child

- Perception of hope
- Above all, trust in the healthcare team, the most important factor (8)

From a Parent to a Provider: Tips and Tricks

- Be confident and honest when delivering bad news. Parents will react in different ways, but we all need to start with the realistic truth.
- Learn the first names of your patients' parents and immediate family members, for example, by keeping notes in the patients' charts. Parents like it when you use their first names rather than "mom" or "dad" all the time.
- Treat your patients like they are part of the team. Acknowledge them—include them in decisions—listen to them.
- Family-centered care means including the family in all of the care. Invite and encourage parents to participate in rounds. Practice closed-loop communication. Learn it and live it.
- Be relatable, supportive, kind, and fun.

CAREGIVING DEMAND

Healthcare providers must recognize the tremendous burden and strain borne by those caring for the child with special healthcare needs. This caregiving is vital to the overall well-being of the child.

A few facts about caregivers for children with complex healthcare needs:

- Over 3 million formal and informal caregivers provide care for children who are less than 18 years of age and have special healthcare needs (10).
- The majority of the caregivers are parents or grandparents (10).
- Caregivers of children with complex healthcare needs often spend at least 2 hours per week on care coordination (11).
- Providers should focus on ways to decrease caregiving demand (Table 2.1).
- Overall, parents strive to do the right thing for their child and by doing so, strive to be a good parent.
- Staff working with children with complex chronic conditions should have a working knowledge of family systems and childhood development (1).

*Life as a parent to a medically fragile child is VERY stressful and can lead to depression and anxiety. It has been incredibly important to us that we receive **permission** and **tools for self-care**. Self-care can seem indulgent, but it is easy to overlook the immense value that rest and good health can bring to a very stressful life.*

SUPPORTING THE FAMILY

A child's serious illness impacts the whole family. According to Social Ecological Theory (Figure 2.2), when you support and impact even one family member there will be results for the entire family. Accordingly, it's

Table 2.1 Interventions to Alleviate Caregiving Demand

Category	Potential resources*⁺	Description of resource
Financial	Supplemental Security Income	Provides cash for basic needs such as rent, clothing, food
Fatigue	Respite resources • The ARCH National Respite Network and Resource Center	Transitional hospitals In home respite Community based respite
Employment	Family Medical Leave Act (FMLA) Local resources	Provides up to 12 weeks per year of unpaid leave Some states offer paid leave
Respect for parental role	Shared decision-making model	Parents are provided accurate information
Feelings of isolation	Support groups	Disease-specific online support groups offer connection to other families with similar experiences

Self-care tips from Kate and Brian:
Maintain a journal, use aromatherapy, take a walk, practice yoga, read a book, take a shower, listen to music, color or try art therapy, compliment someone.
Give yourself the love, care, and attention that you so freely give to others. Forgive yourself for what is not accomplished today and try again tomorrow.

*Eligibility requirements vary
⁺ Local, regional and national benefits vary. Not an exhaustive list of resources available. Referral to social work and case management may assist in identifying resources available

extremely valuable for individual members of a multidisciplinary team to attend to each family member. Healthcare providers can support various members of the family by:

• Processing and managing the flow of information
• Adjusting priorities
• Rearranging family roles
• Assigning meaning to the illness
• Managing the treatment of the illness

It is through these activities that families try to normalize their lives (12).

Likewise, working to ensure palliative care services are available to all children will create a reciprocal impact on the child, family, and the healthcare system.

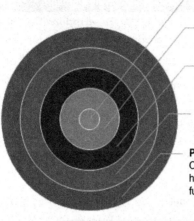

Child

Family, friends, school

Organization
Pediatric palliative care programs available

Community
Pediatric hospice available

Public policy
Concurrent hospice care funding available

Figure 2.2 Social-ecological model.

Supporting the Ill Child

The impact of a child's serious illness extends beyond the family and into the community (13). Attending school and being a student is an important part of a child's life and identity. Friendships, athletic team members, and spiritual and religious communities may play significant roles in addressing psychosocial, spiritual, and emotional needs (14). Accordingly, healthcare providers' reach must extend beyond the walls of the hospital.

Caring for Nolan comes with a range of challenges, including the otherwise ordinary tasks of taking short vacations or trips to visit out-of-town family members. The logistical requirements of making sure that Nolan has an uninterrupted supply of TPN, medications, and supplies can be daunting at times. But Nolan's care team has pulled through time and again so that Nolan can experience traditional family moments. Once, during a trip to a wedding in Chicago (where Nolan was the ring-bearer), one of his TPN bags sprung a leak. We were able to reach his pharmacist over the weekend, who immediately overnighted a replacement bag, which allowed us to finish our trip as planned. Moments like these are so important to Nolan's social and emotional development, and we cannot imagine our lives without them.

A critical component of caring for ill children is understanding and supporting their underlying developmental needs. This includes normalizing their lives as much as possible (Table 2.2), which could mean arranging for a child dying of acute lymphocytic leukemia (ALL) to achieve her dream of going to kindergarten, even if only for a few hours. Or it might mean rearranging treatment to ensure an adolescent makes it to his or her prom. The ultimate purpose is to listen to each child, identify his or her dreams, and promote flexible and creative care plans that seek to achieve those dreams.

Table 2.2 The Illness Experience: The Child and Adolescent

	Infant	Toddler	Preschooler	School-age child	Adolescent
Developmental task	Achievement of awareness of being separate from significant others	Invitation of autonomy	Creation of sense of initiative	Development of sense of industry	Achievement of a sense of identity
Impact of illness	Potential distortion of differentiation of self from parent/significant others	Interference with loss of developing sense of control, independence	Interference/loss of accomplishments such as walking, talking, controlling basic bodily functions	Potential feelings of inadequacy/inferiority if autonomy and independence are compromised	Potential alteration / relinquishment of newly acquired roles and responsibilities
Cognitive age/stage	Sensorimotor (birth through 2 years)	Preoperational thought (2–7 years): egocentric, magical, little concept of bodily integrity	Preoperational thought: egocentric, magical tendency to use and repeat words they don't understand, providing own explanations and definitions. Literal translation of words. Inability to abstract	Concrete operation thought (7–10+ years): beginning of logical thought but tendency to be literal	Formal operational thought (11+ years): beginning of ability to think abstractly. Existence of some magical thinking (e.g., feeling guilty for illness) and egocentrism

(continued)

Table 2.2 The Illness Experience: The Child and Adolescent *(continued)*

	Infant	Toddler	Preschooler	School-age child	Adolescent
Major fears	Separation, strangers	Separation, loss of control	Bodily injury and mutilation; loss of control; the unknown; the dark; being left alone	Loss of control; bodily injury and mutilation; failure to live up to expectation of important others; death	Loss of control; altered body image; separation from peer group
Concept of illness	N/A	Phenomenism (2–7 years): perceives external, unrelated, concrete phenomenon as cause of illness, e.g., "being sick because you don't feel well" Contagion: perceives cause of illness as proximity between two events that occurs by "magic", e.g. "getting a cold because you are near someone who has a cold"	Phenominism; contagion	Contamination: perceives cause as a person, object, or action external to the child that is "bad" or "harmful" to the body, e.g. getting a cold because you didn't wear a hat Internalization: perceives illness as having an external cause but being located inside the body, e.g. "getting a cold by breathing in air and bacteria"	Physiologic: perceives cause as a malfunctioning or nonfunctioning organ or process; can explain illness in sequence of events Psychophysiologic: realizes that psychologic actions and attitudes affect health and illness

(continued)

20

Table 2.2 The Illness Experience: The Child and Adolescent *(continued)*

	Infant	Toddler	Preschooler	School-age child	Adolescent
Interventions	Provide consistent caretakers	Minimize separation from parents/ significant others	Provide simple concrete explanations.	Provide choices whenever possible to increase the child's sense of control	Allow adolescent to be an integral part of decision making regarding care
	Minimize separation from parents/ significant others	Keep security objects at hand	Advance preparation is important: days for major events, hours for minor events	Stress contact with peer group	Give information sensitively, since this age group reacts to content of information as well as the manner in which it is delivered
	Decrease parental anxiety, which is projected on the infant	Provide simple, brief explanations	Verbal explanations are usually insufficient, so use pictures, models, actual equipment, medical play	Use diagrams, pictures, and models for explanations, because thinking is concrete	
	Maintain crib/ nursery as "safe place" in which noninvasive procedures are performed	Explain and maintain consistent limits		Emphasize the "normal" things the child can do, because the child does not want to be seen as different	Allow as many choices and as much control as possible
		Encourage participation in daily care, etc.			Be honest about treatment and consequences
		Provide opportunities for play and play therapy		Reassure child he or she has done nothing wrong; hospitalization, etc., is not "punishment"	Stress what the adolescent can do for himself or herself and the importance of cooperation and compliance
					Assist in maintaining contact with peer group

Source: From Armstrong-Dailey A, Zarbock S. *Hospice Care for Children* 3rd ed. New York, NY: Oxford University Press; 2009:57–59. Reprinted with permission.

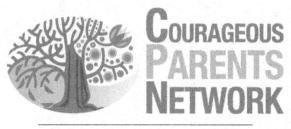

Figure 2.3 Courageous parents network.

Source: https://courageousparentsnetwork.org

Supporting Parents

A parent's definition of being a "good parent" for his or her child is a very personal and influential aspect of medical decision making (15,16). Fear of judgment for making a controversial choice, such as foregoing or withdrawing medically provided nutrition or hydration, may impact important decisions (17). To assist parents with these decisions, it may be helpful to remind them that good parenting includes: focusing on their child's health and spiritual well-being, advocating for their child, making informed decisions, and making sure their child feels loved (16).

We have found the Courageous Parent Network (CPN) (Figure 2.3) to be a valuable source of information. Started by a bereaved family, CPN provides parents and care providers a nontraditional source of online education, community, and advocacy through blog posts and videos of families and providers caring for children with serious medical conditions.

Supporting Siblings

Siblings of children with serious illness can feel excluded and resent being separated from their parent as well as the sick child (18,19). Further, the stress of having a seriously ill brother or sister may manifest as anxiety, depression, or even posttraumatic stress (20). With proper support, however, some studies have shown minimal impact and even posttraumatic growth (21). Accordingly, providers should offer support services to siblings also (20,22). Through developmentally appropriate and supportive care, healthcare providers can promote resilience, enhance coping skills, and prevent psychosocial difficulties.

We each have two siblings and always imagined having several children so that they too could share in the joy of siblinghood. As we discuss the possibility of a brother or sister for Nolan, we cannot ignore the stressors and concerns already mentioned. However, if we decide to grow our family further, we hope that thoughtful parenting, a solid support system, and a bit of luck will enable our children to thrive together.

Ways to Support Siblings

- When the chance arises, talk directly with siblings (using their name) and ask the ill child and the parents how the siblings are doing.
- Provide developmentally appropriate information.

- Maintain consistency where possible (school, extracurricular activities, routine).
- Devote special time for each sibling.
- Enlist the aid of child life specialists or social workers.

Grandparent Perspective

Nolan's grandparents love him dearly and relish their time with him. Their role in his life is fairly traditional in that regard—they offer regular babysitting and Nolan loves trips to their house to play. But they also share our stress. When we are worn down, they feel it too as they seek to comfort and care for us. When Nolan has a prolonged hospital stay, they shuffle their own schedules and take shifts in Nolan's hospital room. When Nolan is not feeling well, it consumes their minds almost as much as it does ours. As critical contributors to our family's well-being, it should be no surprise that they have unique needs of their own.

There is little known about the viewpoints of grandparents caring for seriously ill children. Yet grandparents play important roles in the social networks of their grandchildren. More has been written about the complex relationship of the bereaved grandparents who mourn their own loss while comforting their own child, the grandchild's parent. Grandparents who care for their ill grandchild at the end of life have been found to have posttraumatic stress disorder (PTSD) and depression and suffer

Table 2.3 Suggested Timepoints for Integrating Pediatric Palliative Care

Complex chronic conditions	Oncology	Nolan
Diagnosis	Diagnosis with poor prognosis	Diagnosis of complex chronic condition • Prenatal visit • Birth
Refractory symptoms	Multimodal symptom management	Nausea/vomiting/diarrhea Skin breakdown
Declining health	Worsening Lansky/Karnofsky Frequent admissions for disease- related complications	Frequent re-admissions
Lack of response to treatment	Relapse or recurrence	Inability to advance enteral feedings
Serious change in healthcare	Metastatic or progression of disease Consideration of phase I or phase II trials Bone marrow transplant	ICU admission

prolonged feelings of anger and blame (23). Healthcare providers and researchers must strive to develop and evaluate novel interventions to meet grandparents' needs.

EARLY INTEGRATION OF PALLIATIVE CARE

Families of children with a serious illness define and adjust to their own version of a new normal through processing and managing the flow of information, adjusting priorities, rearranging family roles, assigning meaning to the illness, and managing the treatment of the illness. Early integration of an interdisciplinary palliative care team (Table 2.3) can ease the suffering experienced by families during the illness experience (12).

REFERENCES

1. Himelstein BP, Hilden JM, Boldt AM, Weissman D. Pediatric palliative care. *N Engl J Med*. 2004;350:1752–1762. doi:10.1056/NEJMra030334
2. Feudtner C, Kang TI, Hexem KR, et al. Pediatric palliative care patients: a prospective multicenter cohort study. *Pediatrics*. 2011;127:1094–1101. doi:10.1542/peds.2010-3225
3. October TW, Fisher KR, Feudtner C, Hinds PS. The parent perspective: "being a good parent" when making critical decisions in the PICU. *Pediatr Crit Care Med*. 2014;15:291–298. doi:10.1097/PCC.0000000000000076
4. Institite of Medicine. *When Children Die: Improving Palliative and End-of-Life Care for Children and Their Families*. Washington, DC: The National Academies Press; 2002.
5. Dalberg T, Jacob-Files E, Carney PA, et al. Pediatric oncology providers' perceptions of barriers and facilitators to early integration of pediatric palliative care. *Pediatr Blood Cancer*. 2013;60:1875–1881. doi:10.1002/pbc.24673
6. Johnston DL, Vadeboncoeur C. Palliative care consultation in pediatric oncology. *Support Care Cancer*. 2012;20:799–803. doi:10.1007/s00520-011-1152-6
7. Kennedy RF. *Times to Remember*. New York, NY: Doubleday; 1974.
8. Valdez-Martinez E, Noyes J, Bedolla M. When to stop? Decision-making when children's cancer treatment is no longer curative: a mixed-method systematic review. *BMC Pediatr*. 2014;14:124. doi:10.1186/1471-2431-14-124
9. Popejoy E, Pollock K, Almack K, et al. Decision-making and future planning for children with life-limiting conditions: a qualitative systematic review and thematic synthesis. *Child Care Health Dev*. 2017;43:627–644. doi:10.1111/cch.12461
10. Pilapil M, Coletti DJ, Rabey C, DeLaet D. Caring for the caregiver: supporting families of youth with special health care needs. *Curr Probl Pediatr Adolesc Health Care*. 2017;47(8):190–199. doi:10.1016/j.cppeds.2017.07.003
11. Kuo DZ, Cohen E, Agrawal R, et al. A national profile of caregiver challenges among more medically complex children with special health care needs. *Arch Pediatr Adolesc Med*. 2011;165:1020–1026. doi:10.1001/archpediatrics.2011.172
12. Clarke-Steffen L. Reconstructing reality: family strategies for managing childhood cancer. *J Pediatr Nurs*. 1997;12:278–287. doi:10.1016/S0882-5963(97)80045-0
13. Cabral IE, de Moraes JR. Family caregivers articulating the social network of a child with special health care needs. *Rev Bras Enferm*. 2015;68:1078–1085. doi:10.1590/0034-7167.2015680612i
14. Davis KG. Integrating Pediatric Palliative Care into the School and Community. *Pediatr Clin North Am*. 2016;63:899–911. doi:10.1016/j.pcl.2016.06.013
15. Hinds PS, Oakes LL, Hicke J, et al. "Trying to be a good parent" as defined by interviews with parents who made Phase I, terminal care, and resuscitation decisions for their children. *J Clin Oncol*. 2009;27(35):5979–5985. doi:10.1200/JCO.2008.20.0204
16. Feudtner C, Walter JK, Faerber JA, et al. Good-parent beliefs of parents of seriously ill children. *JAMA Pediatr*. 2015;169:39–47. doi:10.1001/jamapediatrics.2014.2341
17. Rapoport A, Shaheed J, Newman C, et al. Parental perceptions of forgoing artificial nutrition and hydration during end-of-life care. *Pediatrics*. 2013;131:861–869. doi:10.1542/peds.2012-1916

18. White TE, Hendershot KA, Dixon MD, et al. Family strategies to support siblings of pediatric hematopoietic stem cell transplant patients. *Pediatrics*. 2017;139:e20161057. doi:10.1542/peds.2016-1057

19. Murray JS. Siblings of children with cancer: a review of the literature. *J Pediatr Oncol Nurs*. 1999;16:25–34. doi:10.1177/104345429901600104

20. Gerhardt CA, Lehmann V, Long KA, Alderfer MA. Supporting Siblings as a Standard of Care in Pediatric Oncology. *Pediatr Blood Cancer*. 2015;62 Suppl 5:S750–S804. doi:10.1002/pbc.25821

21. Long KA, Lehmann V, Gerhardt CA, et al. Psychosocial functioning and risk factors among siblings of children with cancer: an updated systematic review. *Psychooncology*. 2018;27(6):1467–1479. doi:10.1002/pon.4669

22. Youngblut JM, Brooten D, Blais K, et al. Health and Functioning in Grandparents After a Young Grandchild's Death. *J Community Health*. 2015;40:956–966. doi:10.1007/s10900-015-0018-0

Principles of Palliative Care: Across Age Groups, Settings, and Cultures 3

Meaghann Weaver

INTRODUCTION

Palliative care principles transcend all ages and cultures. By recognizing the shared values of quality of care, symptom management, family-centered care, compassionate communication, and interdisciplinary service, the field of palliative care reaches across life stages and care locations. This chapter depicts the intergenerational nature of palliative care work with the goal of care phrased in developmentally informed steps. Healthcare providers foster dignity when adapting universal palliative care principles to a local community in a participatory and culturally, spiritually, and developmentally informed way.

THE CROSS-CULTURAL VALUES OF PALLIATIVE CARE

The World Health Organization (WHO) and member states were called upon by the World Health Assembly resolution WHA67.19 to improve access to palliative care as a fundamental and core component of community health systems (1).

The Center to Advance Palliative Care defines palliative care as:

- "Palliative care is specialized medical care for people with serious illness. This type of care is focused on providing relief from the symptoms and stress of a serious illness. The goal is to improve quality of life for both the patient and the family" (2).

Both of these definitions can be applied to any infant, child, adolescent, young adult, or an adult advanced in age, regardless of geography, ethnicity, and religion. The adaptation of models of care specific to children and adolescents has been recognized as a research and clinical priority in spirituality and palliative care (3).

PRIMARY AND SECONDARY PEDIATRIC PALLIATIVE CARE

Primary palliative care refers to the fundamental competencies and basic skills required of all healthcare professionals striving to provide quality of life and comfort. Eliciting goals of care and documenting quality of life goals in the patient's medical record represents a primary palliative care competency as a universal skill relevant for all healthcare providers.

Secondary palliative care refers to the subspecialist clinicians, who provide specialty complex care specific to palliative care principles (4). Referrals to subspecialist palliative care providers may occur because of complex symptom management, existential distress, or complex care coordination.

FRAMING PEDIATRIC PALLIATIVE CARE ACROSS SETTINGS

Because of the high remission rates for many childhood cancers and the challenge of prognostic certainty in pediatric illnesses (involving vital organs in young children and advancing medical technologies), many pediatric palliative care teams ground their introduction to families and children as "supportive care" and "symptom management" and "psychosocial support" teams upfront at the time of early integration diagnosis. Goals of care for a child are best determined through longitudinal care of a family across care settings.

Emphasis in pediatric palliative care is on quality of life and optimal living: "How can today be a good day for this dearly loved child?" is a common pediatric palliative care inquiry.

FRAMING PALLIATIVE CARE ACROSS AGES

Even while considering how parents grieve the loss of a child (unique parental bereavement needs), palliative care providers are compelled to also consider how an adult child grieves the loss of his or her aged parents (unique adult child bereavement needs), and how a young child grieves the loss of his or her parents (unique developmental bereavement needs). Palliative providers caring for children and adults recognize a remarkable mutualism that speaks to the beauty of our development, our complex relationships, and the arch of the human trajectory that spans ages. Consider how children develop many of their remarkable milestones (head control, babbling vocalizations, trunk control, ambulation, fine motor skills) in a pattern that is the reverse of how aging adults with advanced dementia lose many of their milestones. This circle-of-life recognition reminds palliative providers that there is no dichotomy between pediatric endings and adult beginnings; this field acknowledges a shared journey with symbiotic knowledge across ages. Adult and pediatric palliative providers can and should learn from each other. For example, in pediatric palliative care, one of the quality of life metrics is "minutes able to engage in meaningful play"—that could and should be a lifelong quality of life metric! Some of what medicine tries to silo is actually shared experiences across developmental and chronological ages.

THE INTERGENERATIONAL NATURE OF PEDIATRIC PALLIATIVE CARE

Consider the following case examples representing one palliative care provider's case list that depicts the vast age array of patients cared for by palliative care teams (Table 3.1).

DEVELOPMENTAL RELEVANCE OF PEDIATRIC PALLIATIVE CARE

Care providers would be wise to familiarize themselves with the cognitive and spiritual developmental stages of childhood, as this empowers a palliative team's interaction with a child so as to be most meaningful for that child's understanding of illness, life, and even death (Table 3.2).

Table 3.1 Pediatric Palliative Care Examples Across Ages

Age	Patient example	Consult goal
Fetal	An yet-to-be-born infant carrying a diagnosis of hypoplastic left heart diagnosed on the echocardiogram in the second trimester of pregnancy	Help pregnant mom and her partner consolidate complex medical information prenatally; focus on surgical decision making and goals of care; establish pregnancy legacy
Neonatal	Peri-viable 25-week infant born with congenital diaphragmatic hernia	Pain management; coordination of communication among multiple subspecialty teams; sibling support from 7-year-old big brother
Infant	3-month-old male with Trisomy 18	Determine goals of care in context of life-limiting illness; hear parental perspectives and narratives on evolving view of medical interventions for children with Trisomy 18
Toddler	18-month-old female from rural community with tracheostomy and G-tube	Discuss transition from extended inpatient stay to home setting; coordination of care for rural community to include training of rural paramedics; engage in ongoing psychosocial support for complex, chronic condition; secretion and spasticity management
Preschool	3-year-old male with hypoxic brain injury from drowning accident	Parental resilience at bedside; spiritual support
Elementary	8-year-old female with cystic fibrosis	Coordination of school support services during recent increase in admissions; pulmonary symptom management

(continued)

Table 3.1 Pediatric Palliative Care Examples Across Ages (*continued*)

Age	Patient example	Consult goal
Junior high	14-year-old female with vertically transmitted HIV and sickle cell disease	Maximize medication adherence during adolescent years; foster peer connectedness via adolescent support group; focus on life goals
High school	17-year-old male with chronic headaches with negative biomedical work-up—currently on opiates	Establish opiate contract with goal to wean off of all opiates; work on functional goals such as returning to school and sports; introduce integrative therapies such as hydrotherapy and acupressure; foster pain diary accountability
Graduated	20-year-old female with osteosarcoma who has had limb salvage surgery and completed radiation/chemotherapy	Transition to adult care team with empowerment of young adult; longitudinal psychosocial needs assessment; employment connectedness; adaptation to new identity as cancer survivor
Young adult	30-year-old male with a toddler and a pregnant spouse newly diagnosed with Huntington's disease	Engage in goals of care conversation; discuss location preferences of care; focus on symptom management; consider legacy opportunities for family and practical realities of advanced care planning
Adult	65-year-old retired, widowed mail clerk diagnosed with advanced pancreatic cancer	Determine goals of care; address symptom management; review social and spiritual support resources; consider practicalities of access to health services; discuss life goals and preferences for family inclusion

Table 3.2 Stages of Development and Supportive Interventions

Age	Stage of cognitive development	Concept of death	Spirituality	Supportive interventions
Infancy: 0–2 years	• Sensorimotor; learning to trust the world • Experience of the world through sensory information • Limited conscious thinking • Limited language • Reality that is based on physical needs being met	• Death is perceived as separation or abandonment	• Undifferentiated • Faith reflects trust and hope in others • Need for sense of self-worth and love	• Provide maximum physical relief and comfort • Provide comfort through sensory input (e.g., touch, rocking, sucking) • Provide comfort with familiar people and transitional objects (e.g., toys)
Early childhood: 2–6 years	• Stage of preoperational thought; imaginative and egocentric • Prelogical • Development of representational or symbolic language • Egocentric orientation • Magical thinking	• Death is reversible or temporary • May equate death with sleep • May believe they can cause death by their thoughts (e.g., wishing someone would go away and thus cause the death of the person) • May not express personal emotion, but may associate death with the sorrow of others • May see death as a punishment	• Intuitive • Faith is fantasy-filled, imitative, and imaginative • Emphasis on participation in ritual	• Minimize the child's separation from usual caregivers (e.g., parents) or provide reliable and consistent substitutes • Ask open-ended questions about their feelings and spiritual experiences • Dispel misconceptions about death as punishment for bad thoughts or actions • Provide concrete information about state of death (e.g., a "dead person no longer breathes or eats")

(continued)

Table 3.2 Stages of Development and Supportive Interventions (*continued*)

Age	Stage of cognitive development	Concept of death	Spirituality	Supportive interventions
Middle childhood: 7–12 years	• Stage of concrete operations • Logical • No abstract reasoning • Orientation is egocentric	• Death is irreversible but is unpredictable • Aware that death is personal and can happen to them • May have great interest in details • May be interested in what happens after death • Can understand the biologic essentials of death	• Mythic: Takes on stories and beliefs of community • Faith is literal and concerns right and wrong • Connects ritual with personal identity	• Don't assume, exercise curiosity. Listen actively. Evaluate for fears of abandonment, destruction, or body mutilation • May benefit from specifics about the illness and treatments and reassurance that treatments are not punishments • Maintain the child's access to peers and spiritual support persons • Foster the child's sense of mastery and sense of control

(continued)

Table 3.2 Stages of Development and Supportive Interventions (*continued*)

Age	Stage of cognitive development	Concept of death	Spirituality	Supportive interventions
Adolescence and adulthood: Older than 12 years	• Stage of formal operations; adopting new ideas; working out identity • Development of abstract thought and advanced logical functions (e.g., complex analogy, deduction)	• Death is irreversible, universal, personal, but distant • Has the ability to develop natural, physiological, and theological explanations of death	• Approaches synthesis: more conventional • Formation of a personal faith, incorporating environment and experience • Evolution of relationship with God or higher power • Searches for meaning, purpose, hope, and value of life	• Reinforce comfortable body image, self-esteem • Allow expressions of anger • Provide privacy for the child • Support reasonable measures for the child to achieve independence • Maintain the child's access to peers • Explore spiritual meaning • Consider peer support groups

Source: From Steven M. Psychological adaptation of the dying child. In: Doyle E, Hanks GWC, Cherny N, Calman K, eds, *Oxford Textbook of Palliative Medicine.* 3rd ed. London: Oxford University Press; 2005; Rando TA. *Grief Dying and Death: Clinical Implications for Caregivers.* Champaign, IL: Research Press; 1984:385–391; Fowler JW. *Stages of Faith: The Psychology of Human Development and the Quest for Meaning.* New York, NY: Harper Collins; 1981; Himelstein BP, Hilden JM, Boldt AM, Weissman D. Pediatric Palliative Care. *New Engl J Med.* 2004;350:1752–1762.

THE SPIRITUAL NATURE OF PALLIATIVE CARE

Palliative care providers benefit from familiarity with what brings patients meaning, joy, strength, and hope. A spiritual assessment tool well-investigated and applicable to palliative practice includes the F-I-C-A scale (Copyright, Christina M. Puchalski, MD, 1996), a scale that reminds us of the need to allow patients of varying ages and walks of life and religious or nonreligious traditions to define their spirituality.

F - Faith and Belief
I - Importance
C - Community
A - Address in Care

THE FAMILIAL AND COMMUNITY NATURE OF PALLIATIVE CARE

Pediatric palliative teams recognize that while the patient is the unit of treatment and care, the family is the unit of understanding and extended care. A patient's wellness affects the family unit. The patient and family define the members of their family unit and the roles of those members.

- Parents—Children are held within the context of a parental unit, whether co-parents, single parent, or married parental units. Each parent brings a "lens" of insight into the child's needs and their hopes for the child. Pediatric palliative care teams are privileged to assess each parent's individual perspective in addition to a coupled unit perspective. Pediatric palliative care providers often have an opportunity to recognize parents, where each parent may hold shared values in addition to nuanced differences in view/role, and to engage in support for parents not just as individuals but as co-providers for a loved child. When illness impacts adult children, parents often resume the parental role or face the impact of witnessing someone they have attempted to protect from suffering now face frailty sooner than seems biologically acceptable (adult parents expect to experience personal illness/death sooner than their adult children).

- Grandparents—Grandparents are known to be "double grievers" as they feel the impact of illness to their own child (as parent) and they feel the impact of illness to their own grandchild (as grandparent). Thus, many palliative care teams recognize the double-duty to support grandparents through listening to grandparent narrative and attending to grandparent bereavement. This must be balanced by a professional commitment to not reveal confidential medical information to grandparents and to allow the child/child's parents to define grandparent inclusion.

- Siblings—Siblings of patients with chronic medical conditions feel the impact not only in terms of sensing the absence of their playmate, if this is a pediatric-age patient, but also in feeling their parents' "torn" wish to be present at home with the sibling and present at the hospital with the ill child. Young siblings sometimes act out in response or sometimes become "the perfect child"—both are a form of attention gathering. Older siblings may now be carrying additional duties as "aunty" stepping into a maternal role for the children of an adult patient or "uncle" stepping forward to provide guidance even if there is geographic or relational distance historically. Siblings warrant specific attentiveness for child life specialists and palliative care teams for psychosocial needs assessment, developmentally appropriate support, honest presence, and special recognition.

- Peers—Peers, known to the pediatric patient, are often forming their view of illness, and even death, through the pediatric patient's medical experiences. Peers note physical changes in an ill child and disabilities; this can be an opportunity for mentored adaptability in accepting to avoid bullying or alienating an ill child. Many pediatric palliative care programs offer Internet or in-person outreach to schools or community groups to foster education and peer adaptation. Adult peers of older patients often struggle with not knowing what to say or how best to direct support; palliative care teams can help adult patients consider how they may wish to protect their privacy or communicate their needs with neighbors/colleagues/friends.

THE RICH DIVERSITY OF PALLIATIVE CARE

Palliative care brings humanistic principles that transcend into all cultures and settings. The basic principles of palliative care include:

- An attentiveness to family function
- A stance of loving kindness and positive regard for the patient
- A listening presence that prioritizes patient voice/patient perspective
- A maximization of symptom management
- A commitment to quality of life
- A coordination of communication
- A desire to alleviate suffering
- A recognition of the dignity and worth of each patient

These principles are relevant for all patients and their families.

REFERENCES

1. World Health Organization. Strengthening of Palliative Care as a Component of Comprehensive Care Throughout the Life Course. WHA67.19. 2014. Sixty-Seventh World Health Assembly Agenda Item 15.5. 2018. http://apps.who.int/medicinedocs/documents/s21454en/s21454en.pdf
2. Center to Advance Palliative Care. Pediatric Palliative Care. 2018. https://www.capc.org/topics/pediatric-palliative-care
3. Balboni TA, Fitchett G, Handzo GF, et al. State of the science of spirituality and palliative care research Part II: screening, assessment, and interventions. *J Pain Symptom Manage*. 2017;54(3):441–451. doi:10.1016/j.jpainsymman.2017.07.029
4. Von Gunten CF. Secondary and tertiary palliative care in US hospitals. *JAMA*. 2002;287(7):875–881. doi:10.1001/jama.287.7.875

The Palliative Care Team and Care Coordination—Healing Versus Curing

4

Lisa C. Lindley and Jessica Keim-Malpass

INTRODUCTION

Patients with cancer and their families often require ongoing care from different healthcare professionals and services, in both the community and the hospital, which has led to an increasing need for care coordination to ensure high quality care (1). These patients have unique physical, psychosocial, financial, and spiritual/existential needs that affect the quality of life (2). Care coordination for patients with cancer remains a challenge as they are high utilizers of the healthcare system, have a high symptom load, have numerous specialist providers overseeing their care, and often place a significant burden on their primary caregivers (3–6). Strategies to improve care coordination for cancer patients and their families are frequently developed to ensure high-quality care even at end of life. Although care coordination approaches are often present within cancer care, there are significant barriers to cancer care coordination including recognition of health professionals' roles and responsibilities, transitions of care, inadequate communication between specialists and primary care providers, inequitable access to health services, and poor information exchanges (7,8). To address these gaps in care coordination, palliative care coordination has emerged as an approach that offers patients with cancer and their families a unique strategy for coordinating the complex nature of cancer care (9–11).

DEFINITION OF PALLIATIVE CARE COORDINATION

Palliative care is an interdisciplinary medical specialty that focuses on preventing and relieving suffering, while supporting quality of life for patients facing serious illness including cancer and their families (12). The primary tenets of palliative care are:

- Symptom management
- Establishment and implementation of care plans
- Consistent and sustained communication between patients and all those involved in their care
- Support for patients and their caregivers
- Coordination of care across sites of care (12)

Care coordination is a complex phenomenon with multiple existing definitions. The definition developed by the Agency for Healthcare Research and Quality (AHRQ) is "the deliberate organization of patient care activities between two or more participants (including the patient) involved in a patient's care to facilitate the appropriate delivery of health-care services" (13, p. 41). The primary tasks of care coordination entail:

- Benefit coordination
- Service use coordination
- Coordination of transitions between care settings
- Clinical information sharing between participants in the care of a cancer patient (14)
- Care planning and collaborations with other participants (15)

Therefore, effective care coordination involves an interdisciplinary approach to ensuring access to healthcare and social support services through which a care coordinator manages and monitors the patient's needs, goals, and preferences based on a plan of care (16,17). The ultimate goal of care coordination is to improve health-related quality of life for patients and their families.

Within the context of palliative care, care coordination is defined as the management of care activities to meet the needs of patients with serious illness and that of their families (18,19). Palliative care coordination assists patients and their families in understanding and regaining control over their care plans (12). The interdisciplinary approach of palliative care enables coordination with numerous participants to ensure that patients receive the most appropriate care based on the patient's needs and available resources, especially during transitions to other care settings (12).

FRAMEWORK OF PALLIATIVE CARE COORDINATION

The palliative care coordination conceptual framework created for this chapter is derived from the Donabedian Quality Framework (Figure 4.1) (13,20–23). Using this framework, palliative care coordination for cancer patients and their families is conceptualized as a process of care that depends on the operational, market, and financial structures of the palliative care program. The process of delivering palliative care coordination includes specific activities such as:

- Information transfer
- Facilitation of transitions across settings
- Alignment of resources with patient needs

Ultimately, the process of palliative care coordination should improve outcomes including healthcare utilization and satisfaction, while reducing costs for cancer patients and their families.

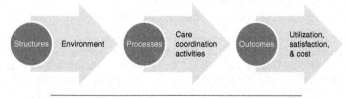

Figure 4.1 Framework of palliative care coordination.

STRUCTURES OF PALLIATIVE CARE COORDINATION

More than 60% of hospitals in the United States have a palliative care program (9,24). A distinctive profile of palliative care programs has emerged in the past decade. These programs operate in an environment with specific operational, market, and financial structures.

Operational Structures

- Older and larger hospitals (9,25,26)
- High case-mix index (9)
- Teaching hospitals (24,26)
- Electronic medical record present with a majority using one of five systems: Epic, Cerner, Allscripts, Suncoast, or McKesson (27)
- Not-for-profit and public hospitals (9,26,28)
- Staff includes physicians, social workers, registered nurses, and chaplains with average staff size of approximately 2.33 full-time equivalent (FTE) personnel per patient (24,26)

Market Structures

- Markets are those with high per-capita income and competition among hospitals (25)
- Penetration is highest in the New England region and lowest in the West and South Central regions of the United States (9,24,28)
- States with high percentage of programs include Montana, New Hampshire, and Vermont, while states with low percentages are Alaska, Alabama, and Mississippi (9)

Financial Structures

- Low return-on-assets (25)
- High occupancy rate (25)
- High total margin (25)
- Internally financed by the hospital (24,26)

PROCESSES OF PALLIATIVE CARE COORDINATION

The process of palliative care coordination includes specific activities aimed at organizing care for cancer patients and their families. Although there is no documented best way to deliver palliative care coordination (19), the care coordination and palliative care literature was reviewed for the most prevalent care coordination activities offered by palliative care programs (13,19,20). There are seven primary palliative care coordination tasks (Box 4.1).

An initial, key task in palliative care coordination is establishing responsibilities for care coordination with the care teams, patient, and family. This includes identifying personnel who will be coordinating care, negotiating specific care coordination duties among the participants in the patient's care, and acknowledging when these responsibilities will be transferred to other care participants. As an example, the palliative care coordinator may identify and communicate durable equipment needs

---

Box 4.1 7 Process Steps of Palliative Care Coordination

1. Establishing accountability or negotiating responsibility
2. Communicating and sharing information
3. Facilitating transitions
4. Creating a plan of care
5. Assessing and monitoring needs and goals
6. Supporting self-management goals
7. Aligning resources with needs

---

with vendors and the family may be responsible for ensuring that someone is present when the equipment is delivered.

Communication among participants in a cancer patient's care includes:

- Interpersonal communication—the two-way exchange of knowledge through personal interactions, or the give-and-take of ideas, preferences, goals, and experiences through personal interactions (e.g., face-to-face interactions, telephone conversations, emails, letters).
  - For example, communicating timely and relevant clinical, social, emotional, psychological updates that could influence the family-centered plan of care.
- Sharing information is the transfer of data such as medical history, medication lists, test results, and other clinical data, from one participant in a patient's care to another.
  - For example, delivery of shared care plans among numerous providers and interprofessional provider types.
- Transition of care handoff communication, or when the team, who was acting as the family-centered medical home, transitions the activities of the medical home model to another team.
  - For example, when the oncology team who was acting as the primary team for care coordination transitions the care coordination to the palliative care team. All teams of care are still involved, but one team is assuming care coordination responsibilities to reduce redundancy and plan of care confusion.

In the case of pediatric patients, a child may have a variety of care coordination agencies or groups involved in their care including a Medicaid Targeted Care Manager, Child Welfare Caseworker, and/or patient-center medical home provider (29). A task of the palliative care coordinator would include contacting the agencies' coordinators when a child is discharged from the hospital and sharing information on discharge medications.

A critical activity in palliative care coordination is facilitating healthcare transitions of care at the end of life. Transitions can occur across settings such as transitions from the inpatient hospital setting to the outpatient setting (i.e., hospice) or transitions between ambulatory care settings (i.e., primary care) to the cancer care clinic. Information about or accountability for some aspect of a cancer patient's care is transferred between two or more healthcare entities. Furthermore, as coordination needs change over time, facilitation of transitions may be warranted. For example, a pediatric cancer patient may transition from a pediatric to an adult provider, which may require sharing information with the new adult provider.

Establishing and maintaining a plan of care is the hallmark of palliative care coordination. The care plan outlines the cancer patient's current and longstanding needs and goals for care and identifies coordination gaps. It will be used as a roadmap to plan the care coordination.

Palliative care coordination activities also include:

- Determining the cancer patient's needs for coordination
- Monitoring those needs over time
- Making adjustments

At the onset of a cancer diagnosis, a patient and family may need care coordination focused on managing pain and symptoms at home. However, at the end of life the needs may change to coordinating bereavement.

Activities in support of self-management include tailoring education and support that align with the cancer patient's capacity and preferences for involvement in his or her own care. This includes providing information, training, and coaching to patients and families that promote understanding and the ability to perform self-care tasks.

A final task of palliative care coordination is to align resources with the needs of cancer patients and their families. Palliative care coordinators provide information on the availability of resources and, if necessary, coordinate access to those resources. Resources can be in the community or within the acute care settings that help support the cancer patients meet their care goals. Community resources include services or programs outside the healthcare system such as financial resources (e.g., food stamps), social services, educational resources, schools for pediatric patients, support groups, or support programs (e.g., Meals on Wheels). Aligning resources in the acute care setting with patient needs might include assisting a cancer patient in obtaining and understanding the state physician order for life-sustaining treatment (POLST) forms during the hospital admission.

OUTCOMES OF PALLIATIVE CARE COORDINATION

Recent evidence suggests that palliative care coordination improves outcomes including healthcare utilization, healthcare transitions, satisfaction, and costs (Figure 4.2; 2,30,31):

Research has shown that palliative care coordination processes (e.g., common assessment tools, collaborative care plans, symptom management guidelines) improves healthcare utilization among cancer patients (32), including a decrease in emergency department visits and acute care hospital admissions. According to adult and pediatric palliative care research, care coordination affects healthcare transitions. In a randomized trial of patients with metastatic, non–small-cell lung cancer, researchers found that palliative care patients had longer enrollments in hospice

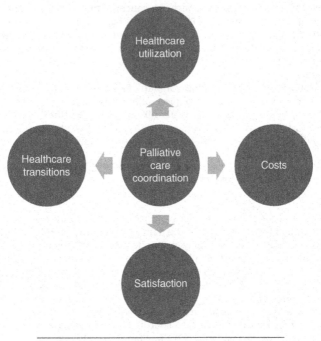

Figure 4.2 Outcomes of palliative care coordination.

care (33). A study of pediatric patients receiving palliative care coordination revealed a similar result (34). In this study, the lengths of stay in a hospice increased by a factor of 5.61 for children receiving palliative care coordination, compared to their peers who did not. Other data have suggested that palliative care coordination may increase patient satisfaction and reduce costs. Researchers examined palliative care coordination among patients with lung cancer (18) and reported that patients valued the coordination between and within clinical settings, along with referrals to end-of-life services and assistance with financial issues. The evidence among caregivers, however, has been inclusive. A recent study found no change in caregiver satisfaction when palliative care coordination was implemented (32). From a cost perspective, a 2012 study of children receiving community-based palliative care with an assigned care coordinator found that Medicaid spending was decreased by 11% when care was shifted from a hospital setting to in-home community-based care (35).

EMERGING MODELS OF PALLIATIVE CARE COORDINATION

Several care coordination models have emerged within palliative care programs (30,32,33,36–43). These models highlight a variety of structures and processes in providing palliative care coordination. Six model types are shown in Table 4.1.

Table 4.1 Models of Palliative Care Coordination

Name	Features	Example
Comprehensive Team Model	• Integrated, interdisciplinary team approach • Designed to meet the physical, psychosocial, and spiritual needs of patients and families • Composed of advanced practice registered nurses, social workers, and a spiritual care counselor • Conducts baseline assessment • Plans care, on-going support according to patient needs • Initiates advance care planning • Conducts monthly contact between patient and team • Conducts regular monthly meetings with oncologists • Refers to and coordinates with community providers (e.g., home care, hospice care), when appropriate	University Hospitals Case Medical Center, Seiden Cancer Center in Cleveland, Ohio
Navigator Model	• Includes a patient navigator from the palliative care team, typically a registered nurse • Functions independently and acts as an intermediary among patients, providers, nurses, interdisciplinary team members, and ancillary services • Directs the interdisciplinary team daily • Provides palliative education to patients, families, and medical staff • Triages need-based consults • Conducts family meetings independently • Facilitates goals of care conversations • Works with the emergency department to avoid hospital admissions, when appropriate	Novant Health Forsyth Medical Center in Winston Salem, North Carolina

(continued)

Table 4.1 Models of Palliative Care Coordination (*continued*)

Name	Features	Example
Staff Model	• Designated team member coordinates care for the patient; often the physician, nurse, or social worker • Provides patient education and care coordination via tele-health and clinic visits • Coordinates care with outpatient clinics • Conducts follow-up discharge phone calls to ensure that patients have transitioned effectively from the hospital • Works with patients and families on problems of symptom management and accessing resources once they have returned to their home • Conducts goals of care conversations with patients.	Mayo Clinic in Rochester, Minnesota
Community-Based Model	• Includes special palliative care coordination mechanisms financed through Medicaid that permit children to receive supportive services (e.g., hospice care services, expressive therapies, bereavement support) together with their curative treatments • Is state-mandated and provides home-based and community-based services for children and families from the time of diagnosis through bereavement • Identifies, enrolls, and manages eligible children in concurrent curative and palliative therapies	Florida program entitled, "Partners in Care; Together for Kids"

(*continued*)

Table 4.1 Models of Palliative Care Coordination *(continued)*

Name	Features	Example
Care Transitions Intervention Model	• Is a 4-week program that encourages patients to take a more active role in their healthcare • Provides specific tools and skills that are reinforced by a "transition coach" (a nurse, social worker, or trained volunteer) • Follows patients across settings for the first 4 weeks after leaving the hospital • Focuses on the tools and skills for patients and their families around medication self-management • Use of a patient-centered health record to help guide patients through the care process • Educates patient to understand "red flag" indicators of a worsening condition and to take appropriate next steps	University of Colorado Health Sciences Center in Denver, Colorado
Integration Model	• Is embedded into an existing care coordination structure often within the acute care setting • Uses a multidisciplinary team-based care coordination program • Facilitates navigation through the healthcare system • Integrates tablet-based bio-psycho-social screening to address patient and caregiver needs and goals proactively • Optimizes medications to improve symptom management and recovery • Empowers patients with teach-back education • Maintains collaborations among multidisciplinary providers across settings	City of Hope National Medical Center in Duarte, California

Table 4.2 Palliative Care Coordination Challenges and Opportunities

Challenges	Opportunities
1. Care fragmentation and difficulties initiating referrals	1. Care pathways, data analytics, and integration
2. Providing quality home and community-based palliative care	2. Medical home models of care and evidence-based policy solutions
3. Palliative care knowledge gaps	3. Increasing palliative care literacy

CHALLENGES AND OPPORTUNITIES

There are several challenges and opportunities for palliative care coordination (Table 4.2).

Challenges

There have been notable challenges in integrating palliative care referrals and treatment plans into existing pathways of care for patients with serious illness and medical complexity. Late referral to palliative care remains a significant barrier for care coordination, and ultimately, for optimal quality outcomes and family-centered care (44–47). There has been an increased recognition of the need to deliver palliative care in home- and community-based settings, so that patients and families can remain in their home and out of the hospital care setting; however, numerous challenges exist in terms of access to care delivery, quality of care, and reimbursement (10,11,48–51). Additionally, there is a shortage of palliative care providers in rural settings (52–55). Members of the general public, as well as some healthcare providers, do not know the meaning and availability of palliative care (56–58). As such, patients are often referred late to palliative care services, which limits the ability to promote effective care coordination (2).

Opportunities

Integrated care pathways are documents or clinical protocols that outline the multidisciplinary care elements that are needed to address a specific clinical problem based on certain screening criteria that initiates the care pathway (59). One strategy to identify relevant patients to include is to devise a screening approach where patients would be considered for an automatic consult based on their meeting specific criteria, also known as a *trigger* (60). Despite an increased use of triggers to initiate palliative care referrals in a variety of adult care settings (60–62), there are currently no validated triggers or instruments in existence that assist interdisciplinary team members in objectively screening children for palliative care needs, and it still remains an area of much needed attention (57). Thus, establishing triggers might promote more timely initiation of palliative care coordination.

The family-centered medical home (FCMH) model of care can be an optimal strategy to deliver quality care in home- and community-based settings (63). Largely started in pediatric primary care settings, the FCMH model consists of the following components of care delivery: accessibility, family-centeredness, continuity of care, comprehensiveness, coordination, compassion, and cultural effectiveness (64). The central premise of a FCMH is that a patient has a coordinating provider who can facilitate continuity care plans across a variety of care settings (including home and community-based settings; 65). The concept borrows key elements from each of the six model types described previously, and while the attributes have been discussed in the context of palliative care delivery, the FCMH model has not been fully realized except in certain high risk subpopulations (63,66,67). Thus, care coordination with a FCMH might provide palliative care teams with creative means of development and enhance their care coordination processes.

In the United States, and globally, a need for public health awareness campaigns to general awareness about palliative care (58) has been recognized. The initiatives "Project on Death in America" in the United States and the "Dying Matters" campaign in the United Kingdom are two such examples (58). In Australia, there is an annual day to generate discussions on death and dying as a part of a "death literacy" movement (58). On the provider side, there is a defined need for ongoing educational opportunities on the goals of palliative care, different palliative care models that may be available, and opportunities for integration into practice (57). For palliative care to be able to offer impactful care coordination, there must be public and provider-specific awareness of the utility of approach to enhance earlier uptake and subsequent outcomes.

SUMMARY

In conclusion, there are specific structures, processes, and outcomes associated with palliative care coordination. Several key palliative models of care coordination highlight the unique contribution palliative care makes to ensuring that cancer patients and their families receive high-quality care. There are opportunities and challenges for palliative care teams developing or expanding their palliative care coordination function.

REFERENCES

1. Nekhlyudov L, Levit L, Hurria A, Ganz PA. Patient-centered, evidence-based, and cost-conscious cancer care across the continuum: translating the Institute of Medicine report into clinical practice. *CA Cancer J Clin.* 2014;64(6):408–421. doi:10.3322/caac.21249
2. Kavalieratos D, Corbelli J, Zhang D, et al. Association between palliative care and patient and caregiver outcomes: A systematic review and meta-analysis. *JAMA.* 2016;316(20):2104–2114. doi:10.1001/jama.2016.16840
3. Bischoff K, Weinberg V, Rabow MW. Palliative and oncologic co-management: symptom management for outpatients with cancer. *Support Care Cancer.* 2013;21(11):3031–3037. doi:10.1007/s00520-013-1838-z
4. Fox K. The Role of the Acute Care Nurse Practitioner in the Implementation of the Commission on Cancer's Standards on Palliative Care. *Clin J Oncol Nurs.* 2014;18(1):39–44. doi:10.1188/14.CJON.S1.39-44
5. Knapp C, Baker K, Cunningham C, et al. Pediatric palliative care and the medical home. *J Palliat Med,* 2012;15(6), 643–645. doi:10.1089/jpm.2012.0075
6. Smith CH, Graham CA, Herbert AR. Respite needs of families receiving palliative care. *J Paediatr Child Health.* 2017;53(2):173–179. doi:10.1111/jpc.13324

7.   Sondergaard EG, Grone BH, Wulff CN, et al. A survey of cancer patient's unmet information and coordination needs in handovers: a cross-sectional study. *BMC Res Notes*. 2013;6:378–390. doi:10.1186/1756-0500-6-378

8.   Walsh J, Harrison JD, Young JM, et al. What are the current barriers to effective cancer care coordination? A qualitative study. *BMC Health Serv Res*. 2010;10:132–141. doi:10.1186/1472-6963-10-132

9.   Dumanovsky T, Augustin R, Rogers M, et al. The growth of palliative care in the U.S. hospitals: a status report. *J Palliat Med*. 2016;19(1):8–15. doi:10.1089/jpm.2015.0351

10. Kamal AH, Currow DC, Ritchie CS, et al. Community-based palliative care: the natural evolution for palliative care delivery in the U.S. *J Pain Symptom Manage*. 2013;46(2):254–264. doi:10.1016/j.jpainsymman.2012.07.018

11. Spetz J, Dudley N, Trupin L, et al. Few hospital palliative care programs meet national staffing recommendations. *Health Aff*. 2016;35(9):1690–1697. doi:10.1377/hlthaff.2016.0113

12. Meier DE, McCormick E. Benefits, services, and models of subspecialty palliative care. *UpToDate*. 2017. https://www.uptodate.com/contents/benefits-services-and-models -of-subspecialty-palliative-care

13. McDonald KM, Sundaram V, Bravata DM, et al. *Closing the quality gap: A critical analysis of quality improvement strategies*. Volume 7: Care Coordination. 2007. https://www. ahrq.gov/downloads/pub/evidence/pdf/caregap/caregap.pdf

14. Leutz WN. Five laws for integrating medical and social services: lessons from the United States and the United Kingdom. *Milbank Q*. 1999;77(1):77–110. doi:10.1111/1468-0009.00125

15. Denboba D, McPherson MG, Kenney MK, et al. Achieving family and provider partnerships for children with special health care needs. *Pediatrics*. 2006;118(4):1607–1615. doi:10.1542/peds.2006-0383

16. Chan WC, Nichols J. Improving the coordination of palliative care. *Int J Med Med Sci*. 2011;2(11):1225–1234.

17. O'Malley AS, Cunningham PJ. Patient experiences with coordination of care: The benefit of continuity and primary care physician as referral source. *J Gen Intern Med*. 2009;24(2):170–177. doi:10.1007/s11606-008-0885-5

18. Epiphaniou E, Shipman C, Harding R, et al. Coordination of end-of-life care for patients with lung cancer and those with advanced COPD: are there transferable lessons? A longitudinal qualitative study. *Prim Care Respir J*. 2014;23(1):46–51. doi:10.4104/pcrj.2014.00004

19. van der Plas AGM, Onwuteaka-Philpsen BD, van de Waterling M, et al. What is case management in palliative care? An expert panel study. *BMC Health Serv Res*. 2012;12:163–171. doi:10.1186/1472-6963-12-163

20. Agency for Healthcare Research and Quality. *Care Coordination Measures Atlas Update*. 2014. https://www.ahrq.gov/professionals/prevention-chronic-care/improve/coordination/atlas2014/index.html

21. Donabedian A. The quality of care: How can it be assessed? *JAMA*. 1988;260(12):1743–1748. doi:10.1001/jama.1988.03410120089033

22. Nuckols TK, Escarce JJ, Asch SM. The effects of quality care on costs: a conceptual framework. *The Milbank Quarterly*. 2013;91(2):316–353. doi:10.1111/milq.12015

23. van Houdt S, Heyrman J, Vanhaecht K, et al. An in-depth analysis of theoretical frameworks for the study of care coordination. *Int J Integr Care*. 2012;13:1–8.

24. Feudtner C, Womer J, Augustin R, et al. Pediatric palliative care programs in children's hospitals: A cross-sectional national survey. *Pediatrics*. 2013;132(8):1063–1070. doi:10.1542/peds.2013-1286

25. Spaulding A, Harrison DA, Harrison JP. Palliative care: a partnership across the continuum of care. *Health Care Manag*. 2016;35(3):189–198. doi:10.1097/hcm.0000000000000115

26. Pantilat SZ, Kerr KM, Billings JA, et al. Palliative care services in California hospitals: Program prevalence and hospital characteristics. *J Pain Symptom Manage*. 2012;43(1):39–46. doi:10.1016/j.jpainsymman.2011.03.021

27. Lindley LC, Rotella JD, Ast K, et al. The quality improvement environment: Results of the 2016 AAHPM/HPNA membership needs assessment survey. *J Pain Symptom Manage*. 2017;54(5):766–771. doi:10.1016/j.jpainsymman.2017.07.031

28. Goldsmith B, Dietrich J, Qingling D, Morrison RS. Variability in access to hospital palliative care in the United States. *J Palliat Med.* 2008;11(8):1094–1102. doi:10.1089/jpm.2008.0053

29. Nageswaran S, Ip EH, Golden SL, et al. Inter-agency collaboration in the care of children with complex chronic conditions. *Acad Pediatr.* 2012;12(3):189–197. doi:10.1016/j.acap.2012.02.007

30. Hauser J, Sileo M, Araneta N, et al. Navigation and palliative care. *Cancer.* 2011;117:3585–3591. doi:10.1002/cncr.26266

31. LeBlanc TW, Currow DC, Abernathy AP. On golidilocks, care coordination, and palliative care: Making it "just right." *Prim Care Respir J.* 2014;23(1):8–10. doi:10.4104/pcrj.2014.00017

32. Dudgeon DJ, Knott C, Eichholz M, et al. (2008). Palliative care integration project (PCIP) quality improvement strategy evaluation. *J Pain Symptom Manage.* 2008;35(6):573–582. doi:10.1016/j.jpainsymman.2007.07.013

33. Greer JA, Pirl WF, Jackson VA, et al. Effect of early palliative care on chemotherapy use and end-of-life care in patients with metastatic non-small-cell lung cancer. *J Clin Oncol.* 2012;30(4):394–400. doi:10.1200/JCO.2011.35.7996

34. Lindley LC. The effect of pediatric palliative care policy on hospice utilization among California Medicaid beneficiaries. *J Pain Symptom Manage.* 2016;52(5):688–694. doi:10.1016/j.jpainsymman.2016.05.019

35. Gans D, Komonski GF, Roby DH, et al. Better outcomes, lower costs: palliative care program reduces stress, costs of care for children with life-threatening conditions. *Policy Brief UCLA Center for Health Policy Res.* 2012;1–8.

36. Cantwell P, Turco S, Brenneis C, et al. Predictors of home death in palliative care cancer patients. *J Palliat Care.* 2000;16(1):23–28.

37. Coleman EA, Roman SP, Hall KA, Min S-J. (2015). Enhancing the care transitions intervention protocol to better address the needs of family caregivers. *J Healthc Qual.* 2015;37(1):2–11. doi:10.1097/01.JHQ.0000460118.60567.fe

38. Daly BJ, Douglas SL, Gunzler D, Lipson AR. Clinical trial of a supportive care team for patients with advanced cancer. *J Pain Symptom Manage.* 2013;46(6):775–784. doi:10.1016/j.jpainsymman.2012.12.008

39. Furner S, Goldsmith B. Effective use of nurse navigator role in palliative care. At the 2017 Center to Advance Palliative Care National Seminar. Phoenix, AZ; 2017.

40. Knapp C, Madden V, Curtis C, et al. Partners in care: Together for kids: Florida's model of pediatric palliative care. *J Palliativ Med.* 2008;11(9):1212–1220. doi:10.1089/jpm.2008.0080

41. Parrish MM, O'Malley K, Adams R, et al. Implementation of the care transitions intervention: Sustainability and lessons learned. *Prof Case Manag.* 2009;14(6):282–293. doi:10.1097/NCM.0b013e3181c3d380

42. Relias.*Integrating palliative care in case management can work*.2016.https://www.ahcmedia.com/articles/137512-integrating-palliative-care-in-case-management-can-work

43. Zachariah F, Gallo M, Loscalzo M, Crocitto LE. Embedding palliative care into care coordination. *J Clin Oncol.* 2014;32(31 suppl):62. doi:10.1200/jco.2014.32.31_suppl.62

44. Ferrell BR. Late referrals to palliative care. *J Clin Oncol.* 2005;23(12):2588–2589. doi:10.1200/JCO.2005.11.908

45. Hui D, Kim S-H, Kwon J, et al. Access to Palliative Care Among Patients Treated at a Comprehensive Cancer Center. *Oncologist.* 2012;17:1574–1580. doi:10.1634/theoncologist.2012-0192

46. Kumar P, Casarett D, Corcoran A, et al. Utilization of supportive and palliative care services among oncology outpatients at one academic cancer center: determinants of use and barriers to access. *J Palliat Med.* 2012;15(8):923–930. doi:10.1089/jpm.2011.0217

47. Morita T, Miyashita M, Tsuneto S, et al. Late referrals to palliative care units in Japan: nationwide follow-up survey and effects of palliative care team involvement after the Cancer Control Act. *J Pain Symptom Manage.* 2009;38(2):191–196. doi:10.1016/j.jpainsymman.2008.09.011

48. Carroll JM, Torkildson C, Winsness JS. Issues related to providing quality pediatric palliative care in the community. *Pediatr Clin N Am.* 2007;54(5):813–827, xiii. doi:10.1016/j.pcl.2007.06.002

49. Cozad M, Lindley L, Mixer S. Staff Efficiency Trends Among Pediatric Hospices, 2002-2011. *Nursing Econ*. 2016;34(2):82–90.

50. Lindley LC, Cozad MJ. Nurse knowledge, work environment, and turnover in highly specialized pediatric end-of-life care. *Am J Hosp Palliat Med*. 2016;34(6);577–583. doi:10.1177/1049909116649415

51. Lindley LC, Mixer SJ, Cozad MJ. The influence of nursing unit characteristics on RN vacancies in specialized hospice and palliative care. *Am J Hosp Palliat Med*. 2016;33(6):568–573. doi:10.1177/1049909115575506

52. Evans R, Stone D, Elwyn G. Organizing palliative care for rural populations: a systematic review of the evidence. *Fam Pract*. 2003;20(3):304–310. doi:10.1093/fampra/cmg312

53. Lynch S. Hospice and palliative care access issues in rural areas. *Am J Hosp Palliat Care*. 2013;30(2):172–177. doi:10.1177/1049909112444592

54. Masso M, Owen A. Linkage, coordination and integration: evidence from rural palliative care. *Aust J Rural Health*. 2009;17(5):263–267. doi:10.1111/j.1440-1584.2009.01089.x

55. Pesut B, Robinson CA, Bottorff JL, et al. On the road again: patient perspectives on commuting for palliative care. *Palliat Support Care*. 2010;8(2):187–195. doi:10.1017/S1478951509990940

56. Alper J. *Health Literacy and Palliative Care Workshop Summary*. Washington, DC: National Academies Press; 2016.

57. Keim-Malpass J, Mitchell EM, Blackhall L, DeGuzman PBPB. Evaluating Stakeholder-Identified Barriers in Accessing Palliative Care at an NCI-Designated Cancer Center with a Rural Catchment Area. *J Palliat Med*. 2015;18(7):634–637. doi:10.1089/jpm.2015.0032

58. Seymour J. The Impact of Public Health Awareness Campaigns on the Awareness and Quality of Palliative Care. *J Palliat Med*. 2018;21(S1):S30–S36. doi:10.1089/jpm.2017.0391

59. Chan R, Webster J. End-of-life care pathways for improving outcomes in caring for the dying. *Cochrane Database Syst Rev*. 2013;(11). doi.org/10.1002/14651858.CD008006.pub3

60. Nelson JE, Curtis JR, Mulkerin C, et al. Choosing and using screening criteria for palliative care consultation in the ICU: a report from the Improving Palliative Care in the ICU (IPAL-ICU) Advisory Board. *Critical Care Medicine*. 2013;41(10):2318–2327. doi:10.1097/CCM.0b013e31828cf12c

61. Hui D, Mori M, Meng YC, et al. Automatic referral to standardize palliative care access: an international Delphi survey. *Support Care Cancer*. 2017;26(1):175–180. doi:10.1007/s00520-017-3830-5

62. Hussain J, Adams D, Allgar V, Campbell C. Triggers in advanced neurological conditions: prediction and management of the terminal phase. *BMJ Support Palliat Care*. 2014;4(1):30–37. doi:10.1136/bmjspcare-2012-000389

63. Wallenstein DJ. Palliative Care in the Patient-Centered Medical Home. *Prim Care*. 2012;39(4):627–631. doi:10.1016/j.pop.2012.08.009

64. AAP. Policy Statement: The Medical Home. *Pediatrics*. 2002;110(1):184–186. doi:10.1542/peds.110.1.184

65. Korda H, Eldridge GN. ACOs, PCMHs, and health care reform: nursing's next frontier? *Policy Polit Nurs Pract*, 2011;12(2):100–103. doi:10.1177/1527154411416370

66. Leyenaar JK, O'Brien ER, Finkelstein SM, et al. Families' Priorities Regarding Hospital-to-Home Transitions for Children With Medical Complexity. *Pediatrics*. 2016;139(4):295–301. doi:10.1542/peds.2016-1581

67. Pritchard S, Cuvelier G, Harlos M, Barr R. Palliative care in adolescents and young adults with cancer. *Cancer*. 2011;117(10 Suppl):2323–2328. doi:10.1002/cncr.26044

The Palliative Care Assessment— Clinical Interview Questions for Adults and Children

5

Ann M. Berger, Lori Wiener,
Najmeh Jafari, and Christina M. Puchalski

INTRODUCTION

Performing a palliative care interview involves listening to the patient's life story and learning about what is important to the patient.

This includes addressing the physical, psychosocial, and spiritual dimensions of the patient and his or her family, each of which impacts the quality of life (Figure 5.1).

THE CLINICAL INTERVIEW

An interview is a controlled situation in which one person, the interviewer, asks a series of questions of another person.

Four Tasks

- Build a therapeutic alliance
- Obtain a database
- Interview for diagnosis
- Negotiate a treatment plan with the patient

The Three Phases

- Opening phase
- Body of the interview
- Closing phase

Essential Concepts to be Mastered During the Opening Phase of the Interview

- Be warm, courteous, and emotionally sensitive
- Actively defuse the strangeness of the clinical situation
- Give patient the opening word
- Gain the patient trust by projecting competence

Essential Concepts to be Mastered During the Body of the Interview

- Use open-ended questions and commands to increase the flow of information
- Use continuation techniques to keep the flow coming

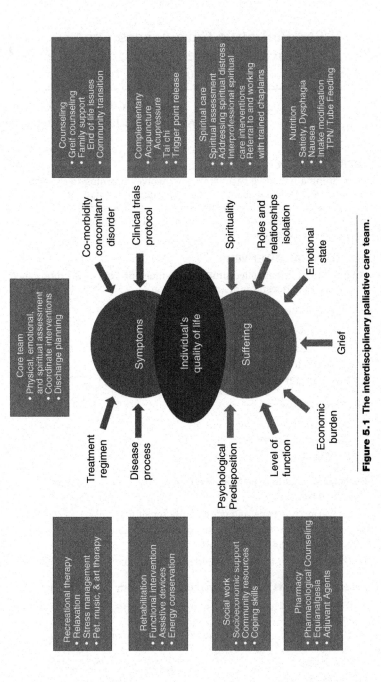

Figure 5.1 The interdisciplinary palliative care team.

- Shift to neutral ground, when necessary
- Suggest that goals/wishes be written down
- Be proactive and anticipate problems
- Identify reliable contacts, such as a palliative care team
- Provide tools to facilitate communication flow with family/friends (before crisis)
- Provide advocacy through education and professional support
- Schedule a second interview, if necessary
- Examine your personal values or agenda

Essential Concepts—Closing Phase

- Listen reflectively
- Assess your own feelings
- Know your biases
- Avoid labeling
- Give importance to your manner of speaking
- Talk the patient's language

Key Areas to be Assessed During the Clinical Interview

- Inquire about perception of disease status and treatment impact on quality of life
- Learn about level of desire for information
- Assess ability to comprehend
- Review cultural or spiritual considerations
- Consider primary communicators in the family, spokesperson, and medical power of attorney
- Ask out about family, hospital, and community support system
- Weigh patient/family goals against anticipated outcomes
- Understand the goals of the primary treating team or teams
- Develop a collaborative plan/goals of care
- Anticipate treatment outcomes
- Appreciate that sooner is better than later when it comes to compassionate conversations

Additional Areas to Explore as Part of a Psychosocial Assessment

- How has your life changed since your diagnosis/treatment?
- How have these changes impacted your everyday life?
- How much distress have these changes caused you and your family/caregiver?
- How do you feel about who you are now ("self"), as compared to who you were before your diagnosis/treatment?
- How do you seem different today than if I had met you a year ago?
- What would make today a good day for you?

Additional Areas to Explore as Part of a Spiritual Assessment

- Has your spirituality or the way you find meaning changed since your diagnosis/treatment?
- If you had spiritual practices before, are those working for you now?
- Are your beliefs and values important to you? Do they impact the way you care for yourself? Do they impact your medical decision making?
- Do you feel there are spiritual issues or goals you want to work on right now?
- Are you able to experience moments of joy or peace or love?
- What are some of your deepest concerns?

Special Considerations for the Pediatric Patient

Similar to the clinical interview with the adult living with a serious illness, identifying what matters most to the child and parent is critical. Domains to be assessed during a clinical interview are:

- Quality of life
  - Food housing, basic needs
  - Physical symptoms that cause suffering
  - Psychosocial strengths and concerns (adaptation to stage of illness, perception of family and peer support/isolation, sleep, anxiety/depression, concerns about body image, hopes and worries)
  - Spiritual strengths and concerns (acceptance, struggle, suffering, deep questions, spiritual practices that are supportive, difficulty doing usual practices)
- Coping and adaptation
  - Parent, sibling, grandparent—coping, adaptation, perceived support
  - Presence of anticipatory grief
  - Quality of communication between child and parent(s); child and sibling(s); sibling(s) and parent(s)
  - Quality of parental marital/partnership relationship
  - Perception of whether one parent feels he or she is parenting the ill child on his or her own (lone parenting)
- Communication
  - How decisions are made, current goals of treatment decisions, consensus on goals of care
  - Perceived regrets, forgiveness needed
  - Whether there have been any conversations with child about death, dying process (and if not, if family would like assistance with this)

Based on what is learned during the interview, several interventions may be suggested, such as:

- Assistance with financial needs, insurance benefits
- Counseling to improve communication, enhance adaptation to progressive illness

- Advance care planning, reassurance of a meaningful life lived
- Legacy building
- Anticipatory guidance on physical symptoms and child's emotional needs, especially as death nears
- Consideration of autopsy
- Funeral planning
- Bereavement care

Facilitating Conversations Between Children and Their Family Members

Ideally, initiation of conversations about serious illness occur before the terminal nature of a child's illness is known definitively.

- Early conversations can be an opportunity to explore values, hopes, and fears as they relate to the future, before the pressure of decision making about end-of-life care is high (1–4).
- Asking children and parents, "What would you want if things don't go as you hope?" reinforces that we value them, their preferences, and their goals of care. They may speak of people they would like to see/speak to, places they may wish to go, ways they may wish to be remembered.

Some parents may want to protect their children from difficult conversations.

- Once therapeutic alliance and trust are established, conversations about ways in which parents can meet their child's needs, alleviate their child's fears, and ultimately protect their child in unanticipated ways can be better heard.
- Understanding a parent's reasoning for including/not including a child in prognostic conversations is important.
- A commitment of honesty is needed if the child asks about his or her condition. Honesty can facilitate later difficult conversations.

Why Are Clinical Palliative Care Interviews so Difficult for Us as Healthcare Providers?

- Medical success is measured by cure, rather than healing.

There's nothing else that can be done for your disease. . .perceived failure of the patient/family/clinician.

- Advanced technology prolongs life, pushing death beyond the realm of probability.

Charging full steam ahead with aggressive treatment and avoiding the discussion of goals in the event that treatment is not effective can result in unrealistic expectations for patient/family/clinician.

- It is a breach of the Hippocratic oath to "first do no harm".

Transitional care discussion can cause emotional distress to patient/family . . . protective avoidance for the patient/family/clinician.

How Do We Get More Comfortable?

- Examine our professional and personal feelings/past experiences/ spiritual or other beliefs, values, and sources of meaning.
- Encourage open communication (fears, concerns, goals) from the onset to promote an environment of security.

  Trust the openness of both optimistic and realistic goals throughout the disease trajectory.
- Communicate with patients as we would want to be communicated with.
- When considering shielding the patient/family from end-of-life facts, consider who we are really protecting. . . the patient/family or ourselves?

THE ASSESSMENT OF PAIN AND OTHER ISSUES (Figure 5.2)

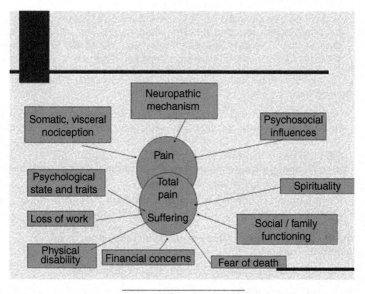

Figure 5.2 Nature of pain.

Along with physical pain (Box 5.1) and the types of pain (Table 5.1) it is necessary to assess for other physical symptoms (Figure 5.3) (4).

Among other things, psychosocial issues (Table 5.2) and other issues (Box 5.2) have to be addressed, and a spiritual assessment (Box 5.3) will also be required.

Box 5.1 Physical Pain Assessment

Where is it most painful now?

How long have you been in pain?

Has this changed from your initial complaint?

What is the temporal pattern of your pain? Is it continuous, or is it intermittent?

What are the characteristics of the pain: aching, cramping, burning, throbbing, numbing, tingling, shooting?

What is its intensity: at present, at its lowest, and at its highest level? Scale: 0–10; or mild, moderate, severe.

What is an acceptable or tolerable level of pain?

What factors aggravate the pain, such as moving, standing, or sitting?

What factors relieve pain, such as heat, cold, massage, or medications?

What treatments have you tried, what has been their effectiveness, and what side effects have you experienced? (Include over-the-counter medications and alternative and complementary therapies.)

Table 5.1 Types of Pain			
Type	**Description**	**Examples**	**Treatment**
Somatic	Localized, aching, throbbing	Bone, joint pain Gnawing feeling	NSAIDs, opioids
Visceral	Pressure, tightening, aching	Pleural, hepatic disease Pulling, stretching	NSAIDs, opioids, steroids
Neuropathic	Severe, sharp, shooting, stabbing, burning, hot, numbing, tingling	Peripheral neuropathy Postherpetic neuralgia	Opioids, steroids, neuroleptics, tricyclic antidepressants, acupuncture
Myofascial	Tightness, pulling, spasm	Upper back, neck	NSAIDs, heat, stretching, TENS trigger point release

Note: Suffering and pain issues: Total pain is more than just physical pain. Total pain can involve a suffering component as well as a physical component. Suffering involves psychological and coping factors, social support and loss issues, fear of death, financial concerns, and spiritual concerns.

NSAIDs, nonsteroidal anti-inflamatory drugs; TENS, transcutaneous electrical nerve stimulation.

Memorial symptom assesment scale														
Name:							Date:							

Section 1:

Instructions: We have listed 24 symptoms below. Read each one carefully. If you have had the symptom during this past week, let us know how OFTEN you had it, how SEVERE it was usually and how much it DISTRESSED or BOTHERED you by circling the appropriate number. If you DID NOT HAVE the symptom, make an "X" in the box marked "DID NOT HAVE".

During the past week. Did you have any of the following symptoms?	Did not have	If yes, How OFTEN did you have it?				If yes, How SEVERE was it usually?				If yes, How much did it DISTRESS or BOTHER you?				
		Rarely	Occasionally	Frequently	Almost Constantly	Slight	Moderate	Severe	Very severe	Not at all	A little bit	Some what	Quite a bit	Very much
Difficulty concentrating		1	2	3	4	1	2	3	4	0	1	2	3	4
Pain		1	2	3	4	1	2	3	4	0	1	2	3	4
Lack of energy		1	2	3	4	1	2	3	4	0	1	2	3	4
Cough		1	2	3	4	1	2	3	4	0	1	2	3	4
Feeling nervous		1	2	3	4	1	2	3	4	0	1	2	3	4
Dry mouth		1	2	3	4	1	2	3	4	0	1	2	3	4
Nausea		1	2	3	4	1	2	3	4	0	1	2	3	4
Feeling drowsy		1	2	3	4	1	2	3	4	0	1	2	3	4
Numbness/ tingling in hands/feet		1	2	3	4	1	2	3	4	0	1	2	3	4
Difficulty sleeping		1	2	3	4	1	2	3	4	0	1	2	3	4
Feeling bloated		1	2	3	4	1	2	3	4	0	1	2	3	4
Problem with urination		1	2	3	4	1	2	3	4	0	1	2	3	4

(A)

Figure 5.3   The revised version of the Memorial Symptom Accessment Scale. (*continued*)

Source: From Portenoy RK, Thaler HT, Kornblith AB, et al. The Memorial Symptom Assessment Scale: an instrument for the evaluation of symptom prevalence, characteristics and distress. *Eur J Cancer*. 1994;30A(9):1326–1336. doi:10.1016/0959-8049(94)90182-1

During the past week. Did you have any of the following symptoms?	Did not have	If yes, How OFTEN did you have it?				If yes, How SEVERE was it usually?				If yes, How much did it DISTRESS or BOTHER you?				
		Rarely	Occasionally	Frequently	Almost Constantly	Slight	Moderate	Severe	Very severe	Not at all	A little bit	Some what	Quite a bit	Very much
Vomiting		1	2	3	4	1	2	3	4	0	1	2	3	4
Shortness of breath		1	2	3	4	1	2	3	4	0	1	2	3	4
Diarrhoea		1	2	3	4	1	2	3	4	0	1	2	3	4
Feeling sad		1	2	3	4	1	2	3	4	0	1	2	3	4
Sweats		1	2	3	4	1	2	3	4	0	1	2	3	4
Worrying		1	2	3	4	1	2	3	4	0	1	2	3	4
Problems with sexual interest or activity		1	2	3	4	1	2	3	4	0	1	2	3	4
Itching		1	2	3	4	1	2	3	4	0	1	2	3	4
Lack of appetite		1	2	3	4	1	2	3	4	0	1	2	3	4
Dizziness		1	2	3	4	1	2	3	4	0	1	2	3	4
Difficulty swallowing		1	2	3	4	1	2	3	4	0	1	2	3	4
Feeling irritable		1	2	3	4	1	2	3	4	0	1	2	3	4

(B)

Section 2:

Instructions: We have listed 8 symptoms below. Read each one carefully. If you have had the symptom during this past week, let us know how SEVERE it was usually and how much it DISTRESSED or BOTHERED you by circling the appropriate number. If you DID NOT HAVE the symptom, make an "X" in the box marked "DID NOT HAVE".

During the past week. Did you have any of the following symptoms?	Did not have	If yes, How SEVERE was it usually?				If yes, How much did it DISTRESS or BOTHER you?				
		Slight	Moderate	Severe	Very severe	Not at all	A little bit	Some what	Quite a bit	Very much
Mouth sores		1	2	3	4	0	1	2	3	4
Change in the way food tastes		1	2	3	4	0	1	2	3	4
Weight loss		1	2	3	4	0	1	2	3	4
Hair loss		1	2	3	4	0	1	2	3	4
Constipation		1	2	3	4	0	1	2	3	4
Swelling of arms or legs		1	2	3	4	0	1	2	3	4
"I don't look like myself!"		1	2	3	4	0	1	2	3	4
Changes in skin		1	2	3	4	0	1	2	3	4

**If you had any other symptoms during the past week, please list below and indicate how much the symptom has distressed or bothered you.

Other:						0	1	2	3	4
Other:						0	1	2	3	4
Other:						0	1	2	3	4

(C)

Figure 5.3 (*continued*)

Table 5.2 Psychosocial Assessment

Initial assessment	Reassessment
What are you most hoping for?	How do you feel things are going?
What are your goals, and how can we best achieve it?	What is the hardest part of your treatment?
What do you fear the most?	Are you having good days? Are you finding enjoyment in things?
Who do you turn to for support?	How is your family/spouse/significant other doing?
Why do you think this disease has occurred? What other losses have you endured during your life?	What helps you meet the challenges you endure?
Do you want others to be involved in decision making about your care?	Who would speak on your behalf if complications arise?

Source: From Baker K, Berger A. Cancer Pain Assessment: Where Does It Hurt? In: Berger A, ed. Advances in Cancer Pain: A Bedside Approach. The Oncology Group, CMP Healthcare Media, ©2004, with permission.

Box 5.2 Other Issues to Address in Assessment

- Current mood state
- History of psychiatric disorders
- Social support
- What name do you use
- What sex were you assigned at birth
- What gender do you identify as now
- Financial stress/insurance issues
- Access to healthcare/medications
- Current use of illicit drugs/alcohol
- Past history of substance abuse
- Coping skills
- Home environment (physical layout, who is living in the home)
- Primary language spoken, literacy
- Whom do you consider to be family
- Conflict within the family

(continued)

Box 5.2 Other Issues to Address in Assessment (*continued*)

- Loss/grief issues
- Fears
- What do you know of your diagnosis
- What do you know of your prognosis
- Comorbidities
- Concurrent symptoms (fatigue, nausea, diarrhea/constipation, insomnia)
- Concurrent medications
- Cultural influences/preferences
- Functional status
- Occupation/education
- Recreational Interests, hobbies
- Pets
- Patient goals
- Family concerns/issues

Box 5.3 The Spiritual History

- *Faith*: Is spirituality a part of your life? Do you consider yourself spiritual?
- *Meaning*: What gives your life meaning at this time?
- *Importance*: Are your beliefs important to you? Do they affect the way you are dealing with your illness?
- *Community*: Do you have a supportive spiritual community?
- *Care*: How can we attend to these spiritual needs in your care?

REFERENCES

1. Mack JW, Wolfe J. Early integration of pediatric palliative care: For some children, palliative care starts at diagnosis. *Curr Opin Pediatr*. 2006;18:10–14. doi:10.1097/01.mop.0000193266.86129.47
2. Wiener L, Zadeh S, Wexler L, et al. When silence is not golden: engaging adolescents and young adults in discussions around end-of-life care choices. *Pediatr Blood Cancer*. 2013;60:715–718. doi:10.1002/pbc.24490
3. Wiener L, Feudtner C, Hinds P, et al. Deeper Conversations Need Not Wait Until the End. *J Clin Oncol*. 2015;33(33):3974. doi:10.1200/jco.2015.62.3405
4. Portenoy RK, Thaler HT, Kornblith AB, et al. The Memorial Symptom Assessment Scale: an instrument for the evaluation of symptom prevalence, characteristics and distress. *Eur J Cancer*. 1994;30A(9):1326–1336. doi:10.1016/0959-8049(94)90182-1

Symptom Management of Advanced Cancer and Cancer Treatment

II

Neurologic Symptom Management in the Advanced Brain and Central Nervous System Cancer Patient

Ann H. Lichtenstein

INTRODUCTION

Cancer with primary origin in the nervous system and cancer with intracranial or spinal metastases present specific challenges to medical providers. Both the disease and treatment have significant effects on the cognition of and quality of life for patients. Posttreatment changes after surgery, chemotherapy, and radiation may have positive as well as negative effects due to sensitivity of the nervous system. Symptoms can significantly affect quality of life and function.

PREVALENCE

- According to the American Brain Tumor Association, 80,000 new cases of primary brain tumors will be diagnosed this year (26,000 malignant and 79,000 nonmalignant) (1). 700,000 people in the United States have a primary central nervous system (CNS) tumor and 17,000 people will die from primary CNS tumors this year (1).

Brain and CNS Tumors in Adults

- Most common brain lesions in adults are from metastatic disease (2)
- Most common cancers that metastasize to the brain are lung cancer, breast cancer, renal cancer, and melanoma (2)
- There are more than 100 histologically unique brain and primary CNS tumors (1)
- Primary brain tumors from most common to least common are:
  - Meningiomas, most common benign intracranial tumors: 36.6% of primary brain tumors, 27,110 new cases in 2017
  - Gliomas: 25% of all primary brain tumors and 75% of all malignant tumors
  - Astrocytomas: 75% of all gliomas, including glioblastoma
  - Glioblastoma: 55% of all gliomas, 15% of all primary brain tumors, most likely to be malignant, 12,390 new cases predicted in 2017
  - Pituitary tumors: rarely malignant, 16% of all primary brain tumors
  - Nerve sheath tumors (including acoustic neuromas): 8% of all primary brain tumors
  - Lymphomas and oligodendrogliomas: 2% of all primary brain tumors

- Medulloblastoma/embryonal/primitive tumors: 1% of all primary brain tumors (1)

Brain and Spinal Cord Tumors in Children

- Brain tumors are the second most common cancer in children ages 0 to 14 years old. After leukemia, this is the leading cause of cancer-related deaths in this age group (1)
- 4,800 cases are diagnosed yearly between the ages of 0 and 19 (1)
- Most common types of brain tumors in children are posterior fossa tumors including astrocytoma, medulloblastoma (40%), ependymoma (12%), and brain stem glioma (10%) (1)

Spinal Cord Tumors

- Primary spinal cord tumors are uncommon as overall prevalence is estimated at 1 for every 4 intracranial lesions. In 2017, 10,000 people in the United States will be diagnosed with a primary or metastatic spinal cord tumor (3)
- Most primary spinal cord tumors are benign. Tumors such as meningiomas and neurofibromas account for 55% to 65% of all primary spinal tumors
- Meningiomas are most commonly seen in women between age 40 and 70
- Intramedullary tumors account for only 5% to 10% of all spinal tumors
- Metastatic spinal tumors comprise 70% of all spinal tumors, most commonly found in the thoracic spine
- Metastatic lesions are most commonly found in patients with prostate cancer, breast cancer, and lung cancer
- Pediatric spinal cord tumors are rare in children and there are many different subtypes (3)

NEUROCOGNITIVE IMPAIRMENT

Neurocognitive impairment may occur as an adverse effect of chemotherapy and/or brain radiation. Mechanisms include microvascular damage and inflammation (4).

History and Physical Assessment

- **General**: awake and alert, lethargic, confused, obtunded, agitated (5)
- **Neurologic examination**: cognitive status, alert, awake, oriented x3, following commands
  - Does the patient know his/her own name?
  - Does the patient know place and time?
  - Does the patient understand the reason for being sick and/or in the hospital?
  - Does the patient know his or her medications?
  - Does the patient understand the consequences of treatment options?
- **Cranial nerves**: assessment of II–XII

- **Speech**: intact, slurred, words confused
- **Functional assessment**: can he/she safely ambulate, perform activities of daily living (ADLs), have awareness of safety issues such as turning off stove, locking door, calling emergency services if needed
- **Emotional:** loss of independence for ADLs may cause fear, depression, and anxiety
- **Social:**
  - Patient may require increased level of care and monitoring, which may be an emotional and financial burden on family
  - Patient may not be able to make decisions for hmself or herself, which places responsibility on others
  - Encourage the patients to discuss wishes with family/proxy
  - Have patient complete a Medical Orders for Life Sustaining Treatment form or comparable form which states wishes including CPR, intubation, and life -ustaining therapies
  - Decide on surrogate decision maker for patient; is there a need for a legal power of attorney
  - Discuss making decisions on financial matters, having a financial power of attorney
  - Initiate discussion of palliative care options, including hospice if appropriate (6)
- **Spirituality:**
- Use HOPE questions to conduct a spiritual assessment.
  - Sources of hope: Investigate sources of hope, comfort, and peace. What gives the patient strength in difficult times? (7)

Medical History

- **Seizures** may be caused by tumor growth, edema, or hemorrhage causing increased intracranial pressure (4).
- Take a history of seizures including type, length of seizure, associated symptoms: aspiration, tongue biting, incontinence, injuries sustained, and memory of the event
- Look at the antiepileptic drugs (AEDs) and consider patient compliance with taking medications
- Physical assessment during the acute presentation. Note if the seizure is generalized (affecting the whole body), partial, or absent
- Ocular findings: Note direction and movement of eyes, upward eye deviation, nystagmus, and dilated pupils
- Look out for tongue biting (sides of tongue) and/or increased secretions
- Note rhythmic motor activity: ranges from subtle to dramatic, highest incidence in face, hands, and toes
- Look out for tachycardia, elevated blood pressure, dilated pupils, increased secretions, head turning or limb posturing
- Consider respiratory changes, apnea, cyanosis
- Consider urinary and bowel incontinence

- After seizure (postictal period) there may be decreased responsiveness, confusion, aphasia, postictal or Todd paralysis for minutes to hours (8)

TREATMENT DRUGS

- According to the National Comprehensive Cancer Network (NCCN) guidelines, patients who have not had a seizure should not be treated with phenytoin, phenobarbital, or valproic acid for seizure prophylaxis. In this case newer agents such as levetiracetam, topiramate, lamotrigine, or pregabalin should be initiated (6)
- Certain antiepileptic drugs have effects on the cytochrome p450 system and change the metabolism of chemotherapy agents. These AEDs include phenytoin, phenobarbital, carbamezapine (6)
- Steroids are used if the patient has mass effect, brain edema, or radiation necrosis. For asymptomatic patients steroids are not needed (6)
- If steroids are initiated, the NCCN recommends lowest possible dose for the shortest amount of time and downward titration when possible. Before radiation therapy, patients with extensive mass effect should receive steroids 24 hours before treatment (6)
- A commonly used steroid is dexamethasone. Dexamethasone helps to decrease brain edema and lessen intracranial pressure. This aids in decreasing pain, nausea, vomiting, and seizures (4)
- Adverse effects include gastrointestinal bleeding (give with proton pump inhibitor or histamine receptor blocker), elevated blood sugar (consider sliding scale insulin), insomnia, and psychiatric disturbances. To prevent insomnia, give a dose in the morning and a second dose in the early afternoon (4)
- Chronic adverse effects include weight gain, peripheral edema, myopathy, Cushing's syndrome, osteoporosis, hypertension, cataracts, and increased infections (4)
- For acute seizure management can use rectal diazepam, SC or IV benzodiazepines (lorazepam or midazolam), or phenobarbital (5)
- **Emotional:** Unpredictability of seizures may cause depression and anxiety and low self-esteem due to social stigmatization
- **Social**
  - Patient may need monitoring for a period of time until seizures are controlled by medications
  - Support groups have been shown to help increase self-esteem and provide patients with hope (9)
  - Discuss driving laws in your state with patients and families (6)
  - Refer patients to social services, support groups, and cancer advocacy organizations. Also refer them to services in the community that can assist with financial, insurance, and legal issues (6)
- **Spirituality:** Use HOPE questions for assessment
- **Organized religion:** Does the patient have a religious affiliation? Does it provide strength and how (7)?

HEADACHES

Headaches in patients with primary or metastatic brain tumors are strongly correlated to increased intracranial pressure by intracranial hemorrhage or edema (10). Interventions such as surgery, chemotherapy, or radiation may also cause headaches. Tumor-related headaches have been described as close to tension type headaches or migraine headaches. Alternatively, they may be typically described as severe shooting or throbbing pain (10).

Pediatric brain tumors are more likely to be located in the posterior fossa and therefore cause hydrocephalus. Headaches will be most severe in the morning or after a nap due to increased intracranial pressure from lying down and hypoventilation during sleep. Neonates may have increased irritability and difficulty with handling as well as macrocephaly. Vomiting may relieve the headache. Vision abnormalities such as sixth and third nerve palsies may occur due to pressure on cranial nerves and blurring of vision due to papilledema (11).

- **Assessment questions**
  - Personal and family history of headaches—how many years, getting better or worse?
  - Can you describe the pain: OPQRST (onset, palliation, quality, radiation, severity, and timing)?
  - Is there any associated nausea or vomiting?
  - Does the pain worsen with coughing, exercise, or a change in body position?
  - Does the pain respond to the usual headache remedies?
  - Are there any new neurologic problems (sensation, motor, bowel, bladder changes; 12)?
- **Treatment** depends on etiology and may involve medical, surgical, and radiotherapeutic components. Surgical tumor debulking and whole brain radiation may be considered as therapy. Medical management of edema may include steroids, osmotic therapies, and diuretics. If hydrocephalus is the etiology, diuretics are used and the patient may require ventricular shunting of cerebrospinal fluid. If pain persists, acetaminophen, NSAIDs, antidepressants, anticonvulsants, and opioids may be used as well.
- **Spirituality:** HOPE questions for assessment
- **Personal spirituality and practices:** How would you describe your personal beliefs and spirituality? What gives meaning to your life? (7)

SPINAL CORD COMPRESSION

- **Progressive sensory loss, motor loss, and pain** may result from spinal cord compression (SCC) or epidural metastasis, which is a frequent complication of metastatic cancer. Bowel and bladder incontinence or retention may be associated with sensory and motor deficits. These patients are at risk for progressive functional loss leading to complete paraplegia (13)
- **Pediatric** patients are more likely to experience coordination and difficulties with gait (ataxia) due to tumor location close to the cerebellum (11)

- **Physical examination**
  - Pain: inspect painful region for deformities, palpate to see if pain is elicited, evaluate range of motion of affected area, and check maneuvers that make the pain better/worse
  - Check for strength of and sensation (pinprick and light touch) on the face, and bilateral upper and lower extremities
  - Check tone of the extremities: flaccidity, rigidity, spasticity
  - Check reflexes of the bilateral upper and lower extremities
  - Undertake a rectal examination for sensation and tone, lack of sensation and/or tone indicates upper motor neuron lesion
  - Skin: Check if the patient is warm or cool or flushed. Look for signs of skin breakdown; skin breakdown may be evidence of sensation abnormalities and may be a source of pain
  - Check urinary output: retention or incontinence may be due to upper motor neuron lesion (1)
- **Treatment**
  - New onset SCC is a medical emergency; urgent evaluation by a surgeon is necessary (14)
  - MRI of the cervical, thoracic, and lumbar spine is recommended as patients may have compression at multiple levels (16)
  - High dose steroids may also be given to decrease spinal cord inflammation and edema (14)
  - Radiation therapy is the treatment of choice in patients without spinal instability. Radiation has been shown to decrease pain and preserve neurologic function for a period of time (14)
  - The NCCN recommends physical and occupational therapy for patients with neurologic deficits. It also recommends a multidisciplinary team to integrate diagnosis, treatment, symptom management, and rehabilitation due to the complex nature of the physical, psychological, and social needs of these patients (6)
- **Prognosis:** Median survival in patients with SCC is 3 to 6 months. Prognosis depends on ambulatory status, type of cancer, and number of metastases (16)
- **Emotional:** Patient may have grief, severe loss, and depression due to lack of physical strength, coordination, difficulty in ambulating and performing ADLs
- **Social:** Requires care from others due to difficulty or inability to ambulate and perform ADLs
  - Consider hospice referral as a hospice can aid in management of pain in addition to other services for comprehensive care of the patient (6)
- **Spirituality: HOPE assessment**
- **Personal spirituality and practices:** How do your beliefs affect the kind of medical care you would like to receive? (7)

INFORMATION AND SUPPORT RESOURCES

- National Brain Tumor Society: www.braintumor.org
- Local Department of Social Services or Human Services (for Food Stamps, Medicaid, other financial supports)
- Lots a Helping Hands: http://lotsahelpinghands.com
- Family Caregiver Alliance: https://www.caregiver.org
- Caring Info: National Hospice and Palliative Care Organization http://www.caringinfo.org/i4a/pages/index.cfm?pageid=1

REFERENCES

1. American Brain Tumor Association. 2018. https://www.abta.org/about-brain-tumors/brain-tumor-faqs/brain-tumor-types/
2. Chung C, Laperriere N. Chapter 38: Management of Intracranial Metastases. In: Berger A, Shuster J, Von Roenn J, eds. *Principles of Palliative Care and Supportive Oncology.* 3rd ed. Philadelphia, PA: Lippincott-Raven; 2006; 508–528.
3. American Association of Neurological Surgeons. 2018. http://www.aans.org/Patients/Neurosurgical-Conditions-and-Treatments/Spinal-Tumors
4. Schiff D, Lee EQ, Nayak L, Norden AD, et al. Medical management of brain tumors and the sequelae of treatment . *Neuro-Oncol.* 2015;17(4):488–504. doi:10.1093/neuonc/nou304
5. Sizoo EM, Grisold W, Taphoorn MJB. Chapter 81: Neurological aspects of palliative care: the end of life setting. In: Biller J, Ferro JM, ed. *Handbook of Clinical Neurology,* Volume 121(3rd series), Neurologic Aspect of Systemic Disease Part III. Amsterdam, The Netherlands: Elsevier; 2014: 1219–1225.
6. Nabors LB, Portnow J, Ammirati M, et al. NCCN Guidelines Version 1.2017; Central Nervous System Cancers. Principles of Brain Tumor Management. Brain E, 1–3.
7. Anandarajah G, Hight E. Spirituality and medical practice: using the HOPE questions as a practical tool for spiritual assessment. *Am Fam Physician.* 2001;63(1):87.
8. St. Louis EK, Cascino GD. Diagnosis of epilepsy and related episodic disorders. *Continuum (Minneap Minn).* 2016;22(1):15–37. doi:10.1212/CON.0000000000000284
9. Sawangchareon K, Pranboon S, Tiamkao S, Sawanyawisuth K. Moving the self-esteem of people with epilepsy by Supportive Group: a clinical trial. *J Caring Sci.* 2013;2(4):329–335. doi:10.5681/jcs.2013.039
10. Nelson S, Taylor LP. Headaches in Brain Tumor Patients: Primary or Secondary? *Headache.* 2014;54:776–785. doi:10.1111/head.12326
11. Wilne S, Collier J, Kennedy C, et al. Presentation of childhood CNS tumours: a systematic review and meta-analysis. *Lancet Oncol.* 2007;8(8):685–695. doi:10.1016/S1470-2045(07)70207-3
12. American Brain Tumor Association. 2018. https://www.abta.org/about-brain-tumors/brain-tumor-signs-symptoms/
13. Metastatic Spinal Cord Compression: Diagnosis and Management of Patients at Risk of or with Metastatic Spinal Cord Compression. NICE Clinical Guidelines, No. 75. National Collaborating Centre for Cancer (UK). Cardiff (UK): National Collaborating Centre for Cancer (UK); 2008. https://www.ncbi.nlm.nih.gov/pubmedhealth/PMH0032985
14. Abrahm JL, Banffy MB, Harris MB. Spinal Cord Compression in Patients with Advanced Metastatic Cancer. *JAMA.* 2008;299(8):937–946. doi:10.1001/jama.299.8.937
15. Mehta RS, Arnold R. Fast Facts and Concepts #237: Evaluation of spinal cord Compression. https://www.mypcnow.org/blank-x57p1
16. Mehta RS, Arnold R. Fast Facts and Concepts #238: Management of spinal cord Compression. https://www.mypcnow.org/blank-k4ugz
17. Loghin M, Levin AV. Headache Related to Brain Tumors. *Curr Treat Options Neurol.* 2006;8:21–32. doi:10.1007/s11940-996-0021-y

Heart Failure in Adults and Children With Oncologic Disease

7

Julia Cheringal and David M. Steinhorn

INTRODUCTION

More than 1.6 million new adult cancers are diagnosed annually with 595,690 cancer deaths. Approximately 40% of adults will be diagnosed with cancer during their lifetimes. In children less than 19 years of age, 15,780 new cancers are diagnosed each year with 1 child in 285 developing cancer before age 19 and an annual childhood cancer mortality of 1,960. Heart failure (HF) is not a unique diagnosis but represents inadequate cardiac function to support the body's needs and activities. In the general population, the incidence of HF is increasing, and pre-exisitng cardiovascular disease may play a role as a comorbidity for patients undergoing therapy for cancer in adults although less commonly for children. HF is a well-recognized complication in cancer-directed therapies (1,2) and is progressive in many cases. As cancer survival continues to improve for adults and children, the consequences of therapies, including newer molecular-targeted therapies, create risks for cardiovascular (CV) health (3). For children treated for malignancies, the risk of HF and coronary artery disease is 15- and 10-fold, respectively (vs. healthy peers), with 3- to 10-fold risk of pericardial and valvular disease (3–5).

General mechanisms leading to HF (6):

- Damage to myocytes → apoptosis/remodeling (change in function, shape, size)
- Remodeling and ischemia → electrical instability → diminished cardiac output
- Diminished cardiac output and reserve → systemic organ dysfunction

Symptom etiology in HF (1):

- HF → RAAS activation/↑proinflammatory cytokines/↑norepinephrine
- Catabolic state → Myopathy (skeletal, respiratory, cardiac)
- HF syndrome impacting multiple organ dysfunction and cumulative disability

Impact of cancer and its therapy on the CV system: adult (7) and children (2):

- Toxicity of chemotherapy
- Radiotherapy-related cardiovascular toxicity
- Complications of monoclonal antibody therapies, tyrosine kinase inhibitors

- Pre-existing CV dysfunction
  - Diabetes, hypertension, coronary artery disease
  - Structural: valvular disease, cardiomyopathy, congenital defects
  - Arrhythmias
- Direct tumor involvement or pericardial disease
- Depression, existential distress → decreased activity → deconditioning

SYMPTOMS ASSOCIATED WITH CV DYSFUNCTION IMPACTING QUALITY OF LIFE

In general, the approach to the management of distressing symptoms in patients receiving palliative care must involve continual reassessment of (a) the symptom's impact on the patient's quality of life, (b) the burden of the symptomatic treatment (e.g., inotropes are easy to infuse in the ICU but are typically not provided at home), (c) the goals of care, and (d) the anticipated disease trajectory based upon the primary, underlying disease and complications of its treatment. Each symptom increases psychological distress because the patient views new symptoms as disease progression. Aside from the physical impact of the symptoms presented in this section, the psychological impact is enormous and must be treated along with the physical problem. Any symptom can become a "threat" to one's self-concept or identity. It represents loss of wholeness and can lead to a snowballing of other symptoms, institution of new treatments with associated side effects producing more symptoms, and so on. Thus, the clinician is obligated to evaluate not only the physical symptoms, but also the emotional and spiritual impact of those symptoms in the context of an incurable illness complicated by a failing heart.

(Where not otherwise indicated, approaches for children are similar to adults with medications adjusted per kg body weight. The reader is referred to a reliable source for pediatric dosing or on-line hospital formulary containing pediatric dosing recommendations.)

SYMPTOMS IN ADVANCED HF

Dyspnea—*Present in 61% dying from cardiac disease*
While dyspnea is usually thought to be the most common morbidity seen with advanced HF, pain and fatigue (see the following) are common findings with significant impact on quality of life (8). The symptom of dyspnea is assessed based upon the patient's report and caregiver's observations. Because the intensity of dyspnea is quite variable, it may wax and wane. Functional limitations due to dyspnea are particularly distressing, requiring attempts at symptomatic management. The inability to "catch one's breath" is a particularly disturbing symptom, creating tremendous emotional suffering. Many patients have a fear of suffocating and insist that their care providers do everything possible to reduce that sensation. Meditation-based stress reduction (MBSR) may be useful for patients who have already been instructed in it to improve self-regulation.

Pain—*Present in 78% with advanced HF*
Patients with advanced malignancies and concomitant heart failure have frequently experienced pain previously. As in other situations, pain is

frequently quantified using visual analog scales or other age-appropriate tools in young children. The nature and cause of the pain in oncologic patients with HF are typically multifactorial involving altered organ perfusion as well as the other causes seen in chronically ill patients including osteoarthritis and old injuries. Pain has both physical and psychological components, leading to patients fearing their disease is progressing. The overlay of anxiety and fear as well as spiritual distress over the realization that the disease is getting worse require care and timely attention from chaplains, psychotherapists, volunteers, and other personnel. Psychoactive medications may benefit these patients, but the somatic pain must be simultaneously managed. Integrative modalities are important adjuncts in managing pain.

Fatigue and Weakness—*Common finding often with progression to anorexia, cachexia, inanition*
Fatigue, weakness, anorexia, and ultimately inanition are common final pathways the body goes through as death approaches. Depending on the patient's goals, where they are estimated to be in the trajectory of their terminal illness, and the degree of physical disability already present, fatigue and weakness are often difficult to treat effectively. Beyond attempts at improving cardiac function and reducing the work of breathing, stimulants such as methylphenidate may be of benefit. Exploring depression as a comorbidity is important with consultation for use of antidepressants, as indicated. Integrative modalities will provide comfort and relief and may allow opportunities for expression of existential or spiritual concerns.

Depression—*Present in 59% with advanced HF*
Depression is common in some patients with cancer and advancing HF. It can be a debilitating symptom and limit a patient's ability to take advantage of the time remaining. The assessment of depression should follow standards for evaluating a patient's psychological state of well-being including appropriate questioning of social supports, suicidal thoughts, and other sources of anxiety and concern. The severity of depression is often proportional to general symptom burden, thus the optimal treatment of other physical symptoms may help to reduce the depression. Psychotherapeutic consultation, spiritual support, and volunteers to provide conversation and distraction are important adjuncts to the management of depression.

Nausea/Vomiting—*Present in 32% with advanced HF*
One of the most debilitating symptoms is nausea with vomiting, which limits a patient's ability to attend to family members, engage in activities, enjoy food, and find pleasure in life. This leads to depression, anger, feelings of isolation, and distrust of medical providers, and undermines a patient's ability to cope with his or her illness. Most often, nausea/vomiting stems from medication effects, including opiates, or impaired gut perfusion. When all attempts to correct the organic and pharmacologic causes are unsuccessful, antiemetic and antacid therapies are frequently used. Occasionally, prokinetic agents are used; however, their use in the face of intestinal "claudication" is not recommended.

Constipation—*Present in 37% with advanced HF*
As in many adults and children with advanced disease, oral intake reduces intake of food with high fiber content, and constipation may ensue. Opiates play a large role in decreasing gut motility and producing constipation. This condition is not only painful but embarrassing and degrading when enemas and other invasive means are needed for relief. A proactive approach to such patients with an effective bowel regimen is the proper course of action.

Anorexia/Cachexia—*Present in 43% with advanced heart failure*
As in the case of fatigue, anorexia and the ensuing cachexia leading to inanition is a common pathway in the process of dying. Many patients are not disturbed by the loss of appetite. Because eating is a social activity in our society, the absence at the dinner table and loss of routines that eating together provides may be a great source of distress for family members. Assessment should look for treatable causes and see whether the family and/or patient is disturbed by the lack of appetite. Depending upon the goals of care and where the patient is in the trajectory of his or her disease, one can consider appetite stimulants or artificial/tube feedings, if that is consistent with the patient's wishes and goals (Table 7.1).

PALLIATIVE CARE EMERGENCIES IN PATIENTS WITH ADVANCED HF

- Consider a pre-emptive discussion of resuscitation status based on patient goals and values.
- Leaving a pacemaker on to provide better cardiac output is consistent with hospice goals.
- Plan with the cardiologist for deactivating the implantable cardioverter defibrillator (ICD) device to prevent terminal shocking.
  - A large, donut magnet placed directly over the ICD will temporarily inactivate the defibrillator function and prevent painful shocks in a dying patient. A pacemaker programming device is required to permanently change the ICD settings.
- As in all other areas of palliative care, pain and inadequately relieved symptoms constitute emergencies and deserve expert involvement.

Table 7.1 Symptoms Commonly Seen in Patients With Advanced Heart Failure

Symptom	Goal	Recommended treatments (9)	Consideration in HF

Dyspnea
• Perception of difficulty in breathing, awareness of uncomfortable breathing, commonly referred to as "shortness of breath"
• Hallmark of advanced heart failure, pleural disease, pulmonary disease; bronchospasm
• Rule outneuromuscular causes
• Frequent finding as complicating factor in pericardial disease, lung metastases, COPD
	• Maintenance of euvolemia/minimize fluid overload
	• Optimize medical HF regimen
	• Treat life-threatening sources, e.g. bronchospasm, arrhythmia, tamponade, airway compression (all of which may be fatal in the short term)
	• Do not overfeed
		• Diuretics
		• Sodium and fluid restriction
		• ACE/ARB (systolic HF)
		• Beta-blocker
		• Mineralocorticoid antagonist
		• IV inotrope infusion (refractory symptom)
		• Opioids
		(usually effective at half the analgesic dose; starting dose depends on recent opiate use)
		Morphine
		  Adults—5 to 15 mg oral
		  1–5 mg SC/IV q10m
		  Child—*orally*
		  0.1–0.25 mg/kg/dose
		  every 4 hours
		  IV 0.02–0.08 mg/kg prn q 10m
		• Alternates
		(Dose adjusted as needed)
		  ○ Hydromorphone
		  ○ Fentanyl
		  ○ Methadone
		• Supplemental oxygen adjusted to symptom needs, ***not*** SaO_2
		• Benzodiazepine (not first line; used as adjunct, n.b. may add to respiratory depression)
		• Fan for cool air to face
		• Consider high-flow or BIPAP for sleep disordered breathing
		Integrative modalities:
		• MBSR
		• Pulmonary rehab
			• Monitor renal function and electrolytes
			• Titrate dose hold if hypotensive or bradycardic
			• Monitor electrolytes
			• Consideration if hypotensive and overloaded, inpatient
			• Dose for renal insufficiency (convert to fentanyl or methadone)
			• Constipation
			  ○ Use bowel regimen
			• Potential for long QTc

(continued)

Table 7.1 Symptoms Commonly Seen in Patients With Advanced Heart Failure (*continued*)

Symptom	Goal	Recommended treatments (9)	Consideration in HF

Pain
• Attempt to identify source: osteoarthritis, neuropathy, chest tube/surgical sites; will exacerbate other symptoms
	Ischemic pain
	Other
	• Surgical sites
	• General
	• Neuropathic pain (from cancer therapies)
		Antianginal therapy
		• Beta-blockers
		• Opiates
		  ○ Wound care
		  ○ Local analgesia
		  ○ Regional blocks
		Acetaminophen
		• Antiepileptics
		• TCA (low-dose)
		• SSRIs (low-dose)
		Topical NSAID
		(avoid systemic due to impact on renal function)
		Medical marijuana
		Opioids
		Tramadol
		Oxycodone, hydromorphone fentanyl
		Integrative Modalities:
		• Acupuncture
		• Massage
		• Exercise
		• MBSR
			• Dose adjust in hepatic insufficiency
			• Dose adjust in renal insufficiency
			• Monitor for hypervolemia (possible systemic absorption)
			• Fluid retention, GI upset, renal dysfunction
			• Dose adjust for renal and hepatic dysfunction
			• Monitor for serotonin syndrome when used in combination with serotonergic medication
			• Constipation (bowel regimen)
			• QTc prolongation (as above)

(*continued*)

Table 7.1 Symptoms Commonly Seen in Patients With Advanced Heart Failure (*continued*)

Symptom	Goal	Recommended treatments (9)	Consideration in HF
Fatigue and weakness • Multifactorial	Reverse/address treatable underlying causes: • Anemia • Thyroid dysfunction • Depression • Sleep-disordered breathing • Insomnia • Cardiac insufficiency • Loss of muscle mass • Deconditioning	• Continuous positive airway pressure (for LV afterload reduction, ↓respiratory work) • Nocturnal oxygen • NIPPV therapy • Trazodone • Melatonin • Behavioral changes (ii.e., sleep hygiene) • Optimize cardiac performance and regular exercise in those who can exercise Stimulant therapy • Methylphenidate Integrative modalities: • MBSR • Acupuncture • Massage • Aromatherapy	• If patient unable to tolerate may exacerbate heart failure • Monitor for QT prolongation • Monitor for heart failure exacerbation, arrhythmia, hyper-/hypotension

(continued)

Table 7.1 Symptoms Commonly Seen in Patients With Advanced Heart Failure *(continued)*

Symptom	Goal	Recommended treatments (9)	Consideration in HF
Depression Correlates with higher symptom burden and increased risk for adverse outcomes Sense of hopelessness, loss of purpose, under-treated pain, existential distress	Establish improved self-worth, discover achievable goals, optimize personal relationships	• Cognitive behavioral therapy and psychotherapy • Spiritual support • SSRI • Citalopram • Fluoxetine • Fluvoxamine • Paroxetine TCA • Mirtazapine • Desipramine • Nortriptyline Psychostimulant • Methylphenidate Integrative modalities • MBSR • Acupuncture • Massage	• Inquire about suicidal ideation • Monitor for hyponatremia, fluid retention • Risk of serotonin syndrome • Monitor for QT prolongation • Monitor for worsening heart failure with increasing doses (side effect: fluid and sodium retention)

(continued)

Table 7.1 Symptoms Commonly Seen in Patients With Advanced Heart Failure (*continued*)

Symptom	Goal	Recommended treatments (9)	Consideration in HF
Nausea/vomiting • Usually due to combination of reduced gut perfusion and medication side effects in advanced HF	Relieve nausea/vomiting to allow some oral intake for social interaction	Discontinue non-essential medications • Low-dose aspirin given with food or discontinue 5-HT3 receptor antagonist • Ondansetron Phenothiazines • Promethazine • prochlorperazine Prokinetic agents • Metoclopramide Dronabinol/medical marijuana Integrative modalities: • MBSR • Acupuncture • Aromatherapy	• Monitor for QT prolongation • Monitor for psychoactive effects and sleep disturbance
Constipation *Present in 37% with advanced HF* • Secondary to decreased food intake, physical inactivity, medication side effects		Consumption of high fiber foods (challenging for many patients) • Stool softener • Osmotic laxatives • Stimulant laxatives • Opioid antagonists, if related to opiates use • Prokinetic agents Integrative modalities: • Acupuncture • Pre-/probiotics	• Some require 8 ounces of fluid • Monitor for abdominal cramping • Monitor for QT prolongation

(continued)

Table 7.1 Symptoms Commonly Seen in Patients With Advanced Heart Failure (*continued*)

Symptom	Goal	Recommended treatments (9)	Consideration in HF

Anorexia/cachexia
• Advanced HF is often associated with increased catabolism in conjunction with anorexia, leading to cardiac cachexia
		• Mirtazapine
		• Optimize HF therapy (positive effects on cardiac cachexia)
		  ○ Carvedilol
		  ○ ACE inhibitor
		  ○ Enalapril
		• Corticosteroids
		• Medical marijuana
		• High energy nutritional supplement
		Integrative modalities:
		• Ginseng
		• Acupuncture
		• Hypnosis/MBSR
		• Aromatherapy
			• Monitor for worsening HF symptoms at doses ↑15 mg
			• Monitor for fluid retention (Loprinzi)

ACE, angiotensin-converting enzyme; ARB, angiotensin receptor blockers; COPD, chronic obstructive pulmonary disease; HF, heart fiailure; MBSR, mindfulness based stress reduction; NIPPV, nasal intermittent positive pressure ventilation; NSAIDs, nonsteroidal anti-inflammtory drugs; SSRI, selective serotonin reuptake inhibitors; TCA, tricyclic antidepressant

REFERENCES

1. Goodlin SJ. Palliative care in congestive heart failure. *J Am Coll Cardiol*. 2009;54(5):386–396. doi:10.1016/j.jacc.2009.02.078

2. Bansal N, Akam-Venkata J, Franco VI, Lipshultz SE. *Heart Failure in Pediatric Oncologic Disease*. In: Jeffries JL, Chang AC, Rossano, et al., eds. *Heart Failure in the Child and Young Adult*. Cambridge, MA: Academic Press; 2018:425–443.

3. Oeffinger KC, Mertens AC, Sklar CA, et al. Chronic health conditions in adult survivors of childhood cancer. *N Engl J Med*. 2006;355(15):1572–1582. doi:10.1056/NEJMsa060185

4. Armstrong GT, Kawashima T, Leisenring W, et al. Aging and risk of severe, disabling, life-threatening, and fatal events in the childhood cancer survivor study. *J Clin Oncol*. 2014;32(12):1218–1227. doi:10.1200/JCO.2013.51.1055

5. Bhakta N, Liu Q, Yeo F, et al. Cumulative burden of cardiovascular morbidity in paediatric, adolescent, and young adult survivors of Hodgkin's lymphoma: an analysis from the St Jude Lifetime Cohort Study. *Lancet Oncol*. 2016;17(9):1325–1334. doi:10.1016/s1470-2045(16)30215-7

6. McMurray JJ. Clinical practice: Systolic heart failure. *N Engl J Med*. 2010;362(3):228–238. doi:10.1056/NEJMcp0909392

7. Bloom MW, Hamo CE, Cardinale D, et al. Cancer Therapy-Related Cardiac Dysfunction and Heart Failure: Part 1: Definitions, Pathophysiology, Risk Factors, and Imaging. *Circ Heart Fail*. 2016;9(1):e002661. doi:10.1161/CIRCHEARTFAILURE.115.002661

8. Reisfield G, Wilson G, Marks S. *Palliative Care Issues in Heart Failure*. 2015, Palliative Care Network of Wisconsin: Fast Facts and Concepts #144.

9. Hamo CE, Bloom MW, Cardinale D, et al. Cancer Therapy-Related Cardiac Dysfunction and Heart Failure: Part 2: Prevention, Treatment, Guidelines, and Future Directions. *Circ Heart Fail*. 2016;9(2):e002843. doi:10.1161/CIRCHEARTFAILURE.115.002843

Pulmonary Symptom Management in Adults and Children With Oncologic Disease

David M. Steinhorn

INTRODUCTION

The symptoms of dyspnea, which is a subjective experience of breathing discomfort (1), breathlessness, a subjective sensation of not being able to catch one's breath, wheezing, and chronic cough are common findings in up to 70% to 80% of adults and children with advanced oncologic disease (2–7). Airway obstruction from mediastinal disease or intrinsic airway tumors may present as a medical emergency requiring expert airway management skills to avoid loss of patency during sedation for procedures and intubation. When the source of the pulmonary symptoms cannot be eliminated or controlled, unrelieved respiratory symptoms may have a devastating and demoralizing impact on a patient's quality of life and will to live, requiring assiduous management through pharmacologic and nonpharmacologic measures.

This chapter provides recommendations for the palliative management of:

1. Dyspnea and breathlessness
2. Airway compression from mediastinal masses
3. Cough
4. Malignant pleural effusion
5. Hiccups
6. Noninvasive ventilation considerations

PALLIATIVE MANAGEMENT

General Guidelines

- Oxygen therapy should be used in palliative care in two situations:
  - When it provides demonstrable symptomatic relief from dyspnea or air hunger
  - When it provides time to undertake thoughtful evaluation, goals of care discussions, or to achieve a short term important goal (e.g., family gathering)
- When patients are actively dying, oxygen may prolong the process of dying without providing greater relief than cool air to the face, for example, from a fan
- In contrast to acute care medicine with curative intention, the goals of respiratory support in palliative care are to achieve comfort, allow alert time for social interaction, and smooth out the process leading to death

- Monitoring of saturations has a limited role in palliative care but comforts the staff

Diagnosis Versus Symptomatic Management in Patients With Advanced Cancer

- Weigh the burden of diagnostic evaluation versus the likelihood of discovering a treatable cause
- Greater probability for survival warrants a more aggressive diagnostic pursuit
- Symptomatic management to improve quality of life takes precedence over diagnosis, when treatment is elusive and life expectancy is limited
- Impending airway obstruction mandates high level expertise to prevent suffocation or inadvertently worsening the patient's situation (8)

Pulmonary Symptom Management

- Respiratory effort is driven by (a) abnormal acid-base and blood gas status, or (b) mechanoreceptor input from the lung or chest wall. Ascending signals from the chest elicit both physical responses (depth and rate of respirations) as well as the perception of difficulty in breathing. Opioids remain the mainstay for the symptomatic management of many respiratory symptoms (discussed separately in the following text)
- The use of noninvasive ventilation (BIPAP, CPAP, high-flow nasal cannula) as a palliative support tool as well as withdrawal of artificial ventilator support is covered after specific symptom management

Considerations for opioid use in patients with respiratory distress:

- Irrational concerns for respiratory depression lead clinicians to undertreat symptoms
- Effective opioid doses are typically less than 1/2 of the typical analgesic dose
- Consider drug interactions and altered kinetics related to hepatic (CYP3A4 and CYP2D6) and renal elimination (9)
- Initial dosing should be based upon the patient's recent opioid use, known allergies (e.g., itching with morphine), and previous reaction to opioids
- Codeine is *no longer recommended for children* due to deaths reported in children who were rapid metabolizers

Dyspnea

Chronic, refractory dyspnea and breathlessness impact all aspects of a patient's life and lead to fear, social isolation, and depression for the patient and caregivers. While dyspnea and breathlessness occur commonly in all ages with advanced cancer (3,6,7), clinicians must also consider other sources such as cardiac failure (65% incidence of dyspnea), neuromuscular disease (weakness, deconditioning), or exacerbations of chronic pulmonary conditions such as COPD (90% incidence of dyspnea).

Table 8.1 Adults—Medical Research Council (MRC) Breathlessness Scale (12)	
Grade	Degree of breathlessness related to activities
1	Not troubled by breathlessness except on strenuous exercise
2	Short of breath when hurrying on the level or walking up a slight hill
3	Walks slower than most people on the level, stops after a mile or so, or stops after 15 minutes walking at own pace
4	Stops for breath after walking about 100 yds or after a few minutes on level ground
5	Too breathless to leave the house, or breathless when undressing

Source: From Stenton C. The MRC breathlessness scale. *Occup Med.* 008;58:226–227. doi:10.1093/occmed/kqm162

- *Dyspnea should be screened* using validated tools in all patients with advanced disease (Table 8.1).
  - Assessment should be based upon the patient's report and caregiver's observations.
  - Intensity of dyspnea can be quite variable—may wax and wane.
  - Assess functional limitations.
  - Patients may fear suffocating and insist that their care providers do everything possible to reduce that sensation.
- Sources of dyspnea in advanced cancer:
  - Complications of cancer-directed therapies, for example, chemo- and radiotherapy, cardiac toxicity, pulmonary fibrosis; complications of hematopoietic stem cell transplantation (HSCT; 10) leading to fibrosis, bronchiolitis obliterans, chronic graft-versus-host disease, and ultimately death in many patients
  - Opportunistic infections due to immunosuppression
  - Chest wall and airway involvement, malignant pleural effusions
  - Fluid overload, cardiac decompensation, massive ascites
  - Psychological and social factors leading to perceptions of breathlessness, for example, anxiety
- **Screening Tools (11)**

Visual-Analog or Numeric Scales (Similar to Pain Assessment) (13)
Dyspnea: Ask patient frequently: How much breathing discomfort (shortness of breath) do you have right now? (assessing response to intervention) Is it better better or worse?

0	1	2	3	4	5	6	7	8	9	10	N/A
None		Mild		Moderate			Severe	Unbearable			Can't Respond

For children, the *"Fifteen-count breathlessness score"* and the pictorial Dalhousie dyspnea scale are reliable and easy to use (14,15).

Fifteen-Count Breathlessness Score (14)

The subject takes a deep breath and counts out loud to 15, taking about 8 seconds to do so. The number of breaths needed to complete the count, including the initial breath, is the score (the minimum score is one).

Treatment Strategies

These will *depend on where the patient is, in the dying trajectory.*

- Non-pharmacologic
  - Positioning for optimal comfort, open airway
  - Use of relaxation techniques (e.g., mindfulness-based stress reduction [MBSR]), pulmonary rehabilitation
  - Reduce fluids in imminently dying
  - Increase air movement (fan toward face)
  - Trial of oxygen (room air *equally* effective) via nasal cannula or mask (may enhance sense of self-control) → titrate to comfort and not SaO_2 in dying patient
  - Use of noninvasive ventilation to reduce symptom burden *(see following text)*
- Pharmacologic—*Opioids are mainstay for adults and children (16)*
  - Starting dose depends on recent opioid use
  - For children less than 6 months, contact pediatric consultant, especially for those less than 1 month
  - Specific agents
    - Morphine:*   Adults: ***orally*** 5–15 mg *(usually effective at ~½ analgesic dose)* SC/IV 1–5 mg q10–60 min until comfortable

      *Nebulized opioids best studied in COPD and not superior to SC in an adult study
    - Children: *(usually effective at ~ 1/4 to 1/2 analgesic dose)*

      orally 0.1–0.25 mg/kg/dose q 4 hours (onset ~30–45) IV 0.02–0.08 mg/kg prn q 10–60 min as needed
  - Alternates – *Adjust dose based upon conventional opioid equivalency*
    - Hydromorphone, fentanyl, methadone, oxycodone
  - Benzodiazepines: adjunct to opioids *to reduce anxiety component*
    - Lorazepam: Adults: 1–2 mg PO/NG q 8 hr
      - Children: 0.025–0.05 mg/kg PO/NG q 6 hr
    - Midazolam: Adults: N/A
      - Children: 0.25–0.5 mg/kg PO/NG max 20 mg q 4 hr

        0.2–0.3 mg/kg intranasal q 2 hr

○ Diazepam: Adults: 10–25 mg daily in 2–3 divided doses

Children: 0.25–0.5 mg/kg PO/NG q 6–8 hrs max 10 mg

- Drying agent to reduce excess oral/pharyngeal secretions (also known as "death rattle"; restrict fluid in dying patient—moisten mouth)
  ○ Scopolamine: Adults/children: 1 patch every 3 days
  ○ Glycopyrolate: Adults: 1–2 mg PO/NG q 8 hr prn max 8 mg/day

  Children: 0.04–0.1 mg/kg q 4–8 hr prn max 8 mg/day

  ○ Atropine: 1% ophth gtt *Infants*: 2 drops sublingual q 2 hrs (17)

Airway Compression Due to Mediastinal Masses (8)

Compression of the trachea, bronchi, esophagus and cardiac structures are recognized complications of anterior mediastinal masses arising from both benign and malignant sources as well as vascular anomalies. Signs may consist of cough, wheezing, and dyspnea, SVC syndrome, dysphagia, and cardiac tamponade. The airway signs may be positional with supine positioning creating the greatest compromise.

- Intubation of patients with anterior mediastinal mass requires *high level expertise*
- Determine patients position of optimal comfort, "rescue position," for example, sitting, decubitus
- Intubation may require rigid bronchoscopy, ear/nose/throat, and anesthesia
- Patients may sense impending suffocation leading to anxiety, hyperpnea, and upper airway obstruction
- Sedation can lead to loss of airway and should only be used in dying patients or with expert airway support at hand
- Determine goals of care and establish an emergency airway plan

Cough

Cough may be a distressing symptom disrupting sleep, creating fatigue, and detracting from daily activities and social interactions. It is present in up to 40% of advanced cancer due to upper and lower airway disease (asthma and chronic obstructive pulmonary disease [COPD]), lung cancer or lung/airway metastases, interstitial pulmonary disease, pulmonary edema, gastroesophageal reflux, aspiration, and drugs (e.g., angiotensin converting enzyme [ACE] inhibitors, nonsteroidal anti-inflammatory drugs [NSAIDs], and inhalant medications).

Treatment Strategies

- Nonpharmacologic
  - Eliminate underlying cause, for example, post-nasal drip, gastroesophageal reflux disease [GERD], bronchospasm

- Sweet syrups, for example, honey, plain syrups—controlled trials absent (but widely touted as effective with no known toxicity)
- Optimize GERD management with anti-reflux measures
- Over-the-counter antitussive agents
  - Typically, antihistamines and mucolytics—poor evidence for efficacy
  - Potential for additive sedation and side effects
  - Actively discouraged for pediatric patients due to lack of beneficial evidence
- Pharmacologic—*opioids are mainstay but no evidence that one is superior to another*
  - Hydromorphone: Adults: **orally** 5–10 mg every 4–6 hr
    - Children: limited evidence/morphine preferred
  - Dextromethorphan: Adults: **orally** 10–20 mg every 4–6 hr *(risk of serotonin syndrome)*
    - Children: **orally** 5–10 mg every 4–6 hr
  - Codeine Adults: **orally** 10–20 mg
    - Children: *not recommended*
- Centrally acting non-opioid antitussives
  - Gabapentin (18): Adults: doses up to 1,800 mg/day
    - Child: *not studied for cough*
- Nebulized lidocaine (2%) and bupivacaine (0.25%)
  - 5 mL nebulized every 6 to 8 hours for refractory cough
  - Weak evidence base, but published anecdotal benefit

Malignant Pleural Effusions (19)

Malignant pleural effusions may present with cough, dyspnea/breathlessness, hypoxia, and decreased exercise tolerance. Up to 50% of malignancies may present with pleural effusion.

- Diagnosis based upon clinical exam, chest x-ray, CT, or ultrasound
- Common with lymphomas and cancer of the breast, lung, and ovary
- Life expectancy typically 4 to 6 months
- Need to rule out other causes, for example, heart failure, infection, as appropriate
- Treatment depends on stage of disease trajectory

Treatment Strategies for Malignant Pleural Effusions

- Ascertain goals of care, that is, extended survival versus comfort during dying process
- Oxgyen therapy to minimize hypoxia, evaluation and goals of care planning, unless imminently dying, then only if oxygen increases comfort
- Noninvasive ventilation support to reduce work of breathing until a definitive plan and goals of care are established, **avoid intubation unless extended survival likely**

- Therapeutic challenge with thoracentesis to determine whether fluid removal will improve symptom burden
  - Trial removal of 20 mL/kg (adult or child) via simple thoracentesis
  - Placement of a pleural drainage device, e.g., Pleurex™ or pigtail catheter, as access for repeated drainage for symptomatic management, then access and draining of fluid as needed for comfort (20)
    - Tunneled or nontunneled depending on expected duration
    - Patients can go home with instructions on how to drain intermittently
  - May need to replace some volume intravenously to prevent hypovolemia
- Chemosclerosis with talc or other agents *(contact thoracic surgery)*
- Palliative chemo/hormone therapy for treatment of sensitive tumors *(contact oncology)*

Hiccups (21)

A hiccup is a distressing symptom involving vagal and phrenic nerve leading to spasmodic activity of the diaphragm and chest wall.

- More than 48 hours = prolonged; more than one month = intractable
- Wide range of causes in patients with cancer: brain stem, mediastinum, GI tract
- No reliable, consistent remedy
- Acupuncture, home remedies, coughing/sneezing to interrupt cycle
- Anti-psychotics

Chlorpromazine:	Adults:	25–50 mg PO tid
	Children:	0.5–1 mg/kg/dose q 4–6 hrs
Haloperidol:	Adults:	1–4 mg PO tid
	Children:	0.05–0.15(max) mg/kg/d ÷ tid

- Anti-convulsants

Gabapentin:	Adults	300–400 mg tid
	Children:	10–15 mg/kg tid

Noninvasive Ventilation Techniques for Patients With Advanced Malignancy

- Noninvasive positive pressure ventilation (NIPPV) widely used in acute medicine
  - BIPAP, CPAP, high-flow nasal cannula (HFNC)
  - Reduce inspiratory work of breathing; createpositive end-expiratory pressure (PEEP) to maintain airway and lung patency (functional residual capacity [FRC])
  - Reduces the incidence of intubation and improves quality of life in acute care
  - Use of NIPPV *can create ambiguity about goals of care and priorities* for patients with incurable, advanced disease

- NIPPV can be frightening and uncomfortable for many, disrupting sleep and interactions with loved ones. So it should be stopped, if not benefiting the patient
- Contraindications to NIPPV
  - Perforation of a hollow viscus, ileus, or vomiting risk (due to aspiration risk especially with full face mask)
  - Nasopharyngeal to intracranial connections (following trauma or surgery)
  - Patients who cannot tolerate the interface
- The application of NIPPV in the palliative care and hospice setting should meet one of several goals:
  - Extending life for as long as possible while rejecting intubation (*typically with a Do Not Intubate order which* implies *Do Not Resuscitate because effective CPR generally requires intubation*)
  - Temporizing while goals of care can be determined or other measures, for example, diuresis, can improve the dyspnea (especially for the patient who rejects intubation)
  - Reducing symptom burden and improving quality of life with reduced sedation requirement during the dying process (22)
- During the **acute dying process, opioids are the symptom treatment of choice**
- Goals of care and indications for stopping NIPPV must be *defined before initiating*
- NIPPV can delay death in the imminently dying patient to provide time for loved ones to get to the bedside or to achieve other meaningful, short-term goals
- Nasal interfaces may make BIPAP/CPAP more acceptable than a mask, especially children
- NIPPV may allow a tenuous, hospitalized patient to be transported home to die
- NIPPV is logistically challenging to initiate in the home or hospice setting
  - Requires respiratory therapy, durable medical equipment supplier, experienced hospice team

High-Flow Nasal Cannula (HFNC) in the Palliative Care Setting

- Originally developed for adults with obstructive sleep apnea
- Good evidence it can reduce the need for intubation and make patients more comfortable
- Widely used for young children in whom a BIPAP interface is not always available
- May provide some minimally invasive symptom relief

Death in Patients With Advanced, Incurable Disease Requiring Artificial Respiratory Support

- Death defined by loss of cardiac function (asystole) occurs through:

- - Decreased myocardial perfusion (oxygen delivery) → asystole
  - Non-perfusing rhythms or intractable hypotension → asystole
  - Respiratory failure → hypoxia → poor myocardial oxygen delivery → asystole
  - Cerebral herniation → cardiac stun → asystole
- Commonly, inadequate myocardial oxygen delivery leading to death, that is, asystole
  - Therefore, *all measures that continue oxygenation will delay death or prolong the process of dying*
- If goals of care do not include extending life, artificially supporting oxygenation should cease
- In the hospitalized patient, artificial means of support include mechanical ventilation, supplemental oxygen, and cardiovascular agents
- Ethically, physicians are entitled to discontinue a therapy that is no longer achieving the intended goal
- When the medical team and the family, ideally with the participation of the patient, accept that further therapy is no longer beneficial, then discontinuation of the artificial life support should be considered

Discontinuation of Artificial Life Support [Detailed Discussion in (23)]

- Have a clear discussion with family of goals, expected outcome, and process
  - Discuss sedation plan and approach to distress (alertness may not be possible)
  - Consider compassionate sedation protocol
    - Propofol or dexmetetomidine infusions planned with ICU/anesthesia
    - Continue or increase narcotic and sedative infusions
- Consider location and timing of discontinuation (ICU, ward, home, hospice)
- Make sure that family is present and all have had an opportunity to say goodbye
- Arrange for family rituals, traditions, celebration of life
- Make sure that support staff are available (nursing, respiratory therapy, chaplain)
- Have multiple doses of chosen sedative at bedside
  - Stop paralytics and ensure patient can manifest signs of distress, if present
    - IV glycopyrrolate IV 30 min before, if intubated
  - Administer morphine and lorazepam bolus, if anxiety/agitation/distress anticipated
  - Decrease FiO_2 → 21% assessing for signs of dyspnea

- Wean BIPAP/ventilator rate and pressures over 5 to 10 min observing for signs of distress in face or breathing pattern; agonal gasping is physiologic but disturbing for family to watch, explain process in advance, sedate patient
- If extubating, deflate endotracheal tube (ETT), have suction for oral secretions, and towel to wrap removed ETT in during withdrawal
- Administer IV bolus sedation as needed for signs of distress
  - Distress most common within the first few hours
- Physician should remain with patient/family talking about what is happening and assuring expert symptom management. *Do not delegate this step to the nurse*
- Be prepared to remain available until death occurs—it means a lot to the family
- Physician and medical staff self-care is important to process the stress created by assisting a patient in leaving his or her life
  - Debrief staff, use chaplain and social worker for support

REFERENCES

1. American Thoracic Society. Dyspnea. Mechanisms, assessment, and management: a consensus statement. *Am J Respir Crit Care Med*. 1999;159:321–340. doi:10.1164/ajrccm.159.1.ats898
2. Star A, Boland J. Updates in palliative care – recent advancements in the pharmacological management of symptoms. *Clin Med*. 2018;18:11–16. doi:10.7861/clinmedicine.18-1-11
3. Singer A, Meeker D, Teno JM, et al. Symptom trends in the last year of life from 1998 to 2010: a cohort study. *Ann Intern Med*. 2015;162:175–183. doi:10.7326/M13-1609
4. Kreher M. Symptom Control at the End of Life. *Med Clin N Am*. 2016;100:1111–1122. doi:10.1016/j.mcna.2016.04.020
5. Mahler D, Selecky PA, Harrod CG, et al. American College of Chest Physicians consensus statement on the management of dyspnea in patients with advanced lung or heart disease. *Chest*. 2010;137:674–691. doi:10.1378/chest.09-1543
6. Wolfe J, Grier HE, Klar N, et al. Symptoms and suffering at the end of life in children with cancer. *N Engl J Med*. 2000;342(5):326–333. doi:10.1056/NEJM200002033420506
7. Wolfe J, Orellana L, Ullrich C, et al. Symptoms and distress in children with advanced cancer: prospective patient-reported outcomes from the PediQUEST study. *J Clin Oncol*. 2015;33(17):1928–1935. doi:10.1200/JCO.2014.59.1222
8. Blank RS, de Souza DG. Anesthetic management of patients with an anterior mediastinal mass: continuing professional development. *Can J Anaesth*. 2011;58(9):853–859, 860–867. doi:10.1007/s12630-011-9539-x
9. Smith H. The metabolism of opioid agents and the clinical impact of their active metabolites. *Clin J Pain*. 2011;27:824–838. doi:10.1097/AJP.0b013e31821d8ac1
10. Pena E, Souza CA, Escuissato DL, et al. Noninfectious pulmonary complications after hematopoietic stem cell transplantation: practical approach to imaging diagnosis. *Radiographics*. 2014;34:663–683. doi:10.1148/rg.343135080
11. Aslakson R, Dy SM, Wilson RF, et al. Assessment Tools for Palliative Care. Technical Brief, No. 30 Agency for Healthcare Research and Quality May 2017 Report No.: 17-EHC007-EF.
12. Stenton C. The MRC breathlessness scale. *Occup Med*. 2008;58:226–227. doi:10.1093/occmed/kqm162
13. Baker KM, DeSanto-Madeya S, Banzett RB. Routine dyspnea assessment and documentation: Nurses' experience yields wide acceptance. *BMC Nurs*. 2017;16:3. doi:10.1186/s12912-016-0196-9

14. Prasad SA, Randall SD, Balfour-Lynn IM. Fifteen-count breathlessness score: an objective measure for children. *Pediatr Pulmonol.* 2000;30(1):56–62. doi:10.1002/1099-0496(200007)30:1<56::AID-PPUL9>3.0.CO;2-R

15. McGrath PJ, Pianosi PT, Unruh AM, Buckley CP. Dalhousie dyspnea scales: construct and content validity of pictorial scales for measuring dyspnea. *BMC Pediatr.* 2005;5:33. doi:10.1186/1471-2431-5-33

16. Pieper L, Zernikow B, Drake R, et al. Dyspnea in Children with Life-Threatening and Life-Limiting Complex Chronic Conditions. *J Palliat Med.* 2018;21:552–564. doi:10.1089/jpm.2017.0240

17. Protus BM, Grauer PA, Kimbrel JM. Evaluation of atropine 1% ophthalmic solution administered sublingually for the management of terminal respiratory secretions. *Am J Hosp Palliat Care.* 2012;30(4):388–392. doi:10.1177/1049909112453641

18. Ryan N, Birring S, Gibson P. Gabapentin for refractory cough: a randomized, double-blind, placebo-controlled trial. *Lancet Glob Health.* 2012;380:1583–1589. doi:10.1016/s0140-6736(12)60776-4

19. Asciak R, Rahman NM. Malignant pleural effusion: from diagnostics to therapeutics. *Clin Chest Med.* 2018;39(1):181–193. doi:10.1016/j.ccm.2017.11.004

20. Mendes MA, Pereira NC, Ribeiro C, et al. Conventional versus pigtail chest tube-are they similar for treatment of malignant pleural effusions? *Support Care Cancer.* 2018;26:2499–2502. doi:10.1007/s00520-018-4171-8

21. Polito NB, Fellows SE. Pharmacologic interventions for intractable and persistent hiccups: a systematic review. *J Emerg Med.* 2017;53(4):540–549. doi:10.1016/j.jemermed.2017.05.033

22. Nava S, Ferrer M, Esquinas A, et al. Palliative use of non-invasive ventilation in end of life patients with solid tumours: a randomized feasibility trial. *Lancet Oncol.* 2013;14:219–227. doi:10.1016/S1470-2045(13)70009-3

23. Downar J, Delaney JW, Hawryluck L, Kenny L. Guidelines for the withdrawal of life-sustaining measures. *Intensive Care Med.* 2016;42(6):1003–1017. doi:10.1007/s00134-016-4330-7

Gastrointestinal Symptom Management in Adults and Children With Oncologic Disease

Shana S. Jacobs, Gleynora J. GilBhrighde, Margaret M. Mahon, and Catriona Mowbray

INTRODUCTION

Symptoms arising from the gastrointestinal (GI) tract are some of the most burdensome that one can experience. Management of those symptoms is often complex, requiring an understanding of the myriad causes that can lead to GI distress. GI symptoms can arise from underlying diseases, from the treatments of diseases, or as a complication of treatment.

Perhaps more than most other systems, some GI symptoms can be minimized by preventive interventions. Even if prevention is implemented, symptoms often still occur, though they may be less severe.

Oral mucositis is a troubling side effect of chemotherapy and radiation therapy that can lead to pain, poor nutrition, and infection. It often causes dose delays in disease-focused treatments, in addition to requiring opioid pain medications and, often, hospital admissions. Up to 40% of patients receiving conventional chemotherapy, 80% of patients receiving high-dose chemotherapy for hematopoietic stem cell transplantation, and nearly all patients receiving head and neck radiation therapy can suffer from mucositis (1).

Both prevention and treatment of oral mucositis are important. Unfortunately, there are few treatments that are proven effective for either in many patients. However, some of the approaches for prevention and treatment are listed in the following (see Figure 9.1).

Prevention of Oral Mucositis

- **Oral care protocols**, such as bland washes, have weak evidence but little downside for patients receiving any type of chemotherapy (2).
- **Cryotherapy** can be highly effective for patients receiving short infusion chemotherapy, such as bolus 5-FU infusion (3). It can also be effective prior to stem cell transplant, as with melphalan (4), as long as the patients are cooperative.
- **Recombinant human keratinocyte growth factor-1 (KGF-1/palifermin)** is an effective preventive measure for transplant patients receiving high-dose chemotherapy and total body irradiation (60 µg/kg per day for 3 days prior to conditioning treatment and for 3 days after transplant).

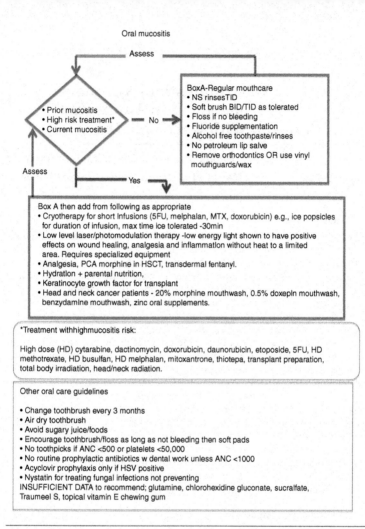

Figure 9.1 Flowchart of mucositis assessment and treatments (4,9–13).

Source: From Sung L, Robinson P, Triester N, et al. Guideline for the prevention of oral and oropharyngeal mucositis in children receiving treatment for cancer or undergoing haemtaopoietic stem cell transplant. *BMJ Support Palliat Care.* 2015;7(1):7–16. doi:10.1136/bmjspcare-2014-000804; He M, Zhang B, Shen N, et al. A systematic review and meta-analysis of the effect of low-level laser therapy (LLLT) on chemotherapy-induced oral mucositis in pediatric and young patients. *Eur J Pediatr.* 2017;177:7–17. doi:10.1007/s00431-017-3043-4; Lalla RV, Bowen J, Barasch A, et al. MASCC/ISOO clinical practice guidelines for the management of mucositis secondary to cancer therapy. *Cancer.* 2014;120(10):1453–1461. doi:10.1002/cncr.28592; Bensinger W, Schubert M, Ang KK, et al. NCCN Task Force Report: prevention and management of mucositis in cancer care. *J Natl Compr Canc Netw.* 2008;6 Suppl 1:S1–S21; quiz S22–S24; Oncology Nursing Society. 2017. https://www.ons.org/practice-resources/pep/mucositis; Chemocare. 2017. http://www.chemocare.com/search.aspx?q=6MP

- **Low-level laser therapy** has been shown to be effective for both prevention and treatment, particularly in patients undergoing stem cell transplant or head and neck irradiation (4–8). As with cryotherapy, patients must be cooperative, which may be a challenge in very young patients.
- **Other specific preventive measures: Benzydamine mouthwash** is effective in patients with head and neck cancer receiving moderate dose radiation therapy. **Zinc supplements** may be effective in oral cancer patients (1).

Treatment of Oral Mucositis

- **Low-level laser therapy** has been shown to be effective for treatment and prevention (see earlier).
- **Pain medications** are really the mainstay of treatment, such as patient-controlled analgesia, transdermal fentanyl, or oral morphine mouth washes; 0.5% doxepin mouthwash may also be effective.
- **Treatment of infection:** In some cases, oral mucositis may be caused by or exacerbated by candidal infection (thrush) or herpetic infection. In these cases, use of nystatin or acyclovir is needed.

XEROSTOMIA

Dry mouth can be a side effect of some medications, such as anticholinergic medications used for nausea, or of treatments such as radiation. Relatively few treatments have been rigorously studied; however, researchers have found some improvement with pilocarpine, artificial saliva, and chewing gum; acupuncture can be tried based on the available data (14).

GASTROESOPHAGEAL (GE) REFLUX

Reflux is often a preexisting condition that is exacerbated by the disease and/or its treatments. A good history, including identifying what has alleviated the symptom, can facilitate management. Reflux may be erosive or nonerosive. It can present with dyspepsia, chest pain, or occasionally cough, irritability or vomiting, especially in young children (15). There are both nonpharmacological and pharmacological ways to treat GE reflux.

- Nonpharmacological
  - Assess for food sensitivities—initiate elimination diets
  - Avoid spicy foods
  - Avoid eating late at night (within 3 hours of reclining)
- Pharmacological management:
  - Initial treatment is H_2 blocker (e.g., famotidine) for 2 weeks
    - If there is no benefit, initiate a trial of proton pump inhibitor (PPI) (16)
    - Can include a combination of a PPI, later adding metoclopramide for prokinesis
  - If the patient has a longer life expectancy, consider a gastroenterology consult

    ◦ If the prognosis is very short, sucralfate (Carafate) may be of more immediate benefit, especially in cases of suspected gastritis/erosive esophagitis (17)

ERUCTATION/GAS

- Air swallowing (aerophagia), a major source of eructation, can occur with food gulping, drinking carbonated beverages, gum chewing, and smoking. Discontinuation or reduction of these behaviors may modify symptoms. Aerophagia may also be a manifestation of anxiety
- Flatulence may result from:
  - Alteration of intestinal motility or microbiome (e.g., following antibiotic treatment, microbial overgrowth)
  - Dietary factors (lactose intolerance, mal-absorption of carbohydrate(s), ingestion of legumes, or ingestion of fructose)
  - Psychological factors that heighten awareness of normal passage of flatus

Dietary evaluation by a nutritionist and dietary changes may be of benefit. Recently, the value of a low FODMAP (**F**ermentable **O**ligosaccharides, **D**isaccharides, **M**onosaccharides, **A**nd **P**olyols) diet has been recognized. FODMAPs are short chain carbohydrates. A low FODMAP diet has been shown to decrease symptoms of irritable bowel syndrome (IBS; 18), as well as discomfort for others with food intolerances. In a subgroup of patients, a low FODMAP diet was associated with a significant decrease in H2 production. Of note, anticholinergic drugs in this patient population may exacerbate symptoms.

If dietary changes do not help, some medications may prove efficacious.

- Beano contains alpha-D-galactosidase, an enzyme that helps metabolize foods with a high alpha linked sugar content, such as grains, seeds, or some vegetables. It might help relieve symptoms for some patients, however, no difference in quality of life was found in a placebo trial, and the experimental group had more drop outs due to abdominal pain and diarrhea (19)
- Bismuth salicylate may reduce odor from eructation and passage of flatus (20)
- Baclofen (adult dose: 10 mg TID) may reduce belching and aerophagia when dietary modifications fail (21)
- Rifamixin (nonabsorbable antibiotic) has shown some benefit in cases of bacterial overgrowth (20)
- Biofeedback offers a nonpharmacological approach that may be of benefit (22)
- Simethicone has not been shown to be of benefit and contradictory evidence exists for use of activated charcoal (20)

If gas is associated with new onset weight loss, diarrhea, abdominal pain, and distension or anorexia, the patient should be referred to GI for work-up (20).

NAUSEA AND VOMITING

Nausea and vomiting are not typically discrete symptoms, in that their presence is often associated with a general sensation of "not feeling well" and decreased quality of life (23,24). Health caregivers often underestimate the burdens that nausea and vomiting cause for patients (24), and treatment is often inadequate to achieve symptom control (23).

Causes (Table 9.1)

As with most symptom management, identification of the cause is critical for optimal management. If possible, the cause should be reduced or eliminated. If this is not possible, then treatment to minimize the symptom is needed. The cause indicates the neural pathway. The neural pathway indicates the neurotransmitter involved. Identification of the neurotransmitter guides decision making about which first-line antiemetic to use, because each antiemetic antagonizes a specific neurotransmitter (25).

Treatment

There are many types of antiemetics. In most cases, knowing the etiology helps to identify the optimal medication class (26) (Table 9.2). Additionally, considering common and significant side effects may be relevant in choosing appropriate antiemetics for a given patient. For example, a patient with known QTc prolongation might not be an appropriate candidate for 5HT3 antagonists or D2 antagonists. Patients with a history of psychosis should avoid dronabinol. Note that some of these medications have not been extensively studied or approved for use in young children, although many are often used off label for children.

Prevention

In addition to treating nausea and vomiting, it is imperative to try to prevent nausea and vomiting when giving medications like chemotherapy that can be emetogenic (27). Chemotherapy can be classified by its emetogenic potential, and the prophylactic antiemetic regimen should be chosen according to the emetogenic potential of the regimen combined with the patient's personal history of nausea and vomiting with prior regimens. Standard preventive regimens are as follows:

- Highly emetogenic regimens: NK1 receptor antagonist + 5HT3 receptor antagonist + dexamethasone + olanzapine
- Moderate or low emetogenic regimens: 5-HT3 receptor antagonist + dexamethasone

Antiemetics other than those listed earlier (lorazepam, cannibinoids, anticholinergics, and prokinetics) can be helpful for treatment or prevention of chemotherapy-induced nausea and vomiting; however, the evidence is weaker. Similarly, many patients find nonpharmacological adjuvants, such as acupuncture and acupressure, ginger, and aromatherapy to be extremely helpful but there is less clear evidence to support their use (27). Recommendations are similar in pediatric patients although olanzapine, and some of the newer NK-1 receptor antagonists, have not been well studied in children (28).

Table 9.1 Causes of Nausea and Vomiting

Causes	Neurotransmitter
Visceral causes (transmitted via vagus nerve to vomiting center) • Distension • Constipation • Irritation	$5HT_3$, D-2, H-1
Chemical causes (via chemoreceptor trigger zone to vomiting center)	$5HT_3$, D-2, NK_1
CNS causes (direct to vomiting center) • Psychological • Limbic • Increased ICP • Increased IOP	H-1
Vestibular causes (direct to vomiting center) • Motion/position • Local tumor • Otic infection	C-M, H-1
Vomiting center to effector organ	C-M, H-1, $5HT_3$
Electrolyte imbalance (e.g., hyponatremia, hypercalcemia, increased ammonia) • Electrolytes affect the CSF, so focus on neurotransmitters approaching the CTZ	$5HT_3$, D-2
Altered liver function • Anatomic distortion: Capsular stretch evokes a visceral cause of nausea/vomiting. • Increased serum ammonia can affect CSF, so focus on neurotransmitters approaching the CTZ	$5HT_3$, D-2
Delayed gastric emptying (use a prokinetic agent (e.g., metoclopramide); use simethicone if gas is present	D-2
Others (e.g., UTI, drug levels)	

$5HT_3$, serotonin; C-M, cholinergic/muscarinic; CNS, central nervous system; CSF, cerebral spinal fluid; CTZ, chemotherapy trigger zone; D-2, dopamine; H-1, histamine; ICP, intracranial pressure; IOP, intraocular pressure; NK_1, neurokinin 1; UTI, urinary tract infection.

OBSTRUCTION

GI obstructions vary based on location and other factors.

Upper GI Obstructions

These will often present with abrupt symptom onset, nausea, and vomiting as the predominant symptom, with less abdominal distension and

Table 9.2 Targeted Treatments of Nausea and Vomiting and Related Side Effects

Cause	Class	Examples	Select side effects
Chemical (i.e., chemotherapy)	Serotonin (5HT3) Antagonists	Ondansetron Granisetron	Headache, constipation/ diarrhea, dry mouth, QTcprolongation
Chemical	Dopamine (D-2) antagonists	Prochlorperazine Chlorpromazine Haloperidol	Tardive dyskinesia/ extrapyramidal symptoms, QTc prolongation, pancytopenia, hepatotoxicity, somnolence
Chemical	Multiple receptors antagonist (5HT3, D-2, others)	Olanzapine	Extrapyramidal symptoms, pancytopenia, hepatotoxicity, drowsiness
Chemical	NK1 antagonist	Aprepitant	Headache, constipation, somnolence, hiccups
Chemical	Cannibinoid	Dronabinol	Hallucinations, dizziness, somnolence, psychiatric symptoms, dependence
Movement related	Anticholinergics	Scopolamine Hydroxyzine Meclizine	Seizures, glaucoma, dry mouth, dizziness, somnolence, confusion
Movement related, chemical	Antihistamine (H1)	Diphenhydramine Promethazine Hydroxyzine	Pancytopenia, seizures, dry mouth, dizziness, somnolence, constipation, palpitations

(continued)

Table 9.2 Targeted Treatments of Nausea and Vomiting and Related Side Effects (*continued*)

Cause	Class	Examples	Select side effects
Bowel spasm	Antimuscarinic	Hyoscine bromide	Psychosis, dry mouth, constipation, palpitations, dizziness, somnolence
Stasis	Prokinetics	Metoclopramide Domeperidone	Tardive dyskinesia, extrapyramidal symptoms, pancytopenia, psychiatric symptoms, dizziness, confusion
Anticipatory/ anxiety	Benzodiazepines	Lorazepam	Respiratory depression, hypotension, syncope, dependence, sedation, constipation, irritability
Increased ICP, chemical	Corticosteroids	Dexamethasone	Adrenal insufficiency, diabetes, psychosis, myopathy, hypertension, weight gain, emotional lability, insomnia

ICP, intracranial pressure; NK$_1$, neurokinin 1.

commonly less pain. The cause is adhesion in 60% of cases, while 20% is due to neoplasm. Less common causes include hernia, intussusception, volvulus, intra-abdominal abscess, gallstones, or foreign bodies (29).

Lower GI Obstruction Symptoms

These may present more slowly and progressively, and include distension, borborygmi, and pain, with diminished to no passage of stool or flatus and hypoactive bowel sounds (30,31).

Obstructions can be partial or complete, and can be extraluminal or intraluminal, and can occur throughout the GI tract. In one study of cancer patients, 16% occurred in the gastric outlet, 64% in the small bowel, and 20% in the large bowel (30).

In considering the etiology, of particular importance is whether or not the patient has had prior abdominal surgery. In adult patients with known malignancy, approximately one third of obstructions are due to benign adhesions (32). In patients without prior surgical history, obstruction should be presumed to be a tumor unless proven otherwise (33). Other benign etiologies include infectious or inflammatory GI diseases (e.g., abscess, phlegmon), radiation enteritis. Most small bowel obstructions in cancer patients are benign (primarily due to adhesions), while large bowel obstructions are more likely to be malignant. The prevalence of obstruction varies by cancer type, with ovarian and colorectal the most common, followed by gastric cancer and abdominal metastases from other cancers (30). Bowel obstructions are relatively rare in children, but are more common after Wilm's tumor resection (34).

Treatment Recommendations

- Patients with a longer life expectancy— prior to confirmatory imaging, initiate fluid resuscitation, fasting (NPO), nasalgastro tube (NGT) decompression, monitoring of urine output. and correction electrolyte abnormalities, surgical referral (29). May consider self-expanding stent in place of palliative resection in patients with cancer
- Patients with a short life expectancy
  - Prokinetics (e.g., metoclopramide) are contraindicated in complete obstruction, but may be useful if it is pseudo-obstruction or incomplete obstruction
  - Dexamethasone may decrease edema surrounding an intrinsic or extrinsic carcinoma. Adult daily dosage is in the range of 6 to 16 mg, with reasonable starting dose of 4 mg BID
  - Use octreotide
  - Use NGT or venting G-tube
  - **IV haloperidol is the treatment of choice in malignant bowel obstruction** (fewer extrapyramidal symptoms than seen with oral form), in conjunction with octreotide and dexamethasone, if needed
  - Manage pain with opioid medications
  - Glycopyrrolate (minimal blood-brain barrier penetration) can be used (29)

Pseudo-obstruction or ileus may mimic obstruction. On x-ray, pronounced colonic dilatation is present (30,35), but with minimal colonic fluid. Presence of air-fluid levels should raise suspicion of obstruction (30). There are many causes of ileus (29,30).

- Medication side effects (e.g., opioids, tricyclic antidepressants, muscarinics)
- Intra-abdominal infections (e.g., appendicitis, gastroenteritis)
- Metabolic disturbances (e.g., hypokalemia)
- Peritoneal carcinomatosis without extrinsic compression due to involvement of autonomic nerves that innervate the intestine
- Neuromuscular disorders (e.g., Parkinson's disease)
- Scleroderma
- Diabetes mellitus, due to neuropathy of involved autonomic nerve involvement

GI BLEED

Upper GI bleeds may present with bright red emesis or "coffee ground" emesis and melena. Lower GI bleeding may present with varying degrees of hematochezia from maroon stools to frank bleeding.

- Patients with a longer life expectancy require judicious work up by a gastroenterologist
  - If the patient is hemodynamically unstable, requires emergent fluid rehydration, oxygen support, NPO, type and crossmatch, placement of large bore IV catheters or central line and immediate surgical consult
  - If the patient is hemodynamically stable, a less urgent GI referral is warranted and the patient may need endoscopy/colonoscopy
- In patients with a very short life expectancy, transexamic acid (TXA; adult dose 1–2 gm orally 4–6 times a day, or 10 mg/kg IV 3–4 times a day) may be of help. Vasopressin (adult dose 0.1 – 0.4 mg/ hr) may be used with select patients in the hospital setting. Alternatively, octreotide (adult dose 50 –100 mcg SC BID) can be used. Rectal bleeding may be addressed with packing with dressings coated with TXA or sucralfate paste (36)
- Patients at the end of life require a thorough and sensitive explanation to caregivers and the patient (if alert), if there is the likelihood that a catastrophic bleeding event will occur, doing so in a manner that educates without provoking fear. If at all possible, someone should remain with the patient. Dark towels should be present (dark maroon, dark brown) to line emesis basin or plastic tub. Dark colored sheets and blankets, quilts and rugs to minimize distress of visual effect of large bleed. Subcutaneous (or sublingual) benzodiazepine may be of some effect, but likely will not have time in a catastrophic event for administration of medication. Ideally, a grief counselor should be available for family members who witness a catastrophic bleeding event, particularly one that involves massive upper GI bleeding with vomiting.

Lower GI massive bleed may be covered with dark towels or blankets to be less distressing to the patient and family members. Patient and family may choose inpatient admission as the situation declines (36)

CONSTIPATION

Constipation is extremely common. The development of constipation may be due to medications, disease, dehydration, weakness, electrolyte imbalances, or other factors. Constipation frequently leads to decreased quality of life, and causes some patients to discontinue treatments that cause constipation (e.g., disease-ocused therapies, opioids, other medications). Prevention of constipation is key to its management.

Steps in Managing Constipation

- Review any drugs or other treatments for constipating potential
- Screen at-risk patients daily, asking directly about constipation and most recent bowel movement
- Addressing the question directly and routinely can help decrease patient embarrassment
- It is especially important to consider the role of opioids as contributing to constipation. The gut has the highest concentration of opioid receptors outside of the CNS; thus the rate of constipation in patients on opioids is extremely high. Though several opioid side effects attenuate with time, constipation will remain a risk throughout the course of treatment. Every patient on an opioid should be on a bowel regimen
- The abdomen may be nontender, but the patient may have distension, or palpation may be uncomfortable (37)
- Digital rectal exam should include evaluation for hypotonia, masses, stricture, and fecal impaction (37) but should be avoided in patients who are neutropenic
- Obtaining a flat plate abdominal film can often clarify the presence or extent of constipation

Although prevalent in the population of those living with serious illness, constipation is frequently overlooked. The index of suspicion of constipation should be low. Consider a rectal exam in patients who are not neutropenic.

The presence of diarrhea does not rule out constipation. Bowel flora will liquefy colonic stool, resulting in the leakage of liquid stool as it passes around the fecal mass. This process is known as overflow diarrhea.

Treatments

Table 9.3 provides the details of medications and their side effects.

In a Cochrane review, the authors reported that, in the general adult population, polyethylene glycol was better than lactulose for resolving constipation. In a population of people receiving palliative care, the authors found no difference between senna, docusate, or lactulose, but polyethylene glycol was not included in most of the studies reviewed (38).

Table 9.3 Treatments for Constipation and Related Side Effects

Class of laxatives	Examples	Side effects/concerns
Osmotic agents	Sorbitol Lactulose Polyethylene glycol Milk of magnesia Magnesium citrate	• Sorbitol and lactulose taste very sweet, which some patients may not like. • PEG may require daily intake of up to 2 liters for optimal effect. • Avoid magnesium products in people with heart or renal failure.
Stimulants (avoid if the patient might have an obstruction)	Sennosides Bisacodyl	May cause cramping.
Bulk forming	Methylcellulose Psyllium	
Softeners	Docusate	
Peripheral opioid agonists	Methylnaltrexone	Expensive, usually a later option for patients. Time limited.
Rectal agents: suppository	Bisacodyl --------------- ---- Glycerin	May cause cramping --------------------------- May be ineffective as sole agent; may be irritating
Enemas	Tap water Saline Mineral oil	

DIARRHEA

Diarrhea in cancer patients may be caused by several different factors, and identifying the cause is essential for treatment. It is also important to determine whether the diarrhea is acute or chronic. Note that diarrhea may be overflow diarrhea related to fecal impaction. Or constipated patients may have taken too much laxative, resulting in diarrhea, so a careful medication history is important.

Acute Diarrhea Management

- Infectious causes are common, especially when patients are myelo-suppressed. In particular, providers should be on alert for *Clostridium difficile* infections, which are more common in patients with neutropenia and after receiving broad spectrum antibiotics (39). If infection is found, treat the cause
  - If present with blood or mucus, most likely infection of large bowel
  - Ask about resent exposures, travel, sick contacts

■ Stool culture should be obtained in cases of severe illness, blood in stool, fever—if grossly bloody test for Shiga toxin. Note that entero-hemorrhagic *Escherichia coli* and Shiga toxin infections should NOT be treated with antibiotics

Treatment

- Volume repletion by oral route with water, salt, sugar solution. If severe dehydration, IV rehydration (40)
- Loperamide may be of some benefit if NOT viral. Counseling patients and families on importance of letting viral illness "run its course" prevents lengthening course or worsening sequelae of viral and infectious diarrhea (41)
- Glycopyrrolate or cholestyramine can add bulk to liquid stool
- Codeine may slow peristalsis, but risks/side effects may outweigh benefits
- For severe cases, paregoric may be of help. However, it is of utmost importance to not confuse paregoric with tincture of opium. **Paregoric contains 0.4 mg/mL of morphine, whereas opium tincture contains 10 mg/mL.** This is a situation that invites serious medication error (42)

Chronic Diarrhea Management

- Common causes are IBS, inflammatory bowel disease, malabsorption syndromes, and chronic infections (as seen in immune compromised patients)
  - ■ Recommend GI referral (41)

Chemotherapy-Related Diarrhea (CRD)

In some cases, diarrhea can be caused by radiation to the abdomen or certain chemotherapy agents, such as irinotecan or flurouracil.

- Dietary accommodations are often necessary both to avoid foods that may aggravate diarrhea (those high in spice or fat, lactose-containing foods, alcohol, caffeine) and to ensure adequate hydration
- Some patients may require IV fluids, electrolyte replacement—oral fluids with water, salt, and sugar (e.g., Gatoraid, broth)
- Medication treatment includes loperamide (adult dose 4 mg initially, then 2 mg every 2 hr or after each loose stool). If diarrhea is refractory to loperamide, use octreotide (adult dose 100–150 mcg subq or IV TID, can titrate rapidly up to 500 mcg TID or higher if needed) (43)
- Tincture of opium or budesonide may be added if the above treatments are ineffective (44)

ANAL AND PERINEAL PAIN

- Continuous pain is usually tumor related. There may be a role for ganglion impar block (lower) or hypogastric plexus block (higher)
- Rectal spasm (proctalgia fugax) can cause severe pain that can last seconds to minutes. The patient is free of pain between episodes (45). Rectal spasms can occur in adults without cancer as well as cancer

patients; most commonly middle-aged women (45). This is a diagnosis of exclusion that requires ruling out hemorrhoids, anorectal abscesses, anal fissures, rectocele, rectal cancer, IBS, pelvic inflammatory disease (PID), chronic benign prostatitis, coccydynia, levator ani syndrome

- Suspected mechanism of action is spasm of the internal anal sphincter. No commonality of trigger events has been reported
- If infrequent, treatment or prevention may not be practical. Reassurance and explanation may be of benefit
- If events are frequent and debilitating, can try (46):
  - Topical glyceryl trinitrate 0.2% prn
  - Salbutamol inhalation 200 g prn
  - Warm water enemas
  - Clonidine (adult dose150 mcg BID)
  - Local anesthetic block
  - Botox injection into anal sphincter.
  - Diltiazem 2% or nitroglycerine for acute attack
  - Biofeedback
  - Inhaled albuterol (helpful in a small randomized study) (47)
- With refractory symptoms (45):
  - Oral clonidine, pudendal nerve block, and botulinum toxin may be tried

Anal Fissure

This is described as a longitudinal tear within the anal canal, usually from the dentate line toward the anal verge. Typical causes include constipation and diarrhea. The primary symptom is pain, often caused by defecation and lasting for several hours. Bleeding may accompany defecation and lead to the incorrect diagnosis of hemorrhoids.

First line treatment incorporates nonoperative measures—sitz baths, psyllium fiber or similar bulking agents and potentially the use of topical anesthetics and/or topical steroids. Improved pain relief is generally observed in patients who use sitz baths and psyllium fiber. Fiber maintenance is also associated with lower recurrence rates of the fissure as opposed to placebo.

Topical nitrate may be used but side effects may limit usefulness. Primary side effect is headache and leads to cessation of use in up to 20%. Topical calcium channel blockers (CCBs) such as diltazem or nifedipine may result in less headache and possibly increased frequency of cure rate. CCBs may also be used orally, but side effect is greater in patients treated with oral as opposed to topical CCBs.

In patients who do not respond to less invasive intervention, botulinum toxin injection or lateral internal sphincterotomy may offer relief and healing, although a Cochrane review demonstrated only marginal superiority to placebo with botulinum toxin. In comparison, lateral internal sphinctoerotomy demonstrated healing rates of 88% to 100% (48).

Anal Abscess and Fistula

Anal abscess is the obstruction of the anal gland and fistula is chronic infection and epithelialization of abscess drainage tract (49).

- Abscess
  - Differential diagnosis includes fissure, thrombosed hemorrhoid, pilonidal disease, hidradenitis, anal cancer and precancerous conditions, Crohn's disease and sexually transmitted diseases
  - Abscesses are more common in men than women
  - Peak incidence is among 30 to 40 year olds
  - Requires incision and drainage
  - Antibiotic therapy is not routinely ordered, with the exception of patients with cellulitis, systemic signs of infection, or underlying immune suppression
- Fistula-in-Ano and Rectovaginal Fistulas
  - In patients with very shortened life span, the use of Flagyl powder may assist with control of odor from the wound (36)
  - If life expectancy is longer, it requires referral to surgeon (48)

Psychological Dimensions

GI disorders are often very disruptive to a person's daily living. The effects of GI disorders, including nausea, vomiting, diarrhea, constipation, and others, may require a person to stay close to home, or at least near a bathroom with which the person is comfortable. GI distress can lead to social isolation, particularly because of the accompanying smells and sounds.

Stress can cause or exacerbate GI symptoms; stress can stimulate gastric emptying and increase colonic transit time (50). Though neurotransmitters are likely involved in these processes, precise mechanisms remain unclear.

Psychological interventions may improve symptoms in patients with GI symptoms. Cognitive behavioral therapy (CBT) has been effective in treating people with IBS, pain, fecal incontinence, and children with functional abdominal pain (51,52). Biofeedback has been beneficial for patients with dyssynergic constipation (51).

Understanding the range of interventions that may benefit people with functional GI disorders informs the overall treatment processes used by palliative providers. However, the difference in causative factors prevents wholesale adoption of these interventions. Some interventions, such as biofeedback, have tremendous anecdotal support, but a less strong evidence base. More study is needed to strengthen the evidence base for a range of interventions.

Patients with GI symptoms may benefit from specific suggestions about how to manage symptoms. These include:

- Prophylactic use of medications
- Altering the timing of treatments that cause GI distress
- Identifying in advance the locations of bathrooms
- Familiarity with over-the-counter interventions to decrease the smell of stools

Perhaps of greatest important is the provider's willingness to engage in specific, albeit occasionally uncomfortable, discussions about the messiness of GI distress.

Spiritual Considerations

All palliative care should include an assessment for spiritual distress. In people with a GI symptom burden, the cost to their daily lives may be so great as to lead to questioning of the meaning of life. Any physical symptom can lead not only to physical distress, but also to psychosocial and to spiritual distress. Treatment modalities may include:

- Prayer
- Labyrinth
- Mandalas
- Art
- Music
- Mindfulness

A chaplain, rabbi, minister, imam, priest, or pastoral care consultant may be supportive to many individuals' search for spiritual comfort. Recreation therapy, psychiatry, or other therapists will help others find meaning and support. Others may choose to pursue peace or meaning on their own. The palliative care provider should be familiar with the resources available at the institution. This will allow the inclusion of those who can provide the greatest benefit to the patient.

CONCLUSION

GI symptoms, whether related to disease or its treatments, may be more burdensome than the underlying disease. The effects of GI symptoms are often extremely disruptive, even leading to other symptoms such as fatigue and social isolation. In this chapter we reviewed common problems experienced by many oncology patients such as mucositis, nausea and vomiting, and constipation, as well as more rare disorders like small bowel obstruction and fistulas. Over recent years, knowledge of how to manage these symptoms has advanced. Many GI symptoms can be minimized or prevented through medical or nonpharmacological means, so awareness of the risks of these symptoms, preventive measures, and early treatment are critically important.

REFERENCES

1. McGuire DB, Fulton JS, Park J, et al. Systematic review of basic oral care for the management of oral mucositis in cancer patients. *Support Care Cancer*. 2013;21(11):3165–3177. doi:10.1007/s00520-013-1942-0
2. McGuire DB, Correa ME, Johnson J, Wienandts P. The role of basic oral care and good clinical practice principles in the management of oral mucositis. *Support Care Cancer*. 2006;14(6):541–547. doi:10.1007/s00520-006-0051-8
3. Riley P, Glenny AM, Worthington HV, et al. Interventions for preventing oral mucositis in patients with cancer receiving treatment: oral cryotherapy. *Cochrane Database Syst Rev*. 2015;23(12):CD011552. doi:10.1002/14651858.CD011552.pub2
4. Sung L, Robinson P, Triester N, et al. Guideline for the prevention of oral and oropharyngeal mucositis in children receiving treatment for cancer or undergoing haemtaopoietic stem cell transplant. *BMJ Support Palliat Care*. 2015;7(1):7–16. doi:10.1136/bmjspcare-2014-000804

5.   Magnus Bjordal J, Bensadoun RJ, Tunèr J, et al. A systematic review with meta-analysis of the effect of low-level laser therapy (LLLT) in cancer therapy induced oral mucositis. *Support Care Cancer*. 2011;19:1069–1110. doi:10.1007/s00520-011-1202-0

6.   Migliorati C, For the Mucositis Study Group of the Multinational Association of Supportive Care in Cancer/International Society of Oral Oncology (MASCC/ISOO), Hewson I, et al. Systematic review of laser and other light therapy for the management of oral mucositis in cancer patients. *Support Care Cancer*. 2013;21;333–341. doi:10.1007/s00520-012-1605-6

7.   Oberoi S, Zamperlini–Netto G, Beyene J, et al. Effect of Prophylactic low level laser therapy on oral mucositis: A systematic review and meta-analysis. *Plos One*. 2014;9(9):107418. doi:10.1371/journal.pone.0107418

8.   Spanemberg J, Figueiredo MA, Cherubini K, Salum FG. Low-level laser therapy: a review of its applications in the management of oral mucosal disorders. *Altern Ther*. 2016;22(6):24–31.

9.   He M, Zhang B, Shen N, et al. A systematic review and meta-analysis of the effect of low-level laser therapy (LLLT) on chemotherapy-induced oral mucositis in pediatric and young patients. *Eur J Pediatr*. 2017;177:7–17. doi:10.1007/s00431-017-3043-4

10. Lalla RV, Bowen J, Barasch A, et al. MASCC/ISOO clinical practice guidelines for the management of mucositis secondary to cancer therapy. *Cancer*. 2014;120(10):1453–1461. doi:10.1002/cncr.28592

11. Bensinger W, Schubert M, Ang KK, et al. NCCN Task Force Report: prevention and management of mucositis in cancer care. *J Natl Compr Canc Netw*. 2008;6 Suppl 1:S1–S21; quiz S22–S24.

12. Oncology Nursing Society. 2017. https://www.ons.org/practice-resources/pep/mucositis

13. Chemocare. 2017. http://www.chemocare.com/search.aspx?q=6MP

14. Hanchanale S, Adkinson L, Daniel S, et al. Systematic literature review: xerostomia in advanced cancer patients. *Support Care Cancer*. 2015;23(3):881–888. doi:10.1007/s00520-014-2477-8

15. Zimmermann AE, Walters JK, Katona BG, et al. A review of omeprazole use in the treatment of acid-related disorders in children. *Clin Ther*. 2001;23(5):660–679; discussion 645. doi:10.1016/s0149-2918(01)80018-7

16. Iwakiri K, Kinoshita Y, Habu Y, et al. Evidence-based clinical practice guidelines for gastroesophageal reflux disease 2015. *J Gastroenterol*. 2016;51:751–767. doi:10.1007/s00535-016-1227-8

17. Scottish Palliative Care Guidelines. Bleeding. 2015. www.palliativecareguidelines.scot.nhs.uk/guidelines/palliative-emergencies/Bleeding.aspx

18. McIntosh K, Reed DE, Schneider T, et al. FODMAPS alter symptoms and metabolism of patients with IBS: a randomized controlled trial. *Gut*. 2017;66:1241–1251. doi:10.1136/gutjnl-2015-311339

19. Hillila M, Farkkila MA, Sipponen R, et al. Does oral alpha-galactosidase relieve irritable bowel symptoms? *Scand J Gastroenterol*. 2016;51:16–21. doi:10.3109/00365521.2015.1063156

20. Abraczinskas D. Intestinal gas and bloating. *UpToDate*. 2017. https://www.uptodate.com/contents/intestinal-gas-and-bloating

21. Blondeau K, Boecxstaens V, Rommel N, et al. Baclofen improves symptoms and reduces postprandial flow events in patients with rumination and supragastric belching. *Clin Gastroenterol Hepatol*. 2012;10:379–384. doi:10.1016/j.cgh.2011.10.042

22. Goldenberg JZ, Brignall M, Hamilton M, et al. Biofeedback for the treatment of irritable bowel syndrome. *Cochrane Database of Systematic Reviews*. 2017;(1). doi:10.1002/14651858.CD012530

23. Vayne-Bossert P, Haywood A, Good P, et al. Corticosteroids for adult patients with advanced cancer who have nausea and vomiting (not related to chemotherapy, radiotherapy, or surgery). *Cochrane Database Syst Rev*. 2017;CD012002. doi:10.1002/14651858.CD012002.pub2

24. Vidall C, Sharma S, Amlani B. Patient-practitioner perception gap in treatment-induced nausea and vomiting. *Br J Nurs*. 2016;25(16):S4–S11. doi:10.12968/bjon.2016.25.S4

25. Harrison C. *A practical approach to nausea and vomiting*. Presentation given to Hospice Nurses meeting, Washington, DC; 2015.

26.   Lau Moon Lin M, Robinson PD, Flank J, et al. The safety of metoclopramide in children: A systematic review and meta-analysis. *Drug Safety*. 2016;39:675–687. doi:10.1007/s40264-0a6-0418-9

27.   Hesketh PJ, Bohlke K, Lyman GH, et al.; American Society of Clinical Oncology. Antiemetics: American Society of Clinical Oncology Focused Guideline Update. *J Clin Oncol*. 2016;34(4):381–386. doi:10.1200/JCO.2015.64.3635

28.   Navari RM. Management of chemotherapy-induced nausea and vomiting in pediatric patients. *Pediatric Drugs*. 2017;19:213–222. doi:10.1007/s40272-017-0228-2

29.   Jackson PG, Raiji MT. Evaluation and management of intestinal obstruction. *Am Fam Physician*. 2011;83:159–165. https://www.aafp.org/afp/2011/0115/p159.html

30.   Mercadante S. Palliative care of bowel obstruction in cancer patients *UpToDate*. 2017. https://www.uptodate.com/contents/palliative-care-of-bowel-obstruction-in-cancer -patients

31.   Jaffe T. Large-bowel obstruction in the adult: Classic radiographic and CT findings, etiology, and mimics. *Radiology*. 2015;275:651–663. doi:10.1148/radiol.2015140916

32.   Moss A, Hodin R. Approach to the patient with intestinal obstruction. Clinical Advisor: Gastroenterology Hepatology. 2017. http://www.clinicaladvisor.com/gas-troenterology-hepatology/approach-to-the-patient-with-intestinal-obstruction/article/596503

33.   Bordeianou L, Yeh DD. Epidemiology, clinical features, and diagnosis of mechanical small bowel obstruction in adults. *UpToDate*. 2017. www.uptodate.com/contents/epidemiology-clinical-features-and-diagnosis-of-mechanical-small-bowel-obstruc-tion-in-adults

34.   Aguayo P, Ho B, Fraser JD, et al. Bowel obstruction after treatment of intra-abdominal tumors. *Eur J Pediatr Surg*. 2010;20(4):234–236. doi:10.1055/s-0030-1253401

35.   Cagir B. Intestinal pseudo-obstruction workup. 2016. https://emedicine.medscape.com/article/2162306-workup#c8

36.   Liao P, Candice J, Rich SE. Bleeding Management in Hospice Care Settings #341. *J Palliat Med*. 2017;20(12):1405–1406. doi:10.1089/jpm.2017.0523

37.   Paquette IM, Varma M, Ternent C, et al. The American Society of Colon and Rectal Surgeons' clinic practice guideline for the evaluation and management of constipation. *Dis Colon Rectum*. 2016;59:479–492. doi:10.1097/DCR.0000000000000599

38.   Candy B, Jones L, Larkin PJ, et al. Laxatives for the management of constipation in people receiving palliative care. *Cochrane Database Syst Rev*. 2015;15:CD003448. doi:10.1002/146518.CD003448.pub4

39.   Hebbard AI, Slavin MA, Reed C, et al. The epidemiology of Clostridium difficile infec-tion in patients with cancer. *Expert Rev Anti Infect Ther*. 2016;14(11):1077–1085. doi:1 0.1080/14787210.2016.1234376

40.   LaRocque R, Harris JB. Approach to the adult with acute diarrhea in resource-rich settings. *UpToDate*. 2017. https://www.uptodate.com/contents/approach-to-the-adult -with-acute-diarrhea-in-resource-rich-settings

41.   Bonis PAL, Lamont JT. Approach to the adult with chronic diarrhea in resource rich settings. *UpToDate*. 2017. https://www.uptodate.com/contents/approach-to-the-adult-with-acute-diarrhea-in-resource-rich-settings

42.   Kelly K, Vaida AJ. *Recurring confusion between opium tincture and paregoric*. Cranbury, NJ: Pharmacy Times; 2003. https://www.pharmacytimes.com/publications/issue/2003/2003-06/2003-06-7241

43.   Krishnamurthi SS, Macron C. Management of acute chemotherapy-related diar-rhea. UpToDate. 2017. https://www.uptodate.com/contents/management-of-acute -chemotherapy-related-diarrhea

44.   Shaw C, Taylor L. Treatment-related diarrhea in patients with cancer. *Clin J Oncol Nurs*. 2012;16(4):413–417. doi:10.1188/12.CJON.413-417.

45.   Barto A, Robson KM. Proctalgia fugax. *UpToDate*. 2017. https://www.uptodate.com/contents/proctalgia-fugax

46.   Wald A, Bharucha AE, Cosman BC, Whitehead WE. ACG clinical guideline: Management of benign anorectal disorders. *Am J Gastroenterology*. 2014;109:1141–1157. doi:10.1038/ajg.2014.190. https://gi.org/guideline/management-of-benign-anorectal-disorders

47.   Eckardt VF, Dodt O, Kanzler G, Bernhard G. Treatment of proctalgia fugax with salbu-tamol inhalation *Am J Gastroenterology*. 1996;91:686–689.

48. Stewart DB Sr, Gaertner W, Glasgow S, et al.Clinical Practice Guideline for the Management of Anal Fissures. *Dis Colon Rectum*. 2017;60(1):7–14. doi:10.1097/DCR.0000000000000735

49. Vogel JD, Johnson EK, Morris AM, et al. Clinical practice guidelines for the management of anorectal abscess, fistula-in-ano, and rectovaginal fistula. *Dis Colon Rectum*. 2016;59:1117–1133. doi:10.1097/dcr.0000000000000733

50. Mertz H. Stress and the gut. *UNC Center for Functional GI & Motility Disorders*. 2018. https://www.med.unc.edu/ibs/files/2017/10/Stress-and-the-Gut.pdf

51. Palsson OS, Whitehead WE. Psychological treatments in functional gastrointestinal disorders: A primer for the gastroenterologist. *Clin Gastro Hepat*. 2013;11:208–216. doi:10.1016/j.cgh.2012.10.031

52. Reed-Knight B, Claar RL, Schurman JV, van Tilburg MAL. Implementing psychological therapies for functional GI disorders in children and adults. *Exp Rev Gastroenterol Hepatol*. 2016;10:981–984. doi:10.1080/17474124.2016.1207524

Genitourinary Symptom Management in Adults and Children With Oncologic Disease 10

Michael H. Hsieh, Jeffrey Villanueva, and Monika Gasiorek

INTRODUCTION

Genitourinary symptoms are common in patients receiving palliative care. One study published in the United Kingdom reported a 14% prevalence of urinary symptoms in the palliative care setting. These symptoms are not always the result of a primary urologic malignancy. Genitourinary pathology in the palliative care setting can occur for a variety of reasons. These include complications of surgery, chemotherapy, or radiation, advanced cancer, an immunocompromised state, or neurologic degeneration. Most importantly, genitourinary symptoms involve an organ system closely associated with a patient's independence, privacy, and intimacy, and therefore have a particular impact on comfort and quality of life. In addressing these components of the patient's well-being, it is important to be aware that more standard or aggressive interventions may not align with the patient's end-of-life goals. A more symptoms-based and practical approach to management may be preferred, keeping in mind patient-centered outcomes.

SYMPTOMS AND TREATMENT: OVERVIEW

In this chapter, we discuss symptoms and treatment of upper and lower urinary tract obstruction, genital (e.g., penile, scrotal, labial) edema, urinary tract infection, iatrogenic urethral catheter injuries, incontinence, fistulae, and bladder and pelvic pain. We also highlight pediatric-specific considerations for the management of these conditions.

Many of the symptoms discussed have similar presentations and clinical courses across etiologies. Common indications of genitourinary pathology include lower urinary tract symptoms such as frequency, urgency, dysuria, nocturia, and incontinence. Obstructive-type lower urinary tract symptoms, including retention, poor stream, hesitancy, or incomplete bladder emptying, are also commonly seen. The location of pain or discomfort may help distinguish between upper and lower urinary tract pathology. Fever, nausea, vomiting, fluid imbalance, or mental status changes in the setting of voiding symptoms or hematuria can indicate chronic and/or progressive disease states.

Although standardized guidelines exist for the diagnostic evaluation and management of each of the discussed topics, these are not necessarily tailored for the palliative care patient. It is important to take into consideration the patient's overall condition, end-of-life goals, life expectancy, and comfort in making decisions surrounding supportive management or more invasive palliative interventions.

Finally, genitourinary symptoms have a significant effect on a patient's psychosocial well-being. Pain, lower urinary tract symptoms, and incontinence can all lead to emotional distress, including frustration, shame, and embarrassment. Patients often lose their sense of independence, which can lead to difficulties in performing activities of daily living and depressive symptoms of decreased mood, hopelessness, and anhedonia. Patients may feel guilty for having to rely on family and friends for their care, and these shifting dynamics place a strain on interpersonal relationships and interactions. Sexual intimacy can become especially challenging due to both practical issues like indwelling urinary catheters, as well as the frequent role of intimate partners as caretakers.

UPPER URINARY TRACT OBSTRUCTION
Symptoms
Physical

- Flank pain
- Nausea, vomiting
- Hemodynamic changes, alterations in volume status (fluid overload)
- Fevers, chills, or dysuria in the setting of infection (pyelonephritis, urosepsis)
- Pelvic or abdominal distension on exam, possibly secondary to severe obstruction
- Signs of uremia secondary to renal failure, including mental status changes

Psychosocial

- Fatigue, drowsiness, decreased alertness
- Emotional distress secondary to physical symptoms
- Decreased mood, hopelessness
- Loss of pleasure from hobbies and interests
- Limited ability and desire for interaction with friends and family
- Inability to perform activities of daily living
- Loss of independence

Treatment
Physical

- Analgesics for palliative pain management
- Antiemetics for nausea/vomiting
- Chronic obstruction typically will not cause acute symptoms
- Pain associated with acute obstruction is well treated with nonsteroidal anti-inflammatory drugs (NSAIDs) in the setting of adequate renal function
- Decompression with either percutaneous nephrostomy tubes or ureteral stent insertion

- Nephrostomy tubes or ureteral stents require replacement every 3 to 4 months, the former under general anesthesia, the latter can sometimes be performed using local anesthesia
- Ureteral stents are completely internal, but can cause urinary frequency and irritation in at least a third of patients. These symptoms often abate spontaneously over time and with antispasmodics such as oxybutynin
- Percutaneous nephrostomy tubes are external and can cause back pain, leak urine, generate an odor, and can be dislodged. Many patients complain of difficulty sleeping with nephrostomy tubes in place
- Antibiotics, if concern for infection/sepsis
- Management of underlying cause of obstruction

Psychosocial

- Ensure physical symptoms are being managed appropriately and patient is not suffering as a result of polypharmacy or drug side effects
- Provide emotional support services as needed, both in the form of psycho- and pharmacotherapy
- Encourage spending time with friends, family, and other patients, as tolerated
- Encourage patient participation in hobbies and interests
- Provide proper support or assistance for activities of daily living

LOWER URINARY TRACT OBSTRUCTION
Symptoms
Physical

- Irritative voiding symptoms such as frequency, urgency, and/or nocturia, incontinence
- Dysuria, particularly in the setting of recurrent secondary infection
- Obstructive voiding symptoms such as poor stream, hesitancy, postvoid dribbling, and incomplete bladder emptying
- Nausea
- Suprapubic pain, discomfort, and/or distension

Psychosocial

- Frustration, particularly from bothersome urinary symptoms
- Emotional distress secondary to physical symptoms
- Shame and embarrassment from incontinence or urinary frequency
- Decreased mood, hopelessness
- Loss of pleasure from or ability to participate in hobbies and interests
- Limited ability and desire for interaction with friends and family
- Inability to perform activities of daily living
- Loss of independence

Treatment

Physical

- Pharmacologic therapy: alpha blockers, 5-alpha reductase inhibitors, if the etiology is an enlarged prostate
- Catheterization for relief of obstruction with indwelling urethral or suprapubic catheter, or clean intermittent self-catheterization
  - Use lidocaine jelly during transurethral insertion
  - Use lidocaine jelly on indwelling urethral catheters to prevent and treat urethral discomfort
  - Use anticholinergics such as belladonna and opium suppositories or oxybutynin to address irritation from indwelling bladder catheter
- Correction of electrolyte imbalance and fluid status in the setting of chronic obstruction or postobstructive diuresis following acute retention
- Management of underlying cause of obstruction

Psychosocial

- Transurethral intermittent catheterization decreases the risk of urinary tract infection (UTI) associated with catheters and avoids the need for any fixed drainage bag
- Ensure physical symptoms are being managed appropriately and patient is not suffering as a result of polypharmacy or drug side effects
- Provide emotional support services as needed, both in the form of psycho- and pharmacotherapy
- Encourage spending time with friends, family, and other patients, as tolerated
- Help patient adapt and incorporate his or her physical condition (including coping with any indwelling catheters) to fit within framework of established social interactions and hobbies or interests
- Provide proper support or assistance for activities of daily living

GENITAL EDEMA

Symptoms

Physical

- Heaviness and discomfort of the affected area
- Bacterial and fungal infection can become superimposed in the affected area. If untreated, it can permanently decrease the elasticity of tissues
- Severe forms can cause skin breakdown

Psychosocial

- Decreased desire to socialize due to body changes
- Embarrassment from not fitting into clothes
- Inability to be intimate with partner

Treatment

Physical

- Spend as much time as possible out of bed
- While lying down, elevate the affected area
- Wear tight fitting undergarments to help compress the affected area
- If a superimposed infection is suspected, then it should be treated if this is within the patient's goals of care

Psychosocial

- Wear loose fitting clothes
- Encourage activities that promote time out of bed
- Provide proper support or assistance for activities of daily living
- Encourage spending time with friends, family, and other patients, as tolerated
- Help patient adapt and incorporate his or her physical condition to fit within framework of established social interactions and hobbies or interests
- Provide proper support or assistance for activities of daily living

HEMATURIA

Symptoms

Physical

- Painful or painless, gross or microscopic blood in the urine, with or without clots
- Bladder spasms
- Lower abdominal, flank, or suprapubic pain
- Irritative lower urinary tract voiding symptoms including urgency, frequency, small volume urination, nocturia, and dysuria
- Hesitancy, weak stream, inability to void, or incontinence
- Weight loss, fatigue
- Fever, chills, and night sweats in the setting of infection

Psychosocial

- Emotional distress secondary to physical symptoms
- Shame and embarrassment
- Decreased mood, hopelessness
- Loss of pleasure from or ability to participate in hobbies and interests
- Limited ability and desire for interaction with friends and family
- Inability to perform activities of daily living
- Loss of independence

Treatment

Physical

- Treat urinary infection, if present

- Consider discontinuation of anticoagulants
- Transurethral fulguration or arterial embolization in the setting of an identified bleeding source/lesion refractory to more conservative measures
- Blood transfusion and angioembolization in the setting of hemodynamic instability
- Surgical excision of involved organ if endoscopic and endovascular source control fails
- Consider radiation therapy if the bleeding is due to a genitourinary malignancy

Treatment of Hemorrhagic Cystitis

- Prevention is the most effective form of treatment
  - Consider hydration (at least 2 liters of fluid/day), suprahydration (IV normal saline infusion and loop diuretics), frequent and/or scheduled voiding, and continuous bladder irrigation (requires urologic consultation for optimal management)
  - Mesna can be given prior to the use of oxazaphosphorine therapy
- Mild hematuria can be treated with hydration and continuous saline bladder irrigation for the extraction and prevention of clots
- Moderate to severe hematuria can be treated with a variety of techniques (the authors strongly recommend urologic consultation at an early stage):
  - Transfusion
  - Cystoscopy for clot evaluation
  - Aminocaproic acid
  - Instillation of astringents (alum, silver nitrate, formalin or phenol)
  - Estrogen
  - Intravesical granulocyte-macrophage colony-stimulating factor (GM-CSF)
  - Pentosan polysulfate
  - Sodium hyaluronate
  - Prostaglandin instillation/irrigation
  - Hyperbaric oxygen
  - Embolization (vesical or internal iliac arteries) and surgery (urinary diversion, cystectomy, percutaneous nephrostomy, cutaneous ureterostomy) indicated in patients with intractable bleeding and hemodynamic instability

Psychosocial

- Ensure physical symptoms are being managed appropriately and patient is not suffering as a result of polypharmacy or drug side effects
- Provide emotional support services as needed, both in the form of psycho- and pharmacotherapy
- Encourage spending time with friends, family, and other patients, as tolerated

- Help patient adapt and incorporate his or her physical condition to fit within framework of established social interactions and hobbies or interests
- Provide proper support or assistance for activities of daily living

URINARY TRACT INFECTION

Symptoms

Physical

- Frequency, urgency, and dysuria
- Suprapubic, flank, or abdominal pain/discomfort
- Incontinence
- Hematuria
- Fever, chills, nausea, and vomiting
- Hypotension, tachycardia, tachypnea
- Lethargy, loss of appetite, decreased cognitive function
- Agitation, altered mental status

Psychosocial

- Emotional distress secondary to physical symptoms
- Shame and embarrassment
- Decreased mood, hopelessness
- Loss of pleasure from or ability to participate in hobbies and interests
- Limited ability and desire for interaction with friends and family
- Inability to perform activities of daily living
- Loss of independence

Treatment

Physical

- Irritative symptoms can be managed with oral pyridium, oral or rectal anticholinergics
- Use empiric antibiotics following local antibiotic resistance patterns for up to 10 to 14 days (shorter courses may be appropriate for less ill patients)
  - Trimethoprim/sulfamethoxazole usually first line, but local antibiograms to be taken into account
  - Other options include amoxicillin/amoxicillin-clavulanate, second- or third-generation cephalosporins, or fluoroquinolones
  - Low dose daily prophylactic antibiotics may be indicated in select patients with recurrent infections
- Removal of indwelling urethral catheter in the setting of catheter-associated infection
  - Substitution with clean intermittent catheterization or suprapubic indwelling catheter, if possible
- Preventive measures in patients with chronic indwelling urinary catheters

- - Catheter exchanges should occur every 3 to 4 weeks, performed with sterile technique
  - Monitoring for unobstructed urine flow, Foley bag hanging below bed with as little tubing as possible looping back up toward bed (air locks form within such loops, and impede urine flow)
- Asymptomatic bacteriuria should only be treated in pregnancy or in patients scheduled for a urologic procedure that may compromise the integrity of the urothelium

Psychosocial

- Ensure physical symptoms are being managed appropriately and patient is not suffering as a result of polypharmacy or drug side effects
- Provide emotional support services as needed, both in the form of psycho- and pharmacotherapy
- Encourage spending time with friends, family, and other patients, as tolerated
- Help patient adapt and incorporate his or her physical condition to fit within framework of established social interactions and hobbies or interests
- Provide proper support or assistance for activities of daily living

IATROGENIC URETHRAL CATHETER INJURIES
Symptoms
Physical

- Suprapubic pain
- Genital pain
- Perineal pain
- Nondraining catheter
- Urethral bleeding

Treatment

- Prevention is key, and protocols to improve nursing catheterization technique have been shown to decrease rates of iatrogenic injury
- Unless the catheter is necessary for palliative or medical reasons, urinary catheterization should be avoided as much as possible
- Most iatrogenic catheterization injuries can be managed conservatively with proper catheter replacement
- If patient has no known anatomic abnormality, provider may deflate the balloon and hub of the catheter during attempted reinsertion. If not possible, then discuss with a urologic provider
- Significant injuries may require urologic intervention, including urethral dilation, placement of a suprapubic tube, or an open urethroplasty. Most palliative care patients are unlikely to proceed to urethroplasty, except possibly perineal urethrostomy as a means to divert urine away from a diseased urethra

INCONTINENCE

Symptoms

Physical

- Urinary frequency, polyuria, urgency, hesitancy, nocturia, or continuous leakage
- Intermittent/slow stream, incomplete bladder emptying, straining
- Stress incontinence: urine leakage or loss with laughing, coughing, and/or sneezing
- Urge incontinence: sudden urge to urinate associated with self-soiling; frequent and small volume voids
- Overflow incontinence: small or large loss of urine without urge or trigger, often associated with frequency, hesitancy, weak stream, and/or incomplete bladder emptying
- Fever, dysuria, pelvic pain, and/or hematuria in the setting of infection
- Neurologic or mental status changes, constipation—etiology dependent

Psychosocial

- Emotional distress secondary to physical symptoms
- Shame, embarrassment, and loss of control
- Decreased mood, hopelessness
- Loss of pleasure from or ability to participate in hobbies and interests
- Limited ability and desire for interaction with friends and family
- Inability to perform activities of daily living
- Loss of independence

Treatment

Physical

- Evaluate for urinary infection or bladder obstruction, which may present with incontinence
- Address underlying or exacerbating factors including medications/treatments
- Suggest lifestyle modifications: timed voiding and pelvic floor muscle exercises
- Encourage use of absorbent pads and garments
- Use external urine collection devices (condom catheter)
- Use male urethral occlusion devices
- Apply estrogen cream in the setting of vaginal atrophy
- Use pessaries in the setting of stress incontinence
- Consider indwelling urethral, clean intermittent, or suprapubic catheterization
- Use traditional* pharmacologic therapy such as alpha blockers and anticholinergics

---

*Often poorly tolerated in the palliative care setting.

Psychosocial

- Ensure physical symptoms are being managed appropriately and patient is not suffering as a result of polypharmacy or drug side effects
- Provide emotional support services as needed, both in the form of psycho- and pharmacotherapy
- Encourage spending time with friends, family, and other patients, as tolerated
- Help patient adapt and incorporate his or her physical condition to fit within framework of established social interactions and hobbies or interests
- Provide proper support or assistance for activities of daily living

FISTULAE (VESICOVAGINAL, VESICOENTERIC)
Symptoms
Physical

- Pneumaturia
- UTI
- Suprapubic pain
- Incontinence
- Feces in the urine, diarrhea, and tenesmus in the setting of vesico-enteric fistulae
- Vaginal leakage in the setting of vesicovaginal fistulae
- Chronic pathology may present with skin changes, including rash and ulcers

Psychosocial

- Emotional distress secondary to physical symptoms
- Shame, embarrassment, and loss of control
- Decreased mood, hopelessness
- Loss of pleasure from or ability to participate in hobbies and interests
- Limited ability and desire for interaction with friends and family
- Inability to perform activities of daily living
- Loss of independence

Treatment
Physical

- Symptom management and control of urinary leakage
- Diversion with urethral or suprapubic catheterization, or bilateral percutaneous nephrostomy tubes
- Diverting colostomy
- Reconstructive repair of the fistula or a urinary conduit diversion in select patients

Psychosocial

- Ensure physical symptoms are being managed appropriately and patient is not suffering as a result of polypharmacy or drug side effects
- Provide emotional support services as needed, both in the form of psycho- and pharmacotherapy
- Encourage spending time with friends, family, and other patients, as tolerated
- Help patient adapt and incorporate his or her physical condition to fit within framework of established social interactions and hobbies or interests
- Provide proper support or assistance for activities of daily living

BLADDER-ASSOCIATED OR PELVIC PAIN

Symptoms

Physical

- Suprapubic or perineal discomfort
- Urgency, frequency, dysuria, and incontinence

Psychosocial

- Emotional distress secondary to physical symptoms
- Shame, embarrassment, and loss of control
- Strain on interpersonal relationships with friends and family due to increasing caregiver burden
- Difficulty navigating sexual intimacy
- Decreased mood, hopelessness
- Loss of pleasure from or ability to participate in hobbies and interests
- Limited ability and desire for interaction with friends and family
- Inability to perform activities of daily living
- Loss of independence

Treatment

Physical

- Management with urethral catheterization or urinary diversion with nephrostomy tubes, if indicated based on underlying etiology
- Pharmacologic therapy
  - Analgesics, antidepressants, or antiepileptics for pain
    - Pentosan polysulphate sodium for cystitis-associated pain
  - Anticholinergics and belladonna or opium suppositories for the management of bladder spasms
  - Intravesical dimethyl sulfoxide, heparin, or hyaluronic acid
- Transurethral resection, surgery, chemotherapy, and/or radiation for tumor-related pain

Psychosocial

- Ensure physical symptoms are being managed appropriately and patient is not suffering as a result of polypharmacy or drug side effects
- Provide emotional support services as needed, both in the form of psycho- and pharmacotherapy
- Encourage spending time with friends, family, and other patients, as tolerated
- Help patient adapt and incorporate his or her physical condition to fit within framework of established social interactions and hobbies or interests
- Provide proper support or assistance for activities of daily living

PEDIATRIC-SPECIFIC CONSIDERATIONS

It can be difficult, if not impossible, for very young children to describe bladder and pelvic pain, whether caused by urinary tract obstruction, infection, or other etiologies. Working with parents to understand when a child's behavior is indicative of acute illness is imperative in the palliative care setting.

Although infants and young toddlers lack genital awareness, older children and adolescents are not only aware of their genitals, but may be particularly shy, ashamed, and/or confused by genital lesions such as edema and catheter-induced injuries. By analogy, non–toilet-trained children may not be embarrassed by fistulae, whereas older children may be ashamed by loss of continence and the presence of urinary fistulae.

The smaller size of the pediatric urinary tract can make it challenging to successfully manage urinary conditions through endoscopic and catheter-based approaches. For instance, adequate drainage of the bladder can be difficult in the setting of hematuria due to the smaller lumens of pediatric catheters.

Collectively, these pediatric-specific considerations make it critical for providers to work with each other, nurses, child life specialists, parents, and children when dealing with palliative urologic care.

CONCLUSION

Genitourinary symptoms in the setting of palliative care pose a significant burden on a patient's comfort and quality of life. It is imperative to recognize signs and symptoms of common genitourinary pathologies affecting these patients. Decision making in terms of diagnostic evaluation and management should align with the patient's and family's values and end-of-life goals, with primary goals of symptomatic management and decreased suffering.

SUGGESTED READING/RESOURCES

Linton KD, Hall J. Obstruction of the upper and lower urinary tract. *Surgery*. 2010;28(7):331–337. doi:10.1016/j.mpsur.2010.03.009

Sountoulides P, Mykoniatis I, Dimasis N. Palliative management of malignant upper urinary tract obstruction. *Hippokratia*. 2014;18(4):292–297.

Up-to-date: Clinical Manifestations and Diagnosis of Urinary Tract Obstruction and Hydronephrosis

Halpern JA, Schlegel PN, Chughtai B. Malignant Ureteral Obstruction. *Urol Nephrol Open Access J*. 2014;1(1). doi:10.15406/unoaj.2014.01.00003

Up-to-date: Cystitis in Patients With Cancer

Manikandan R, Kumar S, Dorairajan LN. Hemorrhagic cystitis: a challenge to the urologist. *Indian J Urol*. 2010;26(2):159–166. doi:10.4103/0970-1591.65380

Up-to-date: Etiology and Evaluation of Hematuria in Adults. Evaluation of Gross Hematuria in Children. Evaluation of Microscopic Hematuria in Children

Kreshover J, Ramasamy R, Singla N. *Hematuria*. AUA University; 2016.

Vasavada SP, Kim ED. Medscape: Urinary Incontinence Treatment and Management. 2017. https://emedicine.medscape.com/article/452289-treatment

Up-to-date: Evaluation of Women With Urinary Incontinence, Treatment of Urinary Incontinence in Women, Urinary Incontinence in Men

Lee OT, Wu JN, Meyers FJ, Evans CP. Genitourinary aspects of palliative care. In: Cherny NI, ed. *Textbook of Palliative Medicine*. 4th ed. Oxford, UK: Oxford University Press; 2015.

Mouton C, Adenuga B, Vijayan J. Urinary tract infections in long-term care. *Ann Longterm Care*. 2010;18(2):35–39.

Walton A. Managing Overactive Bladder Symptoms in a Palliative Care Setting. *J Palliat Med*. 2014;17(1):118–121. doi:10.1089/jpm.2012.0116

Psychiatric Symptom Management in Adult and Pediatric Cancer Patients: Anxiety, Delirium, and Depression

11

Ann H. Lichtenstein, Anna B. Jolliffe, and Rezvan Ameli

INTRODUCTION

Some of the most common symptoms in cancer diagnosis and treatment are psychiatric in nature. Physical changes occur in the body with illness and treatment. In addition, there are psychological effects of suffering and confronting a potentially terminal illness. It is therefore important to screen for depression and anxiety regularly as well as for reversible causes. These psychological responses to illness may affect utilization of treatment and prognosis. Many patients may benefit from pharmacological treatment, complementary therapies (complementary and alternative medicine [CAM]), and behavioral therapies.

BACKGROUND

Symptoms of depression may be seen in 15% to 50% of cancer patients. As per the *Diagnostic and Statistic Manual of Mental Disorders, Fifth Edition (DSM-5)* criteria, 5% to 20% will qualify for the diagnosis of major depressive disorder (1). Depression is undertreated in the cancer population and evidence shows that depression can affect treatment and prognosis (2). Depressed patients are less likely to comply with treatments and have more physical symptoms (2).

CAUSES OF DEPRESSION/ANXIETY

- Disruption of serotonin/dopamine pathways
- Loss or anticipated loss
- Side effects of chemotherapy
- Central nervous system (CNS) tumors
- Uncontrolled pain
- Metabolic abnormalities: hypercalcemia, sodium/potassium imbalance, anemia, vitamin B12 or folate deficiency, fever
- Endocrine abnormalities: hyper or hyperthyroidism, adrenal insufficiency
- Medications: steroids, endogenous and exogenous cytokines (interferon-alfa) and aldesleukin (interleukin-2), methyldopa, reserpine, barbiturates, propranolol, some antibiotics (such as amphotericin B), chemotherapeutic agents (such as procarbazine, L-asparaginase)
- Sleep disruption
- Uncontrolled symptoms such as nausea, vomiting, shortness of breath
- Anemia (3)

Psychosocial spiritual causes include existential distress, demoraliza-tion, fear of dying, not wanting to be dependent on others, losing func-tional abilities, and inability to work and to financially support others (3).

DEPRESSION SCREENING

According to the National Comprehensive Cancer Network (NCCN) guidelines, patients at high risk for distress (depression, anxiety, and other mood disturbances) include younger age patients, those living alone, those with young children and those with trouble communicating (Table 11.1).

The Patient Health Questionnaire-2 (PHQ-2) can evaluate if the patient requires monitoring due to signs of depression:

Over the past 2 weeks how often have you been bothered by:

1. Little interest or pleasure in doing things
2. Feeling down, depressed, or helpless

- Rated from 0 (not at all) to 3 (nearly every day), positive responses to either question indicates that the patient requires monitoring (4).
- NCCN recommends screening for cancer patients using the NCCN Distress Thermometer where 0 is no distress and 10 is extreme dis-tress. Score of 4 or higher is clinically significant and the patient will require monitoring (5).
- According to the NCCN guidelines, it is necessary to assess if the patient may be harmful to self or others. If the patient is, then:
  - Consider hospitalization
  - Order psychiatric consultation
  - Increase monitoring
  - Remove dangerous objects
  - Ensure safety of others
  - Consider referral to social work services or chaplaincy care (5)

Table 11.1 Risk Factors for Depression

Physical/ medical	Psychological/ psychiatric	Social
Severe medical comorbidities	Depression	Younger age
Uncontrolled symptoms	Substance abuse disorder	Living alone
Cognitive impairment	History of abuse (sexual, physical, emotional)	Having young children
		Communication barriers (language)

Source: From National Comprehensive Cancer Network (NCCN) Clinical Practice Guidelines in Oncology Version 2.2018 Distress Management. https://www.nccn.org/professionals/physician_gls/default.aspx

DIAGNOSING DEPRESSION

This is challenging in patients with serious illness as symptoms and signs of depression may also be caused by progressive medical disease (3). Some reactions of sadness to medical illness are normal responses and are not signs of psychiatric illness (3). It is important to be vigilant as depression in this population is underdiagnosed. The criteria for psychiatric diagnoses are defined by the *DSM-5*. Some significant diagnoses, which have similar clinical presentations include **adjustment disorder, major depressive disorder, and anticipatory grief.**

Adjustment Disorder

Adjustment disorder is defined as "the development of clinically significant emotional or behavioral symptoms in response to an identifiable stressor or stressors" (6).

The following are characteristics:

- Lasts less than 6 months and is resolved if the stressor resolves.
- Emotional or behavioral symptoms begin within 3 months of the onset of the stressor(s).
- These symptoms or behaviors are clinically significant.
- There is marked distress that is in excess of what would be expected from exposure to the stressor.
- There is significant impairment in social or occupational functioning.
- The stress-related disturbance does not meet the criteria for another disorder.
- The symptoms do not represent bereavement.
- Once the stressor has resolved, the symptoms do not persist for longer than 6 months (6).

Major Depressive Disorder

Major depressive disorder is characterized by either depressed mood or a loss of interest or pleasure in daily activities consistently for at **least a 2-week period**. Five of the following symptoms must be present nearly every day.

- Depressed mood most of the day. In children and adolescents, this may present as an irritable or cranky, rather than sad, mood.
- Markedly diminished interest or pleasure in all, or almost all, activities
- Significant weight loss or weight gain.
- Insomnia (inability to get to sleep or difficulty staying asleep) or hypersomnia (sleeping too much)
- Psychomotor agitation (restlessness, inability to sit still, pacing, pulling at clothes) or retardation (slowed speech, movements, quiet talking) nearly every day
- Fatigue, tiredness, or loss of energy
- Feelings of worthlessness or excessive or inappropriate guilt

- Diminished ability to think or concentrate, or indecisiveness
- Recurrent thoughts of death (not just fear of dying), recurrent suicidal ideas without a specific plan, or a suicide attempt or a specific plan for committing suicide (6)

Anticipatory Grief

- Feelings of sadness after being told a terminal diagnosis, which may help prepare a patient for death
- Symptoms include: sadness, anxiety, life review, social withdrawal
- Anticipatory grief differs from depression in that patient's depressed feelings lift and change from day to day (7).

Pharmacological Treatment

- Treat other physical symptoms that may be possible causes of depression such as pain, nausea/vomiting, electrolyte abnormalities before starting medication for depression (8).
- Medications are indicated for moderate to severe depression (8).
- Current evidence does not support the relative superiority of one medication over another (8).
- Choice should be made by evaluating side effects, drug interactions, response to previous treatment, and patient preference (8).
- Some side effects such as increased appetite, weight gain, and fatigue (promoting sleep) may also be of benefit (8).
- Onset for antidepressants is 2 to 3 weeks, typical trial for efficacy is 4 to 6 weeks. This time span may be too long in patients with short prognoses. Medications such as methylphenidate, which have shorter onset and duration, can be used (8).
- Medication is more effective when used in conjunction with behavioral or talk therapy (8).
- Common antidepressants used in treatment of depression are given in Table 11.2.

   NCCN guidelines recommend:

- Consider trial of another medication, if first choice is not effective.
- Consult psychiatrist for medication recommendations.
- Re-evaluate psychotherapeutic intervention and consider higher level care with intensive outpatient program (5).

ANXIETY

This is one of the most common psychiatric disorders in the general population and a common symptom in patients with cancer. 29% of the U.S. population has an anxiety disorder at some point in their lifetime. Symptoms of anxiety are thought to occur in more than 70% of medically ill patients (9). Physical symptoms such as difficulty breathing and pain can cause anxiety as well as hospital stays, having cancer treatments, and struggling with a terminal diagnosis.

Table 11.2 Medications for Treatment of Depression		
Medication	**Adverse effects**	**Advantages**
SSRIs: fluvoxamine, sertraline, citalopram, escitalopram, paroxetine,	Nausea, headache, sleep disturbance, sexual dysfunction, citalopram has risk of prolonged QT interval at higher doses	Weight gain, relatively few drug interactions and side effects
SNRIs: venlaxafine, duloxetine		Increased energy Duloxetine: pain management
SNRI: mirtazapine	Weight gain	Appetite stimulant, pain management, sleep aid
TCAs: amytryptiline, nortryptiline, desipramine	Drug interactions, anticholinergic effects (dry mouth, constipation, delirium)	Pain management including neuropathic pain, sleep aid
Psychostimulants: methylphenidate, dextroamphetamine	May worsen anxiety, potential for adverse cardiac events in elderly and patient's with cardiac disease	Increased energy, acts quickly in less than 24 hours

SNRIs, selective norepinephrine reuptake inhibitors; SSRIs, selective serotonin reuptake inhibitors; TCA, tricyclic antidepressants,

Source: Adapted from Irwin SA, Block S. Chapter 33: What Treatments are Effective for Depression in the Palliative Care Setting? In: Goldstein NE, Morrison RS, eds. *Evidence Based Practice of Palliative Medicine*. Philadelphia, PA: Saunders; 2013:181–190.

Symptoms

- Physical: autonomic arousal with associated tachycardia, tachypnea, diaphoresis, diarrhea, dizziness
- Emotional: edginess, terror, feelings of impending doom
- Behavioral: avoidance, compulsions, psychomotor agitation
- Cognitive: worry, apprehension, fear, dread, uncertainty, obsession (9)

During discussions patients may refer to keywords such as feeling "nervous," "concerned," "scared," or "worried" (9).

Diagnosis of Anxiety

- Personal or family history of anxiety
- Medications such as bronchodilators and steroids
- Substance abuse history including alcohol, opioids, and benzodiazepines
- Personal habits including use of caffeine or nicotine

- Evaluation of symptoms: pain, nausea, vomiting, insomnia, and poor concentration
- Using a screening tool such as the Generalized Anxiety Disorder Scale (GAD-7), which utilizes *DSM-5* criteria (10)
- Performing diagnostic tests to rule out medical causes such as pathologies of the neurologic, cardiovascular, pulmonary, and endocrine systems
- Evaluation for electrolyte abnormalities and toxic metabolites
- If patient has prolonged symptoms, assess to identify the following psychiatric disorders by utilizing the *DSM-5* criteria
  - Adjustment disorder with anxious features, panic disorder, posttraumatic stress disorder, and generalized anxiety disorder (11)

Pharmacologic Treatment of Anxiety in the Oncology Population

- Important to keep in mind patient's prognosis (months, weeks, or days), ability to swallow, and time to onset of medication.
- For patients with chronic anxiety and depression and with a prognosis of more than 1 month, SSRIs such as paroxetine, citalopram, and escitalopram are first-line treatments. Trazadone and gabapentin are alternative medications that have some efficacy (9).
- Benzodiazepines are used for treatment of acute anxiety and type is usually chosen by half-life (10).
- Very short acting benzodiazepines such as alprazolam, oxazepam, and triazolam may cause rebound anxiety (10).
- Short acting benzodiazepines such as lorazepam are recommended for the treatment of anxiety and nausea (10).
- More side effects and adverse reactions may occur with long acting agents such as clonazepam and diazepam (10).
- Benzodiazepines must be used with caution in elderly patients as these medications may exacerbate or cause delirium. Also use with caution in patients with liver deficiency (9,10).
- When discontinuing lorazepam, tapering by 25% per week is recommended to avoid withdrawal (10).

NONPHARMACOLOGICAL THERAPIES

- Encouraging sleep hygiene and healthy eating habits
- Limiting caffeine and alcohol
- Music therapy
- Art therapy: encourages self-expression and creativity
- Acupuncture: traditional Chinese medicine may help to alleviate multiple symptoms
- Aromatherapy: essential plant oils that can help calm patients
- Massage
- Exercise and yoga: may help to relieve stress and anxiety (12)

Meditation may be a useful adjunct practice along with medications and therapy. Practitioners learn to focus on breathing, words, or sentences in order to provide distance from feelings. Some goals of practice are cultivating patience, creating an openness to other ideas, trusting, acceptance, gratitude, letting go, and generosity (9).

Psychosocial Interventions Include

- Open communication with oncology team in order to build validation and trust (5)
- Referral to psychologist, social worker, or spiritual counselor (5)
- Social workers help to address needs for housing, food, financial assistance programs, transportation, employment concerns, and caregivers to assist with activities of daily living (5).
- Provide community resources such as support groups, teleconferences, and help lines (5).
- Some useful resources for patients and families:
  - American Cancer Society: www.cancer.org
  - American Institute for Cancer Research: www.aicr.org
  - American Psychosocial Oncology Society: http://apos-society.org/
  - Cancer Support Community: http://www.cancersupportcommunity.org
  - CancerCare: www.cancercare.org
  - National Cancer Institute: www.cancer.gov
  - Cancer.net, sponsored by ASCO: www.cancer.net

PSYCHOLOGICAL TREATMENT IN ONCOLOGY

A diagnosis of cancer challenges patients and their families at all levels, including the psychological, emotional, cognitive, existential, and spiritual. Psychological interventions can be adapted to meet various patient needs during different phases of the illness including diagnosis, treatment, short- and long-term survivorship, palliative care, and end-of-life concerns. Comprehensive oncology care includes a careful assessment of the patient's psychological and psychiatric status and a referral for provision of psychological services when needed. Following are some of the most common psychological treatments that are adapted for use with the seriously ill including oncology and palliative care patients (13).

Supportive Psychotherapy

- This is an integrative approach, and the objective is to reinforce and support the patient's adaptive thoughts, emotions, and behaviors. The therapist engages in a supportive relationship with the patient and draws from a broad range of methods to assist the patient (13).

Group Psychotherapy

- This has many formats including educational, skill training (e.g., problem solving, relaxation, social skills), theoretical (psychodynamic, cognitive behavioral), or support groups with or without a group leader (14–16).

Cognitive Behavioral Therapy (CBT) (17,18)

- CBT is a widely used evidence-based psychotherapy and includes a broad range of interventions that focus on the role of thoughts and beliefs in the development and maintenance of psychological and emotional distress and maladaptive behaviors.
- The therapist's role is to assist the patient in finding and practicing effective strategies to produce change in the patient's thinking, belief system, and behaviors to produce desired emotional change.
- Ten CBT principles: therapeutic alliance, ever-evolving formulation of the problem in cognitive terms, active collaboration and participation, goal-oriented and problem-focused, initially present-focused, educative, time-limited, structured sessions, restructuring of dysfunctional cognitions, and techniques to change thinking, mood, and behavior.

Acceptance and Commitment Therapy (ACT)

- ACT (19,20) is one of the so-called "third wave" and newer CBT approaches, and is considered to be an effective and promising treatment in cancer settings. ACT maintains that an individual's perception of suffering and distress is a normal and healthy response to traumatic and challenging situations and the goal of therapy is to enable the patient to enhance psychological flexibility. Psychological flexibility is affected by acceptance, present moment orientation (mindfulness), cognitive diffusion, self-as-context, values, and committed action.

Mindfulness-Based Therapies (MBT) (21)

- The use of mindfulness approaches in psychotherapy, including mindfulness based cognitive therapy (MBCT) (22) and mindfulness based stress reduction (MBSR) (23) have risen dramatically in the past 15 years (21). Various mindfulness-based therapies incorporate meditation, reflective practices, application of a mindful framework to various activities, and may also include yoga and movement (21).
- The focus of the treatment is to become aware and stay connected to the present moment and allow full experience of the present moment (21).
- Mindfulness is defined by John Kabat-Zinn as paying attention, on purpose, to the present moment, and nonjudgmentally to the unfolding of experience moment by moment (22).
- Attitudinal foundations of mindfulness include being nonjudgmental and having patience, a beginner's mind, trust, and acceptance, being non-striving, and letting go.
- Gratitude and generosity are additional foundational attitudes in the development and practice of mindfulness.
- *Mindfulness-Based Cancer Recovery* by Linda Carlson and Michael Speca and *Mindfulness-Based Cognitive Therapy for Cancer* by Trish Bartley are designed for cancer patients (24,25).

Meaning Centered Psychotherapy (MCP) (26)

- MCP is based on the work of Victor Frankl (27) and is designed to treat psychological, spiritual, and existential distress among patients with advanced cancer. It addresses loss of spiritual wellbeing, sense of meaning, and desire for hastened death. It has also been found to reduce depression and hopelessness.

- It is delivered in a group format and typically includes 8 sessions. It can be modified for individual administration.

Dignity Therapy (28)

- Is designed to address distress and enhance dignity at the end of life.
- It is delivered individually and is typically done in four sessions.
- Includes a semi-structured interview, a typed transcript of the interview, review of the transcript with the patient, and a final document that could be shared with others (28).

SPIRITUALITY

Life-threatening illness brings challenges to patients and families. When facing mortality patients may contemplate the meaning of their lives, go through stages of anger and acceptance, and question previously held religious beliefs. Healthcare providers can help by active listening and allowing for life review. In addition, expressing empathy and normalizing patients' experiences by offering affirming statements will help to build trust. It may be comforting to the patient to reassure him or her that you will be working through this illness together.

Some areas to focus on are listed in the HOPE questions for spiritual assessment:

H: What provides Hope, meaning, and comfort
O: Is the patient affiliated with an Organized religion
P: Spiritual Practices that the patient engages in
E: Effects on decision-making and End of life (29)

Approach other members of your team including the social worker and chaplain for assistance with exploring these topics.

DELIRIUM

Delirium is an acute onset neurocognitive syndrome, often presenting with psychiatric symptoms, marked by a disturbance in attention, awareness and other cognitive deficits, which is secondary to one or more other physiologic disturbances. Development of delirium can be associated with increased mortality, longer intensive care unit (ICU) and total hospital stays (30), increased and early institutionalization and neurotoxicity, evidenced in brain atrophy and white matter changes, long term cognitive decline, and 3.5-fold increase in the development of dementia over 5 years (32). Given the association of delirium with increased severity of illness, the high level of distress it causes patients, families, and caregivers, and its under recognition and treatment, it is a common and challenging problem in the palliative care setting.

Other terms that may be synonymous with delirium include acute confusional state, "ICU psychosis," encephalopathy, acute brain failure or dysfunction, and terminal restlessness.

Prevalence

The prevalence of delirium varies based on clinical factors and illness severity.

- General population: <0.05% to 0.4% (31)
- General medical wards: 21.4% (31)
- General surgical wards: 44% (31)
- Adult ICU): up to 80% (31)
- Pediatric ICU and postoperative settings: 13% to 44% (32)
- Terminal phase, or the days and hours before death: ~88% (33)

Causes

Delirium is caused by an underlying physiological disturbance or disturbances. The development of delirium involves the interaction of underlying patient characteristics, illness factors, and ongoing iatrogenic and environmental factors, which can be thought of as predisposing, precipitating, and perpetuating risk factors (32,33).

Clinical Characteristics and Assessment

The diagnosis of delirium is clinically based on the *DSM-5* criteria given in Box 11.1. There are no specific diagnostic tests for delirium, though

---

Box 11.1 Risk Factors for the Development of Delirium

DSM-5 **Diagnostic Criteria for Delirium (34)**

A. Disturbance in alertness and attention

B. The disturbance is an abrupt change from baseline functioning and has a fluctuation course with waxing and waning of alertness and attention

C. At least one other associated cognitive disturbance:
   - Orientation
   - Memory
   - Visuospatial Ability
   - Perception
   - Language
   - Thought Organization
   - Behavioral Organization

D. The cognitive disturbance cannot be better explained by a pre-existing or established neurocognitive condition, such as dementia or intellectual disability, or be present in a severely reduced arousal state, such as coma.

E. The cognitive disturbances have to be associated with a direct physiologic cause, which may be physical disease, exposure to a toxin, use of a substance (prescribed or illicit substance) or

---

(*continued*)

Box 11.1 Risk Factors for the Development of Delirium (*continued*)

withdrawal from a substance (prescribed or illicit substance). Often times the physiologic cause may be multifactorial.

Risk Factors for the Development of Delirium

Predisposing

- Age (infants/toddlers and the elderly)
- Preexisting developmental, cognitive, or psychiatric disorder
- Preexisting illness
- Visual Impairment

Precipitating

- Illness factors:
  - Most commonly: infectious, inflammatory and autoimmune[mala]
  - Neurologic, such as epilepsy, new onset TBI, encephalitis
  - Oncologic Disease
  - Increased severity
- Toxic ingestion, including alcohol
- Electrolyte derangement
- Metabolic disturbance
- Endocrine abnormality
- Mechanical ventilation
- Use of physical restraints
- Medication exposure, including benzodiazepines, corticosteroids, opiates, anticholinergics, and general polypharmacy

Perpetuating

- Sleep-wake cycle disturbance
- Lack of mobility
- Constipation
- Invasive devices
- Altered fluid status
- Use of physical restraints

Source: From the American Psychiatric Association. *Diagnostic and Statistical Manual of Mental Disorders: DSM-5.* 5th ed. Washington, DC: Author; 2013; Leentjens AF, Rundell J, Rummans T, et al. Delirium: an evidence-based medicine (EBM) monograph for psychosomatic medicine practice, commissioned by the Academy of Psychosomatic Medicine (APM) and the European Association of Consultation Liaison Psychiatry and Psychosomatics (EACLPP). *J Psychosom Res.* 2012;73(2):149–152. doi:10.1016/j.jpsychores.2012.05.009; Malas N, Brahmbhatt K, McDermott C, et al. Pediatric delirium: evaluation, management, and special considerations. *Curr Psychiatry Rep.* 2017;19: 65. doi:10.1007/s11920-017-0817-3

they can be very helpful in evaluation of the underlying cause. Serial physical and standardized mental status examinations should take place at diagnosis and to monitor illness.

Several diagnostic screening tools are available for adults and children to aid in diagnosis and monitoring of illness and are listed in Table 11.3 (30,32,34).

Diagnostic testing to consider for assessment of underlying cause of delirium in order to screen for and treat reversible causes:

- Metabolic panel with electrolytes

Table 11.3 Screening Instruments for Delirium

Tool	Age range	Notes
CAM	Adults	Highest positive and lowest negative likelihood ratio of adult screening measures
CAM-ICU	Adults	Recommended and feasible for routine monitoring in all adult ICU patients; can be completed even with a nonverbal patient
PCAM-ICU	>5 years	Requires interaction/ exam by practitioner; <2 min to complete; "no anchors for hypoactive delirium"; difficult to use in developmental delay
PsCAM-ICU	6 mo-4 years	
CAPD	Birth-21 years	Involves observation of patient over a period of hours; can be completed in <2 minutes by nursing staff or practitioner; addresses hypoactive delirium; developmental anchors for full age range; can be used in developmental delay

CAM, confusional assessment method; CAM-ICU, confusional assessment method for the intensive care unit; CAPD, Cornell assessment of pediatric delirium; PCAM-ICU, pediatric confusional assessment method; PsCAM, preschool or the confusional assessment method for the intensive care unit.

Source: From Leentjens AF, Rundell J, Rummans T, et al. Delirium: an evidence-based medicine (EBM) monograph for psychosomatic medicine practice, commissioned by the Academy of Psychosomatic Medicine (APM) and the European Association of Consultation Liaison Psychiatry and Psychosomatics (EACLPP). *J Psychosom Res.* 2012;73(2):149–152. doi:10.1016/j.jpsychores.2012.05.009; Malas N, Brahmbhatt K, McDermott C, et al. Pediatric delirium: evaluation, management, and special considerations. *Curr Psychiatry Rep.* 2017;19: 65. doi:10.1007/s11920-017-0817-3; APM Delirium Monograph Update. 2014. https://www.apm.org/wp-content/uploads/DeliriumMonographUpdate2014.pdf

- Medication or substance effect/withdrawal: urine and serum drug screens
- Infection: urinalysis and culture, blood culture, lumbar puncture
- Radiography: for possible ileus or bowel obstruction
- CNS events: neuroimaging, EEG
- Other causes including bladder outlet obstruction, uncontrolled pain, hypoxia (35)

Impact of Delirium on the Patient, Family, and Caretakers

In 2012, Partridge, Martin, Harari, and Dhesi completed a review and synthesis of qualitative and quantitative articles dealing with the experience of delirium from the perspective of the patient, relatives, caretakers, and staff. A selection of their findings is summarized in Box 11.2 (37).

Treatment

The treatment of delirium should first and foremost be based on identification and treatment of the underlying physiologic cause(s). Continuous evaluation and intervention for underlying physiologic, environmental, and iatrogenic risk factors should co-occur with any symptomatic treatment of the delirium. Even in the terminal phase, identification of reversible

---

Box 11.2 Delirium as Experienced by Patients and Family/ Caregivers

Patient recall of delirium

- Rate of recall of delirium varies among studies, settings, and populations.
- Increased lack of recall may be associated with poorer baseline cognitive function and more significant short-term memory impairment, delirium severity, and perceptual disturbance during the delirium episode.
- Themes of delirium memories include day-night disorientation; clouding of thought processes; feelings of strong emotions such as fear, anger, insecurity, and hopelessness; lack of control; perceptual disturbances such as delusions, hallucinations, and illusions; and communication problems, especially feeling misunderstood or not heard.

Psychiatric morbidity of delirium

- Recall of delirium associated with higher rates and severity of distress afterwards.
- Presence of memories with delusional content has been associated with increased symptoms of posttraumatic stress disorder, anxiety, depression and higher general distress.

(*continued*)

Box 11.2 Delirium as Experienced by Patients and Family/Caregivers (*continued*)

Family Experience

• There are high rates and severity of distress in family members of patients with delirium.

• Ratings of distress in caregivers can be higher than that of the patient with delirium. One study of caregivers of patients with advanced cancer showed rates of generalized anxiety were 12 times higher in those who perceived their loved one to have recently experienced delirium.

Source: From Partridge JS, Martin FC, Harari D, Dhesi JK. The delirium experience: what is the effect on patients, relatives and staff and what can be done to modify this? *Int J Geriatr Psychiatry.* 2013;28(8):804–812.

causes and contributions may lead to resolution of delirium state and/or decreased distress. During this phase, treatment should be based on goals of care and immediate prognosis, with intervention and palliative sedation both ethically acceptable, depending on goals and prognosis (34).

Nonpharmacological Treatment and Prevention

Many of the nonpharmacological treatment strategies for delirium can also be used prior to onset for prevention of delirium. They are summarized in Box 11.3 (30,32,33,36).

Pharmacological Treatment

Studies of the pharmacological treatment and prevention of delirium have looked at antipsychotics, cholinesterase inhibitors, regional and perioperative anesthesia strategies, gabapentin, and melatonin (31). Previously pharmacologic treatment was often only used in hyperactive delirium, but there is now evidence that many antipsychotics are useful in decreasing symptoms/severity of delirium in both hypoactive and hyperactive subtypes (34) and that those with hypoactive delirium can experience significant distress and undisclosed psychotic symptoms (37). The practitioner should consider use of these medications for any subtype or age range based on clinical factors such as distress, confusion, agitation, prolonged duration, perceptual disturbance, correction of sleep–wake cycle and improved engagement in care (31,32). Dosage ranges of antipsychotics studied in delirium are listed in Table 11.4 (31,32,34,36). When using antipsychotics, you should monitor QTc and transaminases and observe for signs of extrapyramidal symptoms (EPS),, sedation, hypotension, tachycardia, and other toxicities.

Other Pharmacological Considerations

• Review medications and consider decreasing doses of medications dependent on hepatic and renal metabolism (35).

Box 11.3 Nonpharmacological Treatments and Prevention Strategies in Delirium

Provide education on delirium to patient and family.

- Patients have reported reassurance that experiences are common and knowledge of plan of care
- Families feel better able to make medical decisions

  Encourage involvement of family members.
  Advise frequent reorientation and reassurance from family and staff.
  Target modifiable risk factors.

- Monitor hydration status.
- Provide glasses and hearing aids for those with impairment.
- Encourage early mobility.
- Avoid physical restraint use, as able.
- Attempt to normalize daily routine.
- Decrease noise levels, normalize day and night time light levels, and minimize nighttime interruptions to normalize sleep-wake cycle.
- Remove unnecessary tubes and lines.

  Set treatment goals for pain management and level of sedation.

- Monitor frequently.
- Use the least deliriogenic medications possible.
- Monitor for signs of opiate, benzodiazepine, and alcohol intoxication and withdrawal.
- Consider uncontrolled pain, bladder distension, constipation/impaction, and akathisia as causes of agitation, especially in the severely ill.

Source: Leentjens AF, Rundell J, Rummans T, et al. Delirium: an evidence-based medicine (EBM) monograph for psychosomatic medicine practice, commissioned by the Academy of Psychosomatic Medicine (APM) and the European Association of Consultation Liaison Psychiatry and Psychosomatics (EACLPP). *J Psychosom Res.* 2012;73(2):149–152. doi:10.1016/j.jpsychores.2012.05.009; Malas N, Brahmbhatt K, McDermott C, et al. Pediatric delirium: evaluation, management, and special considerations. *Curr Psychiatry Rep.* 2017;19: 65. doi:10.1007/s11920-017-0817-3; Bush SH, Leonard MM, Agar M, et al. End-of-life delirium issues regarding recognition, optimal management, and the role of sedation in the dying phase. *J Pain Symptom Manage.* 2014;48(2):215–230; Hyung-Jun Y, Kyoung-Min P, Won-Jung C, et al. Efficacy and safety of haloperidol versus atypical antipsychotic medications in the treatment of delirium. *BMC Psychiatry.* 2013;13:240. doi:10.1186/1471-244x-13-240.

- Consider possible overtreatment of agitation with opioids, which may worsen delirium. Also consider opioid rotation (35)

Table 11.4 Antipsychotic Doses to Consider for Use in Delirium

Medication	Dose children	Dose adult	Notes
Haloperidol	0.1–5 mg/day; initial dose 0.1–0.25 mg	0.25–10 mg/day	Higher EPS risk; IV infusion (only) associated with prolonged QTc and arrhythmia
Risperidone	0.1–3 mg/day; initial dose 0.1–0.25 mg	0.25–4 mg/day	Higher EPS risk than other SGAs, but lower than haloperidol
Olanzapine	2.5–15 mg/day; initial dose 0.625–2.5 mg	1.25–20 mg/day	
Quetiapine	6.25–200 mg/day; initial dose 6.25–25 mg daily	25–200 mg/day	

The FDA has not approved the use of antipsychotics for use in delirium in children or adults, so all use is off label.

EPS, extrapyramidal symptoms; SGA, second generation antipsychotics.

Source: From Leentjens AF, Rundell J, Rummans T, et al. Delirium: an evidence-based medicine (EBM) monograph for psychosomatic medicine practice, commissioned by the Academy of Psychosomatic Medicine (APM) and the European Association of Consultation Liaison Psychiatry and Psychosomatics (EACLPP). *J Psychosom Res.* 2012;73(2):149–152. doi:10.1016/j.jpsychores.2012.05.009; Malas N, Brahmbhatt K, McDermott C, et al. Pediatric delirium: evaluation, management, and special considerations. *Curr Psychiatry Rep.* 2017;19: 65. doi:10.1007/s11920-017-0817-3; APM Delirium Monograph Update. 2014. https://www.apm.org/wp-content/uploads/DeliriumMonographUpdate2014.pdf; Hyung-Jun Y, Kyoung-Min P, Won-Jung C, et al. Efficacy and safety of haloperidol versus atypical antipsychotic medications in the treatment of delirium. *BMC Psychiatry.* 2013;13:240. doi:10.1186/1471-244x-13-240.

- Evidence of antipsychotic treatment on duration of delirium data are mixed, but data that suggest that second generation antipsychotics (SGA) reduce duration of delirium in ICU patients (34).
- Antipsychotic use for prevention of delirium may be more effective than for the treatment of ongoing delirium with studies of IV haloperidol, oral olanzapine, and oral risperidone showing reduced postoperative delirium compared to placebo (31).
- Cholinesterase inhibitors have not shown superiority to placebo in prevention of postoperative delirium or reduced duration or severity of delirium (31).

- Many studies in adults and children have shown significantly lower rates of delirium in the ICU when sedation is initiated with dexmedetomidine than with midazolam (31,32).
- Significantly greater rates of bradycardia have been seen with dexmedotomedine (31).
- Preprocedural regional blocks may decrease the incidence of delirium, as use of perioperative bupivacaine fascial block showed decreased incidence, severity, and duration of postoperative delirium in hip fracture patients (31).
- Studies are promising for use of melatonin to reduce incidence of delirium in general medical and ICU patients (31,32).
- If there is concern for substance withdrawal, intervention should be targeted toward treatment of the withdrawal syndrome.

Social interventions include reduction of patient and family distress and relief of caregiver burden. In addition, it includes discussing the physical manifestations of the dying process, including hyper and hypoactive delirium, with patient, family, and caregivers. Patient and family may benefit from palliative care consultation. If there is consideration of discharge from the hospital, assess for eligibility for hospice services. Social workers and chaplains should be enlisted to guide patients and families through the process (35).

Spirituality

When a patient enters into end-stage delirium, the family and friends who remain grieve their loss. At this time coping comes in many forms including questioning of their own beliefs, turning to religious practices, and seeking comforting rituals. Suggest that family and friends speak to a trusted and trained individual who can assist with working through this challenging time.

Clinical Pearls

- Delirium is associated with increased morbidity and mortality in all stages of illness.
- Treat the underlying cause of the delirium, including evaluating for and treating substance withdrawal.
- Prevention strategies may be the most effective intervention.
- Routine screening in high risk populations can be easily instituted and can save money and lives.

Online resources for patient/provider education:
- Website of the ICU delirium and cognitive impairment study group of Vanderbilt University Medical Center. Patient handouts for ICU and non-ICU delirium and patient and provider education available:http://icudelirium.org/index.html
- American Academy of Child and Adolescent Psychiatry. Delirium in adolescents and children [A patient/family education flyer]. https://www.aacap.org/App_Themes/AACAP/docs/homepage/headlines/2015/DeliriumFlyer.AACAP.pdf

REFERENCES

1. Warm E, Weissman DE. *Fast Facts and Concepts #7 Assessing Depression in Advanced Cancer* (3rd ed). 2015. https://www.mypcnow.org/blank-hn0yj
2. Caruso R, GiuliaNanni M, Riba MB, Sabato S, Grassi L. Depressive spectrum disorders in cancer: diagnostic issues and intervention. A Critical Review. *Curr Psychiatry Rep*. 2017;19(6):33. doi:10.1007/s11920-017-0785-7
3. PDQ® Supportive and Palliative Care Editorial Board. PDQ Depression. Bethesda, MD: National Cancer Institute; 2017. https://www.cancer.gov/about-cancer/coping/feelings/depression-hp-pdq
4. Kroenke K, Spitzer RL, Williams JB. The Patient Health Questionnaire-2: Validity of a Two-Item Depression Screener. *Medical Care*. 2003;(41):1284–1294.
5. National Comprehensive Cancer Network (NCCN) Clinical Practice Guidelines in Oncology Version 2.2018 Distress Management. https://www.nccn.org/professionals/physician_gls/default.aspx
6. American Psychiatric Association. *Diagnostic and Statistical Manual of Mental Disorders: DSM-5*. 5th ed. Washington, DC: Author; 2013.
7. PDQ® Supportive and Palliative Care Editorial Board. PDQ Grief, Bereavement, and Coping With Loss. Bethesda, MD: National Cancer Institute; 2017. https://www.cancer.gov/about-cancer/advanced-cancer/caregivers/planning/bereavement-hp-pdq
8. Rodin G, Katz M, Lloyd N, et al. Treatment of depression in cancer patients. *Curr Oncol*. 2007;14(5):180–188. doi:10.3747/co.2007.146
9. Irwin SA, Block S. Chapter 33: What Treatments are Effective for Depression in the Palliative Care Setting? In: Goldstein NE, Morrison RS, eds. *Evidence Based Practice of Palliative Medicine*. Philadelphia, PA: Saunders; 2013:181–190.
10. Irwin SA, Hirst JM. Overview of Anxiety in Palliative Care. In: Block SD, ed. *Uptodate*. 2017 https://www.uptodate.com/contents/overview-of-anxiety-in-palliative-care
11. PDQ® Supportive and Palliative Care Editorial Board. PDQ Adjustment to Cancer. Bethesda, MD: National Cancer Institute. 2017. https://www.cancer.gov/about-cancer/coping/feelings/anxiety-distress-hp-pdq
12. PDQ Integrative, Alternative, and Complementary Therapies Editorial Board. Topics in Integrative, Alternative, and Complementary Therapies (PDQ®). In: *PDQ Cancer Information Summaries [Internet]*. Bethesda, MD: National Cancer Institute (US); 2002. https://www.ncbi.nlm.nih.gov/books/NBK131880
13. Holland JC, Breitbart WS, Butow P, et al. eds. *Psycho-Oncology*. New York, NY: Oxford University Press; 2015.
14. Yalom ID, Leszcz M. *The theory and practice of group psychotherapy* (5th ed). New York, NY: Basic Books; 2005.
15. Yalom ID, Greaves C. Group therapy with the terminally ill. *Am J Psychiatry*. 1977;134(4), 396–400. doi:10.1176/ajp.134.4.396
16. Montgomery C. Role of dynamic group therapy in psychiatry. *Adv Psychiatr Treat*. 2002;8(1):34–41. doi:10.1192/apt.8.1.34
17. Beck JS. *Cognitive Behavior Therapy: The basics and beyond*. New York, NY: The Guilford Press; 2011.
18. Levin TT, Applebaum AJ. Acute cancer cognitive therapy. *Cogn Behav Pract*. 2014;14:1077–7229. doi: 10.1016/j.cbpra.2014.03.003
19. Hayes SC, Strosahl KD, Wilson KG. *Acceptance and Commitment Therapy: The Process and Practice of Mindful Change*. New York, NY: Guilford Press; 2011.
20. Hulbert-Williams NJ, Storey L, Wilson KG. Psychological interventions for patients with cancer: psychological flexibility and the potential utility of Acceptance and Commitment Therapy. *Eur J Cancer Care*. 2015;24(1):15–27. doi:10.1111/ecc.12223
21. Ameli R. *25 lessons in mindfulness: Now time for healthy living*. Washington, D.C.: American Psychological Association; 2013.
22. Segal ZV, Williams JMG, Teasdale JD. *Mindfulness-based cognitive therapy for depression* (2nd ed.). New York, NY: The Guildford Press; 2013.
23. Kabat-Jinn J. *Full Catastrophe Living: Using the wisdom of your body and mind to face stress, pain, and illness*. New York, NY: Bantam Dell; 2005.
24. Carlson LE, Speca M. *Mindfulness-Based Cancer Recovery: a step-by-step MBSR approach to help you cope with treatment & reclaim your life*. Oakland, CA: New Harbinger Publications, Inc; 2010.

25. Bartley T. *Mindfulness-based cognitive therapy for cancer: gently turning towards*. West Sussex, UK: Wiley-Blackwell; 2011.

26. Breitbart W, Rosenfeld B, Pessin H, et al. Meaning-centered group psychotherapy: An effective intervention for improving psychological well-being in patients with advanced cancer. *J Clin Oncol*. 2015;33(7):749-754. doi: 10.1200/JCO.2014.57.2198

27. Frankl V. *Man's Search for Meaning*, Beacon Press, Boston: Rider; 1946.

28. Chochinov HM, Hack T, Hassard T, et al. Dignity therapy: a novel psychotherapeutic intervention for patients near the end of life. *J Clin Oncol*. 2005;23(24):5520–5525. doi:10.1200/jco.2005.08.391

29. Owri A, Hight E. Spirituality and Medical Practice: Using the HOPE Questions as a Practical Tool for Spiritual Assessment. *Am Fam Phys*. 2001;63(1):81–89.

30. Leentjens AF, Rundell J, Rummans T, et al. Delirium: an evidence-based medicine (EBM) monograph for psychosomatic medicine practice, commissioned by the Academy of Psychosomatic Medicine (APM) and the European Association of Consultation Liaison Psychiatry and Psychosomatics (EACLPP). *J Psychosom Res*. 2012;73(2):149–152. doi:10.1016/j.jpsychores.2012.05.009

31. Friedman JI, Suleiman L, McGonagall DP, et al. Pharmacologic treatments of non-substance-withdrawal delirium: a systematic review of prospective trials. *Am J Psychiatry*. 2014;171(2);151–159. doi:10.1176/appi.ajp.2013.13040458

32. Malas N, Brahmbhatt K, McDermott C, et al. Pediatric delirium: evaluation, management, and special considerations. *Curr Psychiatry Rep*. 2017;19: 65. doi:10.1007/s11920-017-0817-3

33. Bush SH, Leonard MM, Agar M, et al. End-of-life delirium issues regarding recognition, optimal management, and the role of sedation in the dying phase. *J Pain Symptom Manage*. 2014;48(2):215–230.

34. APM Delirium Monograph Update. 2014. https://www.apm.org/wp-content/uploads/DeliriumMonographUpdate2014.pdf

35. National Comprehensive Cancer Network (NCCN) Clinical Practice Guidelines in Oncology Version I.2014 Palliative Care. https://www.nccn.org/professionals/physician_gls/default.aspx

36. Partridge JS, Martin FC, Harari D, Dhesi JK. The delirium experience: what is the effect on patients, relatives and staff and what can be done to modify this?. *Int J Geriatr Psychiatry*. 2013;28(8):804–812.

37. Hyung-Jun Y, Kyoung-Min P, Won-Jung C, et al. Efficacy and safety of haloperidol versus atypical antipsychotic medications in the treatment of delirium. *BMC Psychiatry*. 2013;13:240. doi:10.1186/1471-244x-13-240

38. National Comprehensive Cancer Network (NCCN). Clinical Practice Guidelines in Oncology Version I. *Palliative Care*; 2014. https://www.nccn.org/professionals/physician_gls/default.aspx

Sleep Disorders, Fatigue, and Sleep Deprivation Management in Adult and Pediatric Cancer Patients — 12

Meaghann Weaver and Jill Bechaz

INTRODUCTION

Disordered sleep ranges from inadequate sleep hygiene to disrupted circadian rhythm to sleep-associated movement disorders to insomnia. Sleep disturbance impacts daytime mood, social functioning, cognitive wellness, and biomedical markers. Sleep disorders often take a toll on not only the patient but also on family sleep patterns and collective energy. This chapter defines sleep disturbances and shares targeted integrative therapies and pharmacologic approaches to interventions.

IMPACT OF DISORDERED SLEEP

Problems with sleep impact mood, social functioning, cognitive wellness, and pain tolerance. Inability to sleep well at night may prevent participation in meaningful daytime activities such as employment for adults and playtime for children. Sleep disorders often take a toll on not only the patient but also on family sleep patterns and collective energy.

DEFINITIONS

- Primary Insomnia is defined in the *DSM-5* as "difficulty initiating or maintaining sleep, or non-restorative sleep, for at least one month." This is further quantified according to more than 3 nights per week; more than 30 minutes to fall asleep; waking more than 30 minutes too early; or feeling unrefreshed in the morning.

- One must consider insomnia for patients in the context of impact on quality of life and overall functioning.

The International Classification of Sleep Disorders (ICSD-2) classifies insomnias into various categories (1):

1. Acute Insomnia: adjustment to an acute stressor that is expected to resolve when the stressor disappears (<3 months); many patients experience acute insomnia in the inpatient setting due to change in environment.

2. Life-Long Insomnia: etiology is unknown, but family history of early infantile and childhood sleep habits may hint at this diagnosis.

3. Learned Insomnia: situation in which the patient no longer associates the bed with sleeping, such as when a child is in a hospital bed all day and play/activities all take place in the bed setting; the child's bed is no longer associated with a sleep expectation.

4. Inadequate sleep hygiene: related to irregular sleep schedule, frequent external nighttime interruptions, use of bright-lights or technology before bed, consumption of caffeinated beverages in the afternoon or early evening.

5. Circadian rhythm sleep disorders: jet lag and shift work

Additional sleep disorders are depicted as:

- Parasomnia: disruption during sleep that may cause awakening or other disturbances such as nightmares, sleep terrors, and sleepwalking
- Sleep apnea: periods of breathing cessation during sleep; obstructive or central in origin
- Restless legs syndrome (RLS): paresthesias and dysesthesias of the legs, which may be relieved by movement (patient aware of sensation)
- Periodic limb movement syndrome (PLMS): involuntary, rhythmic twitches such as ankle dorsiflexion occurring every 20–40 seconds during sleep (patient not aware of kicking sensation)
- Narcolepsy: abnormalities in regulating sleep-wake cycles with subsequent excessive daytime sleepiness and tendency to fall asleep when relaxed during the day; may be associated with sleep paralysis and in some cases episodes of cataplexy (loss of muscle control triggered by strong emotions) (2)

SLEEP HISTORY

- Early sleep patterns
  - Inquire about infant sleep patterns (such as the age when the child first slept through the night, ease of falling asleep and staying asleep as an infant, requirement [or need] to be rocked as an infant, nap and wakefulness pattern in early childhood)
- Sleep chronology
  - Learn about onset, pattern, and duration of sleep through a sleep journal (include daytime nap patterns).
  - Explore whether the difficulty is in initiating sleep or sustaining sleep or both.
- Feelings about sleep
  - History of nightmares or night terrors; whether the patient has dreams
  - Apprehension about falling asleep—explore whether the patient is scared of dying if he or she falls asleep
  - Fear of the dark or fear of "night monsters" (particularly relevant in children or patients with altered mental status/delirium)
  - Desire to stay awake to not miss out on social activity if patient goes to bed earlier than family members
  - Level of personal and familial distress or comfort with current sleep patterns
- Medical symptoms

- Check whether physical symptoms such as cough, dyspnea, pain, central or obstructive forms of apnea, or restless movements are interfering with sleep.
- Ask about any bed-wetting or encopresis patterns.
- Determine the extent to which underlying medical conditions may be impacting sleep pattern, such as prostate enlargement causing frequent awakenings.
- Review pharmaceuticals for possible sleep-impacting medications such as steroids causing evening wakefulness or diuretics causing frequent evening urination.
- Impact of hospitalizations
  - Inquire about recent hospitalizations, particularly in intensive care setting, due to known substantial loss of pediatric sleep and disturbance to sleep-wake cycles in the hospital setting.
- Current sleep hygiene
  - Ask about the sleep environment (whether shared room or independent room, bedding, access to comfort item such as favorite blanket or stuffed animal for a child, room lighting, household noise that may impact sleep, etc.).
  - Inquire about technology use (such as cell phone or television) before bed.
  - Inquire about caffeine intake (amount and time of day).
  - Inquire about sound machine or gentle music.
  - Ask about spiritual rituals such as sharing gratitudes before bedtime, family prayers, or poetry before bed.
- Family impact
  - Ask about family sleep patterns and inquire as to the ways the patient's sleep pattern is impacting partner sleep or family fatigue/family function.
  - Learn about the family's behavioral response to the patient's wakefulness (such as for a pediatric patient whether child is allowed to join the parent bed, whether the parent stays in the room with the child, whether child is allowed to return to kitchen for snacks in the night, etc.; and, for an adult patient whether their partner sleeps in a different room or whether the partner's sleep is disrupted).

SLEEP SCREENING

Insomnia screening tool options for adults consist primarily of the Insomnia Severity Index (ISI) questionnaire, the National Sleep Foundation's Sleepiness Test, and the Epworth Sleepiness Scale. Most practitioners recommend that adults complement sleep screening tools with completion of a sleep diary over a few weeks to provide information about sleep patterns and practices. The "STOP BANG" adult sleep screening questionnaire explores components of obstructive sleep apnea that may be impacting sleep health: Snoring, Tiredness, Observation of stopping breathing, high blood Pressure, Body mass index, Age, Neck size, and Gender.

SLEEP HYGIENE RESOURCES

- National Sleep Foundation (for adults and adolescents). What is sleep hygiene? Sleep Hygiene. 2015. Retrieved from: http://sleepfoundation.org/ask-the-expert/sleep-hygiene
- American Academy of Pediatrics (for younger children). Sleep Tips for Your Family's Mental Health. Retrieved from: https://www.healthy-children.org/English/healthy-living/sleep/Pages/Sleep-and-Mental-Health.aspx

SLEEP EVALUATION

- Sleep diary
- Polysomnography

BEHAVIORAL AND INTEGRATIVE SLEEP INTERVENTIONS

Behavioral interventions for sleep are noted to prove more beneficial than no treatment, placebo, alternative treatments, and frequently used medications (3). Behavioral interventions include sleep hygiene education; cognitive behavioral therapies for insomnia (4,5); and integrative approaches such as aromatherapy (lavender, marjoram, tangerine, ylang-ylang), massage, acupuncture, relaxation therapy, hypnosis, and therapeutic music.

PHARMACEUTICAL INTERVENTIONS

There are no medications that are approved by the Food and Drug Administration (FDA) for the indication of insomnia in pediatric patients; however, there are several medications that may be utilized off-label for this purpose. A list of various medications used to promote sleep in children are provided in Table 12.1.

FATIGUE

Impact

Fatigue is one of the most prevalent, severe, and disabling symptoms in patients, particularly toward natural end of life (6).

Definitions

Fatigue is a subjective feeling of low energy, tiredness, or weakness. Physical fatigue (weakness) may prevent a patient from engaging in everyday activities; cognitive fatigue (tiredness) may prevent patients from engaging in activities such as reading or active conversation. Primary fatigue is due to the underlying diagnosis; secondary fatigue is due to contributing health, psychosocial, or treatment factors (Table 12.2).

Fatigue History

- Assess the intensity and duration of fatigue through the patient's perspective and then include the family's perspective.
- Inquire as to general fatigue, mental fatigue, activity, and motivation longitudinally using patient and family narrative.

Table 12.1 Pharmaceutical Options for Sleep Promotion

Medication	Example and dose	Potential benefit	Clinical caution
Naturally occurring sleep hormone	Melatonin (classified as dietary supplement and thus available OTC): 2–5 mg at bedtime for patients >6 mo; may titrate based on response Ramelteon (melatonin receptor agonist): Adults: 8 mg 30 min prior to bedtime	Melatonin is considered as a first-line intervention; classified as a dietary supplement and available OTC	Melatonin is an endogenous metabolite of tryptophan and serotonin, released cyclically from the pineal gland according to the body's circadian rhythm
Tetracycline antidepressants	Trazodone: 18 mo to <3 y/o: initial 25 mg at bedtime and may increase every 2 weeks by 25 mg intervals to a maximum of 100 mg 3 y/o to 5 y/o: initial 50 mg at bedtime and may increase every 2 weeks in 25 mg intervals to a maximum of 150 mg >5 y/o: initial 0.75–1 mg/kg/dose at bedtime; reported range 0.5–2 mg/kg/dose Adults: initial 50 mg at bedtime; titrate to maximum of 300 mg/day Mirtazapine: Adults: 15 mg at bedtime; titrate to a maximum of 45 mg/day	May help with concurrent depression or anxiety	Recommend consultation with a psychiatrist
Alpha-agonist	Clonidine: 2–5 mcg/kg/dose PO at bedtime; maximum of 200 mcg	May help with concurrent medication withdrawal or cerebral irritability	Risk of hypotension; rebound hypertension if stopped abruptly

(continued)

Table 12.1 Pharmaceutical Options for Sleep Promotion (*continued*)

Medication	Example and dose	Potential benefit	Clinical caution
Benzodiazepines	Lorazepam: Children: 0.05–0.1 mg/kg PO at bedtime; initial maximum of 2 mg; may titrate to a maximum of 4 mg Adults <65 y/o: 0.5–2 mg at bedtime Adults >65 y/o: 0.5–1 mg at bedtime Clonazepam: 0.005–0.01 mg/kg/dose PO at bedtime; initial maximum of 0.25 mg Diazepam: 0.1–0.2 mg/kg/dose PO at bedtime; initial maximum of 1–2.5 mg	May help relieve anxiety or cerebral irritability	Sedating Risk of rebound wakefulness Dependence over time
Neuropathic pain agents	Gabapentin: Children: 5 mg/kg/dose at bedtime; may titrate to 10 mg/kg/dose Adults: 300 mg 2 hr prior to bedtime; titrate to a maximum of 1800 mg/day Pregabalin: Adults: 75 mg 1–3 hr prior to bedtime, titrate to a maximum of 450 mg/day Amitriptyline: Adults: 25–100 mg at bedtime; maximum of 150 mg	May assist with concurrent neuropathic pain	Must be slowly tapered off over time
Atypical antipsychotics	Quetiapine Risperidone	At low doses may be useful in treating agitation in combination with insomnia	Recommend consultation with a psychiatrist

mo, month; OTC, over the counter; y/o, year old.

Table 12.2 Fatigue Evaluation—Grounded in Attentive Physical Exam

Etiology	Evaluation*	Intervention*
Dehydration/ electrolyte imbalance	Electrolytes Orthostatic blood pressures	Hydration; electrolyte supplementation
Anemia	Complete blood count Microcytic anemia may trigger iron studies; macrocytic anemia may trigger folate or vitamin B12 labs	Transfusion Iron/B12 supplements
Untreated pain	Thorough pain assessment	Pain medication and integrative therapies
Sleep disturbance	Sleep diary; sleep hygiene history	Consider sedative agents at bedside; mindfulness practices and quality sleep hygiene at bedtime
Inactivity or deconditioning	Occupational therapy/ physical therapy evaluation	Gentle exercise or passive range of movement; massage
Psychiatric comorbidities (depression or anxiety)	Depression/anxiety screen	Antidepressant medication and counseling as appropriate
Pharmaceuticals (sedating medications or polypharmacy)	Medication review (recent medication changes)	Consider medication rotation; dose adjustments
Hypoxemia or dyspnea	Oxygen saturation evaluation for hypoxemia; subjective questions for dyspnea	Supplemental oxygen for comfort; opiate and benzodiazepine for dyspnea; fan in room
Organ dysfunction	Organ-specific labs such as brain natriuretic peptide (BNP) for heart failure; potential organ specific imaging such as echocardiogram	Level of organ-specific intervention to be grounded in goals of care
Systemic infection	Blood or urine cultures; chest x-ray, if appropriate	Antibiotics

(continued)

Table 12.2 Fatigue Evaluation—Grounded in Attentive Physical Exam (*continued*)

Etiology	Evaluation*	Intervention*
Cachexia/anorexia	Albumin/prealbumin	Very little evidence for nutritional supplementation and appetite stimulants toward natural end of life; respect the body's natural decrease in appetite
Hypothyroidism	Thyroid panel	Thyroid supplementation
Adverse effects of treatment	Chemotherapy, radiation, extended hospitalizations	Evaluate with child and family whether disease-directed treatments are impacting fatigue symptoms; may consider to reduce or discontinue these interventions depending on goals of care
Spiritual distress/ existential suffering	Spiritual screening; thoughtful questions about life meaning and joy	Child-specific spirituality screening tools; chaplain and child life support

*Please note that the work-up and intervention for secondary causes of fatigue will be highly case-dependent; the driving intention should be grounded on goals of care for the child (just because an invasive workup or treatment is available does not automatically mean it is congruent with goals of care for that child).

- Explore the level of distress fatigue has on the patient and family; determine the patient's goals for engagement/activity.
- Screen for depression, anxiety, and sleep quality.
- Ask about whether level of tiredness is relieved by rest.
- Evaluate any change in medications or dosages.

Screening Tools for Adult Fatigue

- Fatigue Questionnaire (FQ)
- Fatigue Severity Scale (FSS)
- Piper Fatigue Scale

- Fatigue Symptom Inventory (FSI)
- Brief Fatigue Inventory
- Epworth Sleepiness Scale (ESS)

Screening Tools Specific to Pediatric and Adolescent Fatigue

- Memorial Symptom Assessment Scale (MSAS)
- Edmonton Symptom Assessment Scale (ESAS)
- Pediatric Quality of Life Scale (PedsQL)
- Childhood Fatigue Scale (CFS)
- Fatigue Scale-Adolescent (FS-A)
- Parent Fatigue Scale (PFS)
- Pediatric Functional Assessment of Chronic Illness Therapy-Fatigue (Peds FACIT-F)

Fatigue Interventions

- Educate—to normalize symptoms and promote adaptation; to work toward energy conservation principles to "save energy" for moments of potential play (without placing pressure on a requirement to have those moments).
- Passive exercise—gentle low intensity exercise to include passive range of movement; focus less on movement expectations and more on helping patients cope and adjust to the impact of fatigue on their ability to enjoy today.
- Dietary supplements—L-carnitine has been investigated in adults but there are suboptimal data in children to recommend at this time (7).
- Integrate therapies—Acupuncture; massage therapy; aromatherapy (lemon, orange, bergamot, peppermint), psychotherapy/relaxation therapy; music therapy.

Fatigue Pharmaceuticals

While these may be considered on a case-by-case basis, there are few data to support psycho-stimulants such as methylphenidate (may cause arrhythmia in children with cardiac vulnerability, nervousness, or agitation); or steroids; or megestrol acetate for fatigue in children. Dosing recommendation of methylphenidate for the indication of narcolepsy in patients more than 6 years old is 5 mg BID before breakfast and lunch; increase weekly as necessary by 5 to 10 mg/day to a maximum of 60 mg/day. Dosing recommendation of methylphenidate for cancer-related fatigue in adults is 5 mg BID, titrated to a maximum of 40 mg/day. Current recommendations are to maximize educational, environmental, and behavioral support interventions.

REFERENCES

1. Sateia MJ. International Classification of Sleep Disorders-Third Edition. *Chest.* 2014;146(5):1387–1394. doi:10.1378/chest.14-0970
2. Arnold R, Miller M, Mehta R. Palliative Care Network of Wisconsin. Fast Facts and Concepts #101 Insomnia. 2017. https://www.mypcnow.org/blank-xwnba

3. Taylor DJ, Roane BM. Treatment of insomnia in adults and children: a practice-friendly review of research. *J Clin Psychol*. 2010;66:1137–1147. doi:10.1002/jclp.20733

4. Siebern AT, Manber RM. New developments in cognitive behavioral therapy as the first-line treatment of insomnia. *Psychol Res Behav Manag*. 2011;4:21–28. doi:10.2147/PRBM.S10041

5. Shatkin JP, Pando M. Diagnosis and treatment of common sleep disorders in adolescence. *Adolesc Psychiatr*. 2015;4:1–13. doi:10.2174/2210676605666150521232247

6. Drake R, Frost J, Collins JJ. The symptoms of dying children. *J Pain Symptom Manage*. 2003;26(1):594–603. doi:10.1016/S0885-3924(03)00202-1

7. Cruciana RA, Zhang JJ, Manola J, et al. L-carnitine supplementation for the management of fatigue in patients with cancer: an eastern cooperative oncology group phase III, randomized, double-blind, placebo-controlled trial. *J Clin Oncol*. 2012; 30(31):3864–3869. doi:10.1200/JCO.2011.40.2180

Cancer Pain and Its Treatment 13

**Sarah M. Verga, Andrew Whitman,
Kevin Adams, and Ambereen K. Mehta**

INTRODUCTION

Pain is a common symptom for patients with cancer that is often distressing to them, their families, and their caregivers. In patients with metastatic or terminal disease, up to 66% reported having pain, with more than one third describing it as moderate or severe. The prevalence of cancer pain has been found to be as high as 55% during cancer treatment and 39% after curative treatment (1). Successful management of cancer pain involves assessment and treatment of all components of total pain (Table 13.1). This includes physical symptoms, emotional pain, social pain, and spiritual/existential distress. The prevalence of psychosocial distress ranges from 29% to 43%, although this varies by cancer type (2). This chapter focuses heavily on the assessment and management of physical pain. Other components of total cancer pain are addressed in more detail in additional chapters of this handbook and are referenced individually in the subsections of this chapter.

SYMPTOMS OF PAIN

Collaboration with spiritual care professionals, social workers, psychologists, pharmacists, patients and caregivers is necessary for a comprehensive pain assessment (3–5).

Physical Pain

Physical pain can be caused by neuropathic, nociceptive somatic, and nociceptive visceral pathways and can be either acute or chronic (Table 13.2 and Table 13.3). It is important to take a detailed physical pain history to appropriately identify the etiology and onset of physical pain as this can guide treatment strategies.

Physical Pain in the Pediatric Population

Pediatric palliative care is child, family, and relationship focused and must address the concerns of the child in the setting of their developmental stage and relationship with their parents. Inadequate identification and treatment of pain in children can not only cause discomfort but can affect a child's future pain events while simultaneously causing distress to their families (9).

Table 13.1 Components of Total Cancer Pain

Physical	Emotional	Social	Spiritual / existential
• Onset + temporal pattern • Location • Intensity • Quality • Provocative factors • Relieving factors • Inferred pathophysiology • Medical comorbidities • Effect on physical function • Current and prior treatments • Extent of disease	• Anxiety • Depression • Grief and preparatory grief • Loss of independence • Fear of death • Sleep disturbance • Fatigue (physical and cognitive) • Psychiatric comorbidities • Substance abuse history • PTSD	• Effect on role functioning • Effect on relationships • Caregiver burden • Communication barriers • Social isolation • Financial stress • Sexual function • Attitudes about opioids • Cultural beliefs • Family dynamics • Isolation	• Lack of meaning • Lack of connectedness • Isolation • Abandonment • Hopelessness • Helplessness • Demoralization • Uselessness
Examples of questions for assessment			
• When is pain the worst? • At what level of pain do you feel you are able to function? • Does pain prevent you from doing things you normally would or things that you enjoy?	• Do you find yourself worrying? • What has helped you cope with difficult situations in the past? • How has your sleep been affected by pain? • What do you enjoy doing? • Do you have the energy to do the things you want to do?	• Who are the most important people in your life? Are you worried about them? • How has your cancer affected your financial situation? • How has your cancer affected your relationships? • What is most important to you?	• Have religious or spiritual practices been previously helpful for you during times of uncertainty, pain, or distress? • What gives meaning to your life? • What in your life are you most proud of? • Do you feel at peace? (6)

Table 13.2 Pathophysiology of Physical Pain		
Neuropathic pain	**Nociceptive somatic**	**Nociceptive visceral**
Direct damage or dysfunction of central or peripheral nervous system or physical compression of nerve	Nociceptive receptors activated by ongoing tissue damage in **muscle, soft tissue, and bone**	Ongoing tissue injury caused by **tension, stretching, ischemia, or inflammation of visceral organs** (thoracic, abdominal, pelvic viscera)
Characteristics of physical pain		
• Burning • Tingling • Stabbing • Searing • Shooting • Numbness	• Superficial (skin/mucosa): • Localized • Sharp • Stinging • Deep (muscle, joint, bone): • Localized • Gnawing • Aching	• Poorly localized • Dull • Pressure • Squeezing • Cramping • If organ capsule involved: • Sharp • Stabbing

Physical Pain in the Geriatric Population (Box 13.1)

25% to 40% of elderly cancer patients have daily pain, which is often undertreated because of age-related communication barriers or reluctance to report (12).

Emotional and Social Pain

Uncontrolled psychological and emotional pain may result in inappropriate escalation of pharmacological treatments without adequate pain relief (7). An interdisciplinary team including psychology, pastoral care, social work, and nursing is helpful and often necessary.

Adults: Total Symptom Assessment Scales

- Edmonton Memorial Assessment Scale (ESAS)—9-item comprehensive symptom assessment including eight symptoms and one well-being item (14)
- Memorial Symptom Assessment Scale (MSAS)—symptom frequency, distress, and severity assessment for 32 physical and psychological symptoms (15)

Pediatrics (9,16,17) (Table 13.4)

- Higher levels of stress and increased depression in parents of children with chronic medical conditions

Table 13.3 Differentiaing Between Acute and Chronic Cancer Pain (7,8)

Acute cancer pain	Chronic cancer pain syndromes

• *New pain* and usually transient
• As healing occurs, pain expected to resolve
• Can be an indicator of disease progression
• Can be caused by cancer treatment:
  ▪ Chemotherapy
  ▪ Radiation
  ▪ Postoperative
• Can be caused by noncancer conditions (which may be exacerbated by cancer treatment):
• Constipation
• Bladder spasms
• Wounds/pressure ulcers
• Falls/injury
• Migraines
• Musculoskeletal pain
	• Pain that
	• Lasts longer than 3 months
	• Lasts more than 1 month after resolution of inciting factor
	• Occurs with a lesion unlikely to heal or resolve
	• Is recurrent over several months
	• Typically caused by effect of tumor
	  ▪ Direct involvement of bone, nerves, viscera
	  ▪ Tumor release of inflammatory mediators
	Also can be caused by
	• Side effects of treatment/intervention
	• Disease progression

Source: From Dalal S, Bruera E. Assessing cancer pain. *Curr Pain Headache Rep.* 2012;16:314–324. doi:10.1007/s11916-012-0274-y; Komatz K, Carter B. Pain and Symptom Management in Pediatric Palliative Care. *Pediatr Rev.* 2015;36(12):527–533; quiz 534. doi:10.1542/pir.36-12-527

- Concept of "mutual care": patient and parent worry about each other and attempt to protect each other
- Themes important to patient, parent, and clinician
  - "Holding to hope"
  - "Honest communication"
  - "Relief from symptoms"
  - "Caring for each other"
- Children (preschool age) may feel shame or guilt; important to emphasize pain or illness is not a punishment to prevent further distress
- Unique concerns: self-esteem, body image concerns, effects on physical growth and development, treatment effects on cognitive growth and development, school/extracurricular participation/performance

Evaluating the Family and Caregiver Population (18–21)

- Addressing family and caregiver needs is essential to minimize the psychosocial distress and total pain of both the patient and the caregivers.
- Patients and caregivers are primarily responsible for administering pain medications and executing pain regimen schedules.

Table 13.4 Objective Pediatric Pain Assessment Scales (Observational/Behavioral) (9–11)

Population	Assessment scale
<37 weeks' gestational age	Premature Infant Pain Profile-Revised (PIPP-R)
Infants up to 1 year	Neonatal Infant Pain Scale (NIPS)
2 months–7 years	Face, Leg, Activity, Cry, Consolability Scale (FLACC)
Nonverbal child with intellectual disability (parent reported)	Individualized Numeric Rating Scale
Subjective pediatric pain assessment scales (Self-reported)	
>3 years	Wong-Baker FACE scale
>7 years	Visual analog scale
>9 years	Numerical rating scale

Source: From Goldstein R, Wolfe J. Chapter 65: What Are Special Considerations for Treating Pediatric Patients and Their Families? In: Goldstein N, ed. *Evidence-Based Practice of Palliative Medicine*. Philadelphia, PA: Elsevier; 2013:377–387. doi:10.1016/B978-1-4377-3796-7.00065-3; Lawrence J, Alcock D, McGrath P, et al. The development of a tool to assess neonatal pain. *Neonatal Netw*. 1993;12(6):59–66. doi:10.1016/0885-3924(91)91127-U; Merkel SI, Voepel-Lewis T, Shayevitz JR, Malviya S. The FLACC: a behavioral scale for scoring postoperative pain in young children. *Pediatr Nurs*. 1997;23(3):293–297. http://www.ncbi.nlm.nih.gov/pubmed/9220806

Box 13.1 Behavioral Indicators of Pain in Patients With Cognitive Impairment (13)

- **Verbal cues:** sighing, groaning, grunting, moaning
- **Facial expressions:** grimacing, wrinkled forehead, tightly closed eyes
- **Body movements:** rigid, tense, guarding, fidgeting
- **Social interactions:** withdrawn, combative, aggressive, decreased interaction
- **Changes in activity pattern or routine:** appetite change, increased wandering, change in sleep pattern

Source: Herr K, Bjoro K, Decker S. Tools for assessment of pain in nonverbal older adults with dementia: a state-of-the-science review. *J Pain Symptom Manage*. 2006;31(2):170–192. doi:10.1016/j.jpainsymman.2005.07.001

- Caregivers may feel helpless, frustrated, and may suffer from spiritual distress.
- Caregivers may have increased psychological distress when patient's pain rating is higher.
- Caregivers desire information, support, communication, self-efficacy, effective coping, and recognition
- Caregiver educational interventions have shown improved knowledge of pain management, increased self-efficacy in pain management, and less distress due to patient pain

Untreated substance abuse, maladaptive chemical coping, and fear of opioid addiction can be barriers to pain control and can contribute to emotional and social pain (Table 13.5).

Chemical Coping and Substance Abuse

- CAGE—alcoholism screening tool, 4-item scale (cut down, anger, guilt, eye opener) (22)
- Opioid Risk Tool—assessment of risk of aberrant opioid behavior, useful prior to opioid prescribing, involves assessment of the following risk factors (23):
  - Family history of substance abuse (alcohol, illegal drugs, prescription drugs)
  - Personal history of substance abuse (alcohol, illegal drugs, prescription drugs)
  - Age between 16 to 45 years

Table 13.5 Chemical Coping and Substance Abuse Definitions (24)	
Concept	**Definition**
Tolerance	Physiological increase in drug requirement to achieve same effect previously attained with lower amount of drug
Physical dependence	Physiological presence of withdrawal symptoms if drug discontinued or dose reduced after chronic use
Addiction	Characterized by tolerance and physical dependence on drug with associated drug-seeking behavior and compulsive use despite adverse consequences
Pseudo-addiction	Perceived drug-seeking behavior that mimics addiction behavior but is a sign of undertreatment of pain. With adequate pain management drug-seeking behavior resolves (unlike in addiction)
Chemical coping	Maladaptive use of drugs to relieve psychological distress

Source: From Jackson LK, Imam SN, Braun UK. Opioids in Cancer Pain: Right or Privilege? *J Oncol Pract.* 2017;13(9):e809–e814. doi:10.1200/JOP.2016.019216

Table 13.6 Assessment of Spiritual and Existential Distress (27)

Spiritual screening: Used to identify patients in need of more in-depth spiritual assessment	Spiritual history: Used to better understand a patient's needs and resources
"Are spirituality or religion important in your life?" "How well are those resources working for you at this time?" (27)	• Guide for spiritual history—Faith and belief, Important, Community, Address in Care (FICA; 28) • SPIRIT • HOPE • Domains of spirituality More formal and in-depth assessments should be performed by chaplains

Source: Puchalski C, Ferrell B, Virani R, et al. Improving the quality of spiritual care as a dimension of palliative care: the report of the consensus conference. *J Palliat Med.* 2009;12(10):885–904. doi:10.1089/jpm.2009.0142

- History of preadolescent sexual abuse
- Psychological disease (ADD, OCD, bipolar, schizophrenia, depression)

Spiritual and Existential Distress (3,25,26)

Spirituality is characterized by the search for meaning and connectedness. Spiritual distress may involve feelings of isolation, abandonment, hopelessness, and helplessness and can increase physiological distress (Table 13.6).

TREATMENT OF PAIN

Physical Pain in Adults and Children

Nonsteroidal anti-inflammatory drugs (NSAIDs) (29,30) (Table 13.7) (Boxes 13.2 and 13.3)

Table 13.7 Adults (NSAIDs for Cancer Pain) (31–33)

Medication	Typical starting dose range	Max daily doses	Clinical pearls
Ibuprofen	PO: 400–800 mg every 6–8 hours PRN	3,200 mg	Analgesic effect limited by dose ceiling; negative GI, cardiac, and renal effects; increased risk of bleeding; **lowest risk of cardiac effects with naproxen**
Naproxen	PO: 500 mg every 8–12 hours PRN	1,500 mg	

(continued)

Table 13.7 Adults (NSAIDs for Cancer Pain) (31–33) (*continued*)

Medication	Typical starting dose range	Max daily doses	Clinical pearls
Ketorolac	IM: 30 mg every 6 hours PRN IV: 15–30 mg every 6 hours PRN PO: 20 mg, then 10 mg every 4–6 hours PRN	IV/IM: 120 mg PO: 40 mg	**Short-term (up to 5 days)**; intrathecal or epidural routes contraindicated; opioid adjunct for painful bony metastasis
Diclofenac	PO: 50 mg every 8 hours IV: 37.5 mg every 6 hours	150 mg	**Proven opioid-sparing effects in cancer patients**
Celecoxib	PO: 400 mg once then 200 mg every 12 hours	400 mg	Monitor cardiac adverse effects
Pediatrics and Infants			
Ibuprofen	Infants >6 months/children (or <60 kg): PO: 5–10 mg/kg every 6–8 hours PRN	40 mg/kg (up to 2,400 mg)	Similar adverse effect profile as adults; suspension formulation for easier dose titration and weight based (mg/kg) dosing
Naproxen	Children ≥2 years old: PO: 5 mg/kg every 12 hours PRN	10 mg/kg (up to 1,000 mg)	
Ketorolac	Infants and children: IV/IM: 0.5 mg/kg every 6 hours PRN	2 mg/kg (up to 120 mg)	**Short-term (up to 5 days)**; intrathecal or epidural routes contraindicated; opioid adjunct for painful bony metastasis

Source: From Angiolillo DJ, Weisman SM. Clinical Pharmacology and Cardiovascular Safety of Naproxen. *Am J Cardiovasc Drugs*. 2017;17(2):97–107. doi:10.1007/s40256-016-0200-5; Joishy SK, Walsh D. The opioid-sparing effects of intravenous ketorolac as an adjuvant analgesic in cancer pain: application in bone metastases and the opioid bowel syndrome. *J Pain Symptom Manage*. 1998;16(5):334–339. doi:10.1016/S0885-3924(98)00081-5; Bjorkman R, Ullman A, Hedner J. Morphine-sparing effect of diclofenac in cancer pain. *Eur J Clin Pharmacol*. 1993;44(1):1–5. doi:10.1007/BF00315271

Box 13.2 NSAID Checklist

- Does the patient have existing or potential renal impairment? If so, is oral or IV hydration appropriate?
- Is the patient on other therapies that may harm the kidneys?
- Does the patient have risk factors for bleeding (e.g., recent GI bleed, low platelets, prolonged NSAID use, elderly)?
- Is the patient on other therapies that may increase bleeding risk (e.g., fish oil)?
- Should the rectal route of administration be avoided (i.e., active bleeding, neutropenic)?
- Does the patient have existing cardiac disease that could be exacerbated by NSAID use?
- Should stress ulcer prophylaxis be considered? (34)
- Is the patient taking any over-the-counter combination products that contain an NSAID?
- Is the type of pain being treated likely to respond to an NSAID?
- If an infant or pediatric patient, is the concentration of the product appropriate for the patient's age?

- Varying selectivity for COX-1 or COX-2 enzymes results in different adverse effect profiles
- Effective for pain due to inflammation, bony lesions
- Effective adjuncts to opioid pain relievers
- Higher risk of bleeding from NSAIDs in patients with hematologic disturbances at baseline
- Ibuprofen, naproxen, and ketorolac are most widely used in the cancer population

Acetaminophen (35) (Table 13.8) (Boxes 13.3 and 13.4)

- Analgesic and antipyretic, no clinically significant anti-inflammatory activity
- Opioid sparing properties when used for cancer related pain

Opioids (Table 13.9) (Boxes 13.5 and 13.6) (Table 13.10)

This is the main treatment modality for cancer-related pain (38–40).

- Most do not have a dose ceiling for analgesic effect.
- Monitor for immune suppression and adrenal insufficiency with chronic use.

Table 13.8 Adults (Acetaminophen for Cancer Pain) (36,37)

Medication	Typical starting dose range	Max daily doses	Clinical pearls
Acetaminophen	PO, PR: 650 mg every 4–6 hours IV: (≥50 kg) 650 mg every 4 hours or 1000 mg every 6 hours	PO/IV: Adults: 4,000 mg Geriatric: 3,000 mg Cirrhosis: 2,000 mg	**Caution with OTC products containing acetaminophen— potential for duplicate therapies**; IV more expensive; reduced dosing if significant dehydration or malnourished
Pediatrics and infants			
Acetaminophen	Infants and children: PO/PR/IV: 10–15 mg/kg/ dose every 6 hours PRN	75 mg/kg (not to exceed 4,000 mg)	Caution with OTC products containing acetaminophen— potential for duplicate therapies

Source: From Lewis JH, Stine JG. Review article: Prescribing medications in patients with cirrhosis - A practical guide. *Aliment Pharmacol Ther*. 2013;37(12):1132–1156. doi:10.1111/apt.12324; Jibril F, Sharaby S, Mohamed A, Wilby KJ. Intravenous versus Oral Acetaminophen for Pain: Systematic Review of Current Evidence to Support Clinical Decision-Making. *Can J Hosp Pharm*. 2015;68(3):238–247. doi:10.4212/cjhp.v68i3.1458. http://www.ncbi.nlm.nih.gov/pubmed/26157186

Box 13.3 Acetaminophen Checklist

- Does the patient have baseline liver impairment?
- Is the patient taking other drug therapies that may impact the liver (e.g., imatinib)?
- Is the patient taking other drug therapies that may interact adversely with acetaminophen (e.g., phenobarbital)?
- Based on patient characteristics, should the maximum total dose be modified?

(continued)

Box 13.3 Acetaminophen Checklist (*continued*)

- Should the rectal route of administration be avoided (e.g., active bleeding, neutropenic)?
- Is the patient taking other therapies (including combination analgesics) containing acetaminophen?
- Has the patient been counseled about being cautious with combination agents (e.g., prescription, over-the-counter products) also containing acetaminophen?
- Has the patient been counseled about limiting alcohol consumption when utilizing acetaminophen as an analgesic?

Box 13.4 Important Points for Caregivers—NSAIDs Acetaminophen

- Always check the ingredients of over-the-counter products.
- Many products contain acetaminophen.
- In most cases, the maximum daily dose of acetaminophen from all sources should be 4,000 mg.
- Liver injury is the most common side effect of acetaminophen.
- Stomach ulcers and kidney injury are the most common side effects of NSAIDs.
- Acetaminophen does not have any meaningful impact on inflammation.
- All NSAIDs have an impact on inflammation.

Table 13.9 Adults (Opioids for Cancer Pain)

Medication	Typical starting dose range	Clinical pearls
Morphine	PO/SL:15–30 mg every 3–4 hours (IR); MS Contin™ - 15 mg every 12 hours (ER) IV: 2.5–5 mg every 3–4 hours	SQ, SL, epidural, intrathecal, and rectal routes available; **avoid repeat dosing in patients with renal dysfunction;** constipation and pruritus may be more troublesome with morphine

(*continued*)

Table 13.9 Adults (Opioids for Cancer Pain) (*continued*)

Medication	Typical starting dose range	Clinical pearls
Hydrocodone	PO (with acetaminophen): 2.5–10 mg every 4–6 hours (IR)	Dosing frequency limited by non-opioid component
Hydromorphone	PO: 2–4 mg every 3–4 hours (IR) IV: 0.2–0.8 mg every 2–3 hours (IR)	Less itching and nausea than morphine
Oxycodone	PO (plain oxycodone): 5–15 mg every 4 hours (IR) OxyContin™ 10 mg every 12 hours (ER) PO (with acetaminophen): 2.5–10 mg every 4–6 hours	Caution in elderly patients with moderate to severe renal dysfunction
Fentanyl	Duragesic (patch)—dose based on daily oral morphine equivalent (OME) every 48–72 hours Actiq™ (lozenge)	**Not first line in opioid naive patients**; avoid direct heat to patches; consider body weight and availability of subcutaneous tissues
Methadone	*Dosing varies by morphine equivalents* Typical starting dose (pain): PO: 2.5–10 mg every 8–12 hours IV: 1–5 mg every 8–12 hours	**Consult palliative care or pain management;** QTc prolongation, liver impairment, serotonin syndrome, and drug interactions; **adjust dose every 4–7 days**
Tramadol	PO: 25–100 mg every 4–6 hours (IR) Maximum daily dose: 400 mg	**Increased risk of serotonin syndrome and seizures; avoid in elderly patients**
Codeine	PO (with acetaminophen): Acetaminophen (300–1,000 mg/dose)/codeine (15–60 mg/dose) every 4 hours Maximum daily dose (codeine): 360 mg	Constipation; **should not be considered first line for cancer-related pain**—other more efficacious therapies are available

(*continued*)

Table 13.9 Adults (Opioids for Cancer Pain) (*continued*)

Medication	Typical starting dose range	Clinical pearls
Pediatrics and Infants		
Morphine	PO: 0.1–0.3 mg/kg every 4–6 hours PRN Older children or adolescents may transition to extended release products when dose/dosage form allows IV: 0.05 to 0.1 mg/kg every 4 hours PRN; or 0.01 to 0.05 mg/kg/hr as a continuous infusion	**Avoid IM (painful);** <3 months age more susceptible to respiratory depression; can cause seizures in newborns
Fentanyl	IV: 1–3 mcg/kg every 1–2 hours PRN or 0.5–2 mcg/kg/hr continuous infusion Duragesic (patch)—dosing based on daily oral morphine equivalent (OME) (~50% OME = starting patch dose)	Same as adult patients
Oxycodone	PO (plain oxycodone): 0.1–0.2 mg/kg every 4 hours PRN (IR) Older children and adolescents may transition to extended release products when dose/dosage form allows	
Hydrocodone	PO (with acetaminophen): 0.1–0.2 mg/kg every 4–6 hours PRN (IR)	**Off-label use in infants and pediatric patients**
Hydromorphone	PO: 0.03 mg/kg/dose every 3–6 hours IV: 0.01 mg/kg/dose every 3–6 hours	

(*continued*)

Table 13.9 Adults (Opioids for Cancer Pain) (*continued*)

Medication	Typical starting dose range	Clinical pearls
Methadone	*Initial dosing will vary based on patient's current morphine equivalents* Typical starting dose (pain): PO: 0.05–0.1 mg/kg every 8–12 hours IV: 0.025–0.05 mg/kg every 8–12 hours	Same as adult patients

---

Box 13.5 Opioid Checklist

- Have nonpharmacological options and nonopioid therapies been considered prior to opioid use?
- Has a bowel regimen been prescribed/ordered (optimize stimulant laxatives)?
- Is the patient opioid naive or opioid tolerant?
- Will the opioid pain reliever respond to the type of pain being targeted? (nociceptive versus neuropathic)?
- Does the dosing interval make sense based on the kinetics of the medication?
- Does the patient have pre-existing liver or hepatic impairment that may help drive opioid selection or adjustment?
- Has the patient been screened for opioid misuse?
- Has the patient been counseled on risk of opioid dependence and addiction?
- Should naloxone be ordered or prescribed concomitantly?
- Codeine and tramadol should be avoided or used cautiously in children due to variable drug metabolism and unpredictable levels of active drug (38).

Box 13.6 Important Points for Caregivers—Opioids

- May cause unwanted harm when used inappropriately or for the wrong patient.
- Commercially available "lock-boxes" (found online or in retail stores) prevent misuse and diversion.
- Prescribe naloxone to all patients on chronic opioids, patients with a history of substance misuse/overdose, or also on benzodiazepines.
- Train caregivers/family/friends on when and how to administer naloxone.

(*continued*)

Box 13.6 Important Points for Caregivers—Opioids (*continued*)

- Dispose of any unwanted or unused opioid medications safely (fire/police departments, mix medications in hot water and mix with kitty litter/coffee grounds/paper towels, place in trash)

Table 13.10 Opioid Adverse Effects (41)

Adverse effect(s)	Practical considerations
Constipation	**Tolerance does NOT develop**; prescribe bowel regimen for all patients; evidence-based treatment—senna, polyethylene glycol; refractory cases—methylnaltrexone, opioid rotation; **no data to support use of docusate**
Sedation	**Tolerance develops over time, most likely with dose or frequency changes**; therapy options—dose reduction, opioid rotation, psychostimulants (i.e., methylphenidate 5–10 mg daily); moderate exercise
Respiratory depression	Sedation prior to respiratory depression; naloxone therapy—ensure patient is not sleeping
Nausea and vomiting	**Not a drug allergy**; more common with morphine and codeine; tolerance develops within 3–7 days; therapy options—dose reduction, opioid rotation, anti-emetics
Pruritus	**Rule out other causes (e.g., renal failure, other medications, allergies)**; therapy options—topical moisturizers/steroids, oral antihistamines, antidepressants (i.e., mirtazapine), and opioid antagonists
Urinary retention	Higher incidence with epidural administration; **rule out other drug-induced causes (e.g., anticholinergic therapies [diphenhydramine, antipsychotics], SSRIs, benzodiazepines, NSAIDs, and calcium channel blockers)**
Neuroexcitation	**Myoclonus is the most described**, hyperalgesia, delirium, hallucinations, or seizures may occur; Therapy options—dose reduction, opioid rotation, opioid sparing techniques with adjuvant therapies, or low dose benzodiazepines
Other effects	Hyperalgesia, sleep disturbances, cognitive impairment, hypotension/vasodilation, QTc prolongation, increased intracranial pressure, opioid endocrinopathy, immunosuppression, hearing loss, depression

Non-Opioid (Adjuvant) Therapies (8,42,43) (Table 13.11) (Boxes 13.7 and 13.8)

- Consider for neuropathic pain, mixed types of pain, and bone pain
- Can be used with opioids for synergistic or opioid sparing effects

Interventional Therapies (48–50)

- Indications: cancer-related pain without satisfactory response to escalating doses of systemic opioids, dose limiting opioid side effects
- May be effective for months and may be repeated
- Epidural and intrathecal drug delivery: delivery of opioids through spinal infusion bypassing systemic circulation
- Nerve blocks: anesthetic block with lidocaine initially, then alcohol for lysis if initial block is successful (Table 13.12)

Symptom Directed Chemotherapy (51)

- This is also known as palliative chemotherapy.
- This is given in the noncurative setting to optimize symptom control (decrease pain, increase physical function, improve appetite, decrease dyspnea, relieve obstructive constipation), improve quality of life, and possibly improve survival.
- Basic tenets of palliative care should be followed—including shared decision making, identifying clear goals of care, and assessing risks and benefits of all therapies offered (Box 13.9).
- Examples of symptom-directed chemotherapy regimens
  - Gemcitabine—pancreatic cancer, lung cancer, ovarian cancer
  - Docetaxel—lung cancer
  - Erlotinib—lung cancer
  - Doxorubicin—breast cancer

Palliative Radiation

- Goal in adults and children—reduce symptoms and improve quality of life using shorter treatment courses with higher fractions (Table 13.13).
- Shorter duration of treatment decreases burden of therapy (travel, hospital time) on patients, families, and caregivers.
- American Society for Radiation Oncology recommends treating bony metastasis with a single fraction of radiation (52).
- Shown to be effective for dyspnea, neurologic symptoms, and bone pain in advanced cancer in children (53).

Emotional Pain

Total pain treatment involves attention to emotional, social, and spiritual aspects in addition to the physical treatment modalities. Many of the therapies listed in Table 13.14 are also used to treat physical pain in addition to having benefits for emotional distress. Emotional distress can include symptoms of anxiety, depression, insomnia, and fatigue.

Table 13.11 Adults (Adjuvant Medications for Cancer Pain) (44–47)

Medication	Typical starting dose range*	Maximum daily doses	Clinical pearls
Ketamine	PO: 10–25 mg every 6–8 hours IV: 0.5 mg/kg daily or 0.1 mg/kg bolus over 1 minute then 0.1 mg/kg/hr infusion (max 0.5 mg/kg/hr)	Not defined	**Opioid-resistant pain, neuropathic pain, hyperalgesia, allodynia, depression**; oral ketamine solution for mucositis pain; potential for neuropsychiatric, urinary tract, and hepatobiliary toxicity
Dexamethasone	PO/IV: 1–8 mg daily	As tolerated	**Inflammatory pain (i.e., spinal, central nervous system., bone metastases, capsular expansion)**; risks of side effects if >2 weeks; consider stress ulcer prophylaxis
Zoledronic acid	IV: 4 mg every 3–4 weeks	4 mg	Multiple myeloma, breast cancer with bony metastases; **adjustment for renal impairment**
Gabapentin	PO: 300 mg every evening Increase by 100–300 mg every 1–3 days Target doses of 900–3,600 mg/day	3,600 mg	Neuropathic pain (cancer, chemotherapy induced); **adverse effects (dizziness, somnolence, and peripheral edema)**; dose adjustment with renal impairment
Pregabalin	PO: 150 mg/day in 2–3 divided doses	600 mg	Neuropathic pain (cancer, chemotherapy induced); **adverse effects (dizziness, somnolence, and peripheral edema)**; dose adjustment with renal impairment

(continued)

Table 13.11 Adults (Adjuvant Medications for Cancer Pain) (44–47) *(continued)*

Medication	Typical starting dose range*	Maximum daily doses	Clinical pearls
Duloxetine	PO: 30–60 mg daily Dose titration can occur after 7 days	120 mg	**Chemotherapy induced peripheral neuropathy,** analgesic effects seen after 1 week, maximum benefit after 4 weeks; increased adverse effects evident >120 mg/day
Venlafaxine	PO: 37.5–75 mg daily (ER) Titrate by 75 mg/week	225 mg	Adverse effects—sedation, headache, dizziness, transient rises in blood pressure
Amitriptyline	PO: 25–50 mg at bedtime Increase by 10–25 mg every 3–7 days	150 mg	Severe neuropathic pain, concomitant insomnia, **avoid in older adults (anticholinergic effects, monitor for bone marrow suppression)**; caution in patients with pre-existing cardiovascular disease
Nortriptyline	PO: 10–25 mg at bedtime	100 mg	
Lidocaine	Topical: 5% patch every 12 hours on and 12 hours off IV: 0.5 mg/minute (continuous infusion)	Topical: 3 patches/single application IV: 1 mg/minute infusion	**Localized neuropathic or mixed pain;** local irritation at site of application; expensive; lidocaine infusions adjunct therapy for refractory neuropathic pain or postoperatively
Pediatrics and Infants			
Gabapentin	PO: Initially 5 mg/kg at bedtime then titrate to maintenance 5 mg/kg 3 times daily. May further titrate as needed.	35 mg/kg (Not to exceed 3,600 mg/day)	**Attempt to use twice daily dosing for school-age children;** use higher dosing at bedtime; titrate to maximum tolerated dose

(continued)

Table 13.11 Adults (Adjuvant Medications for Cancer Pain) (44–47) *(continued)*

Medication	Typical starting dose range*	Maximum daily doses	Clinical pearls
Dexamethasone	PO/IV: 0.1–0.6 mg/kg daily in the morning	As tolerated	Same as adult patients
Nortriptyline	PO: 0.2 mg/kg nightly Titrate after 3 days to 0.4 mg/kg nightly	3 mg/kg/day or 150 mg/**day**	**Increased urinary retention in children**
Amitriptyline	0.1 mg/kg/day at bedtime (max 25 mg), may titrate up to 0.5–2 mg/kg	2 mg/kg (not to exceed 150 mg)	Off-label; may trial in older children or adolescents with severe neuropathic pain
Lidocaine	>5 years old Topically: 5% patch apply 12 hours on and 12 hours off >2 years old and < 40 kg IV: 15 mcg/kg/minute (continuous infusion)	Topically: 3 patches/single application IV: 25 mcg/kg/ minute infusion	Same as adult patients

Source: From Caraceni A, Zecca E, Bonezzi C, et al. Gabapentin for neuropathic cancer pain: a randomized controlled trial from the Gabapentin Cancer Pain Study Group. *J Clin Oncol.* 2004;22(14):2909–2917. doi:10.1200/JCO.2004.08.141; Rao RD, Michalak JC, Sloan JA, et al. Efficacy of gabapentin in the management of chemotherapy-induced peripheral neuropathy: A phase 3 randomized, double-blind, placebo-controlled, crossover trial (N00C3). *Cancer.* 2007;110(9):2110–2118. doi:10.1002/cncr.23008; Mishra S, Bhatnagar S, Goyal GN, et al. A comparative efficacy of amitriptyline, gabapentin, and pregabalin in neuropathic cancer pain: a prospective randomized double-blind placebo-controlled study. *Am J Hosp Palliat Care.* 2012;29(3):177–182. doi:10.1177/1049909111412539; Mañas A, Ciria JP, Fernández MC, et al. Post hoc analysis of pregabalin treatment in patients with cancer-related neuropathic pain: Better pain relief, sleep and physical health. *Clin Transl Oncol.* 2011;13(9):656–663. doi:10.1007/s12094-011-0711-0

Box 13.7 Adjuvant Therapy Checklist

- Does the patient have other symptom clusters for which a specific adjuvant therapy would be effective in addition to pain (e.g., gabapentin for neuropathic pain as well as refractory cough)?
- What is the adverse effect profile for the particular adjuvant agent?
- Does the dose need to be adjusted for hepatic or renal impairment?
- Does the therapy require therapeutic drug monitoring?
- Have drug-drug interactions been reviewed?
- Is the therapy appropriate based on the patient's age (e.g., avoid TCAs in elderly patients [≥65 years])

Box 13.8 Important Points for Caregivers—Adjuvant Therapies:

- Often have more than one use (e.g., pain and seizure prevention)
- Many of these medications come in different dosage forms (consider if difficulty swallowing)
- Very different side effects of each of these medications
- Some of these therapies are used "off-label" to manage difficult to control pain

Table 13.12 Selected Examples of Nerve Blocks in Cancer Pain

Indications	Block
Upper abdominal visceral pain (pancreas, hepatobiliary, small intestine, stomach, spleen, ascending colon, adrenal glands)	Celiac plexus
Pelvic visceral pain (uterus, cervix, ovary, bladder, prostate, descending and sigmoid colon, testes)	Superior hypogastric plexus
Hot flashes, upper extremity pain, phantom limb pain	Stellate ganglion
Perineal pain, coccygeal pain from rectal/anal cancers	Ganglion impar

Box 13.9 Symptom Directed Chemotherapy Checklist ("Palliative Chemotherapy")

- Has an open conversation occurred between the oncologist and the patient about the primary purpose of chemotherapy?
- Does the evidence base support palliative use of the particular regimen for the proposed malignancy?
- What is the response rate of the proposed anti-cancer therapy (i.e., will the therapy meaningfully affect tumor growth)?
- If the patient has a response, how long will this be sustained (median duration of response)?
- What are the potential treatment toxicities?
- What are some logistical concerns regarding palliative chemotherapy (e.g., loss of work, clinic visits, imaging)?
- How much will this therapy cost the patient and healthcare system (quality adjusted life years [QALY])?
- How long will the patient continue this therapy(e.g.., one time dose versus monthly)?
- Which patient reported outcome measures (PROMs) will be used to assess quality of life and symptoms?

Spiritual and Existential Distress (3,25,28)

- Studies support the treatment of spiritual distress with an interdisciplinary team and incorporation of the patient as an equally important contributor to the healing process.
- Complex or unresolved distress—refer to chaplain services.
- Not complex—utilize therapeutic communication techniques, self-care, therapy, meaning making (all or any).

Table 13.13 Palliative Radiation for Cancer Pain

Indications	Important considerations
• Local symptoms (bleeding, ulceration, compression, dysphagia, obstruction, pain, dyspareunia, edema)	• What is the patient's prognosis?
• Pain from bony metastasis	• What are the risks of acute toxicity due to radiation?
• Spinal cord compression	• What are the patient's goals?
• Neurologic symptoms (headache, confusion) from brain metastasis	• Will radiation help to achieve these goals?
• Tumor causing symptomatic obstruction or invasion (e.g., superior vena cava syndrome)	• What is the patient's functional level?

Table 13.14 Selected Examples of Pharmacologic and Nonpharmacologic Therapies for Emotional Pain

Pharmacologic therapies	Nonpharmacologic therapies
Selective serotonin reuptake inhibitors (SSRIs)	Cognitive behavioral therapy
Selective norepinephrine reuptake inhibitors (SNRIs)	Relaxation therapy
Tricyclic antidepressants	Guided imagery
Atypical antidepressants (i.e., mirtazapine, buproprion, trazodone)	Stress management techniques
Benzodiazepines	Psychoeducation techniques
Psychostimulants (i.e., methylphenidate)	Meaning making
Antipsychotics (i.e., olanzapine, quetiapine)	

Complementary Therapies for Total Pain (Physical, Emotional, Social, Spiritual) (54,55)

- Acupuncture
- Music therapy
- Massage therapy
- Use of TENS unit
- Pet therapy
- Support groups
- Mindfulness meditation
- Aromatherapy
- Art therapy
- Tai Chi
- Yoga
- Physical therapy

CONCLUSION

This chapter provides an in-depth review of physical pain assessment and treatment in the context of total pain and an introduction to the psychosocial and spiritual elements. Successful management of total pain requires an interdisciplinary team to address physical pain, emotional pain, social pain, and spiritual/existential distress. These components must be treated simultaneously to prevent delays in relief.

REFERENCES

1. Van Den Beuken-Van Everdingen MHJ, Hochstenbach LMJ, Joosten EAJ, et al. Update on prevalence of pain in patients with cancer: systematic review and meta-analysis. *J Pain Symptom Manage*. 2016;51(6):1070–1090.e9. doi:10.1016/j.jpainsymman.2015.12.340

2. Zabora J, Brintzenhofeszoc K, Curbow B, et al. The prevalence of psychological distress by cancer site. *Psychooncology*. 2001;10(1):19–28. doi:10.1002/1099-1611 (200101/02)10:1<19::AID-PON501>3.0.CO;2-6

3. Handzo G, Meyerson REM. What Are Sources of Spiritual and Existential Suffering for Patients With Advanced Disease? In: Goldstein N, ed. *Evidence-Based Practice of Palliative Medicine.* Philadelphia, PA: Elsevier; 2012:480–483. doi:10.1016/B978-1-4377-3796-7.00081-1

4. Portenoy RK. Treatment of cancer pain. *Lancet (London, England).* 2011;377(9784):2236–2247. doi:10.1016/S0140-6736(11)60236-5.

5. Krajnik M, Zylicz Z (Ben). Pain Assessment, Recognising Clinical Patterns, and Cancer Pain Syndromes. In: Hanna M, Zylicz Z (Ben), eds. *Cancer Pain.* London: Springer Publishing; 2013:95–108. doi:10.1007/978-0-85729-230-8_7

6. Steinhauser KE. Are You at Peace? *Arch Intern Med.* 2006;166(1):101. doi:10.1001/archinte.166.1.101

7. Dalal S, Bruera E. Assessing cancer pain. *Curr Pain Headache Rep.* 2012;16:314–324. doi:10.1007/s11916-012-0274-y

8. Komatz K, Carter B. Pain and Symptom Management in Pediatric Palliative Care. *Pediatr Rev.* 2015;36(12):527–533; quiz 534. doi:10.1542/pir.36-12-527

9. Goldstein R, Wolfe J. Chapter 65: What Are Special Considerations for Treating Pediatric Patients and Their Families? In: Goldstein N, ed. *Evidence-Based Practice of Palliative Medicine.* Philadelphia, PA: Elsevier; 2013:377–387. doi:10.1016/B978-1-4377-3796-7.00065-3

10. Lawrence J, Alcock D, McGrath P, et al. The development of a tool to assess neonatal pain. *Neonatal Netw.* 1993;12(6):59–66. doi:10.1016/0885-3924(91)91127-U

11. Merkel SI, Voepel-Lewis T, Shayevitz JR, Malviya S. The FLACC: a behavioral scale for scoring postoperative pain in young children. *Pediatr Nurs.* 1997;23(3):293–297. http://www.ncbi.nlm.nih.gov/pubmed/9220806

12. Bernabei R, Gambassi G, Lapane K, et al. Management of Pain in Elderly Patients With Cancer. *Jama J Am Med Assoc.* 1998;279(23):1877–1882. doi:10.1001/jama.279.23.1877

13. Herr K, Bjoro K, Decker S. Tools for assessment of pain in nonverbal older adults with dementia: a state-of-the-science review. *J Pain Symptom Manage.* 2006;31(2):170–192. doi:10.1016/j.jpainsymman.2005.07.001

14. Bruera E, Kuehn N, Miller MJ, et al. The Edmonton Symptom Assessment System (ESAS): a simple method for the assessment of palliative care patients. *J Palliat Care.* 1991;7(2):6–9. http://www.ncbi.nlm.nih.gov/pubmed/1714502

15. Portenoy RK, Thaler HT, Kornblith AB, et al. The Memorial Symptom Assessment Scale: an instrument for the evaluation of symptom prevalence, characteristics and distress. *Eur J Cancer.* 1994;30A(9):1326–1336. doi:10.1016/0959-8049(94)90182-1

16. Perrin JM, Gnanasekaran S, Delahaye J. Psychological Aspects of Chronic Health Conditions. *Pediatr Rev.* 2012;33(3):99–109. doi:10.1542/pir.33-3-99

17. Weaver MS, Heinze KE, Bell CJ, et al. Establishing psychosocial palliative care standards for children and adolescents with cancer and their families: An integrative review. *Palliat Med.* 2016;30(3):212–223. doi:10.1177/0269216315583446

18. Meeker MA, Finnell D, Othman AK. Family caregivers and cancer pain management: a review. *J Fam Nurs.* 2011;17(1):29–60. doi:10.1177/1074840710396091

19. Gröpper S, van der Meer E, Landes T, et al. Assessing cancer-related distress in cancer patients and caregivers receiving outpatient psycho-oncological counseling. *Support Care Cancer.* 2015;24:2351–2357. doi:10.1007/s00520-015-3042-9

20. Ferrell BR, Grant M, Chan J, Ahn C, Ferrell BA. The impact of cancer pain education on family caregivers of elderly patients. *Oncol Nurs Forum.* 1995;22(8):1211–1218. http://www.ncbi.nlm.nih.gov/pubmed/8532545

21. Waldrop D, Kutner JS. What Is the Effect of Serious Illness on Caregivers? In: Goldstein NE, Morrison RS, eds. *Evidence-Based Practice of Palliative Medicine.* Philadelphia, PA: Elsevier; 2012:421–428. doi:10.1016/B978-1-4377-3796-7.00072-0

22. Ewing JA. Detecting alcoholism: The cage questionnaire. *JAMA.* 1984;252(14):1905–1907. doi:10.1001/jama.1984.03350140051025

23. Webster LR, Webster RM. Predicting Aberrant Behaviors in Opioid-Treated Patients: Preliminary Validation of the Opioid Risk Tool. *Pain Med.* 2005;6(6):432–442. doi:10.1111/j.1526-4637.2005.00072.x

24. Jackson LK, Imam SN, Braun UK. Opioids in Cancer Pain: Right or Privilege? *J Oncol Pract.* 2017;13(9):e809–e814. doi:10.1200/JOP.2016.019216

25. Wachholtz AB, Fitch CE, Makowski S, Tjia J. A Comprehensive Approach to the Patient at End of Life: Assessment of Multidimensional Suffering. *South Med J.* 2016;109(4):200–206. doi:10.14423/SMJ.0000000000000439

26. Lee Y-P, Wu C-H, Chiu T-Y, et al. The relationship between pain management and psychospiritual distress in patients with advanced cancer following admission to a palliative care unit. *BMC Palliat Care.* 2015;14:69. doi:10.1186/s12904-015-0067-2

27. Puchalski C, Ferrell B, Virani R, et al. Improving the quality of spiritual care as a dimension of palliative care: the report of the consensus conference. *J Palliat Med.* 2009;12(10):885–904. doi:10.1089/jpm.2009.0142

28. Borneman T, Ferrell B, Puchalski CM. Evaluation of the FICA Tool for Spiritual Assessment. *J Pain Symptom Manage.* 2010;40(2):163–173. doi:10.1016/j.jpainsymman.2009.12.019

29. Harirforoosh S, Asghar W, Jamali F. Adverse effects of nonsteroidal antiinflammatory drugs: an update of gastrointestinal, cardiovascular and renal complications. *J Pharm Pharm Sci.* 2013;16(5):821–847. http://www.ncbi.nlm.nih.gov/pubmed/24393558

30. Derry S, Wiffen PJ, Moore RA, et al. Oral nonsteroidal anti-inflammatory drugs (NSAIDs) for cancer pain in adults. *Cochrane Database Syst Rev.* 2017;7(7):12. doi:10.1002/14651858.CD012638.pub2

31. Angiolillo DJ, Weisman SM. Clinical Pharmacology and Cardiovascular Safety of Naproxen. *Am J Cardiovasc Drugs.* 2017;17(2):97–107. doi:10.1007/s40256-016-0200-5

32. Joishy SK, Walsh D. The opioid-sparing effects of intravenous ketorolac as an adjuvant analgesic in cancer pain: application in bone metastases and the opioid bowel syndrome. *J Pain Symptom Manage.* 1998;16(5):334–339. doi:10.1016/S0885-3924(98)00081-5

33. Bjorkman R, Ullman A, Hedner J. Morphine-sparing effect of diclofenac in cancer pain. *Eur J Clin Pharmacol.* 1993;44(1):1–5. doi:10.1007/BF00315271

34. Laine L, Curtis SP, Cryer B, et al. Risk factors for NSAID-associated upper GI clinical events in a long-term prospective study of 34 701 arthritis patients. *Aliment Pharmacol Ther.* 2010;32(10):1240–1248. doi:10.1111/j.1365-2036.2010.04465.x.

35. Israel FJ, Parker G, Charles M, Reymond L. Lack of Benefit From Paracetamol (Acetaminophen) for Palliative Cancer Patients Requiring High-Dose Strong Opioids: A Randomized, Double-Blind, Placebo-Controlled, Crossover Trial. *J Pain Symptom Manage.* 2010;39(3):548–554. doi:10.1016/j.jpainsymman.2009.07.008

36. Lewis JH, Stine JG. Review article: Prescribing medications in patients with cirrhosis - A practical guide. *Aliment Pharmacol Ther.* 2013;37(12):1132–1156. doi:10.1111/apt.12324

37. Jibril F, Sharaby S, Mohamed A, Wilby KJ. Intravenous versus Oral Acetaminophen for Pain: Systematic Review of Current Evidence to Support Clinical Decision-Making. *Can J Hosp Pharm.* 2015;68(3):238–247. doi:10.4212/cjhp.v68i3.1458. http://www.ncbi.nlm.nih.gov/pubmed/26157186

38. Wiffen PJ, Cooper TE, Anderson A-K, et al. Opioids for cancer-related pain in children and adolescents. In: Cooper TE, ed. *Cochrane Database of Systematic Reviews.* Vol 7. Chichester, UK: John Wiley & Sons, Ltd; 2017. doi:10.1002/14651858.CD012564

39. Boland JW, Pockley AG. Influence of opioids on immune function in patients with cancer pain: From bench to bedside. *Br J Pharmacol.* 2017;175:2726–2736. Epub ahead of print. doi:10.1111/bph.13903

40. Wiffen PJ, Wee B, Derry S, Bell RF, Moore RA. Opioids for cancer pain - an overview of Cochrane reviews. *Cochrane Database Syst Rev.* 2017;2017(7). doi:10.1002/14651858.CD012592.pub2

41. Benyamin R, Trescot A, Datta S, et al. Opioid complications and side effects. *Pain Physician.* 2008;11:S105–S120.

42. Lussier D, Huskey AG, Portenoy RK. Adjuvant analgesics in cancer pain management. *Oncologist.* 2004;9(5):571–591. doi:10.1634/theoncologist.9-5-571

43. Kane CM, Mulvey MR, Wright S, et al. Opioids combined with antidepressants or antiepileptic drugs for cancer pain: Systematic review and meta-analysis. *Palliat Med.* 2017;32:276–286. doi:10.1177/0269216317711826

44. Caraceni A, Zecca E, Bonezzi C, et al. Gabapentin for neuropathic cancer pain: a randomized controlled trial from the Gabapentin Cancer Pain Study Group. *J Clin Oncol.* 2004;22(14):2909–2917. doi:10.1200/JCO.2004.08.141

45. Rao RD, Michalak JC, Sloan JA, et al. Efficacy of gabapentin in the management of chemotherapy-induced peripheral neuropathy: A phase 3 randomized, double-blind, placebo-controlled, crossover trial (N00C3). *Cancer*. 2007;110(9):2110–2118. doi:10.1002/cncr.23008

46. Mishra S, Bhatnagar S, Goyal GN, et al. A comparative efficacy of amitriptyline, gabapentin, and pregabalin in neuropathic cancer pain: a prospective randomized double-blind placebo-controlled study. *Am J Hosp Palliat Care*. 2012;29(3):177–182. doi:10.1177/1049909111412539

47. Mañas A, Ciria JP, Fernández MC, et al. Post hoc analysis of pregabalin vs. non-pregabalin treatment in patients with cancer-related neuropathic pain: Better pain relief, sleep and physical health. *Clin Transl Oncol*. 2011;13(9):656–663. doi:10.1007/s12094-011-0711-0

48. Sindt JE, Brogan SE. Interventional Treatments of Cancer Pain. *Anesthesiol Clin*. 2016;34(2):317–339. doi:10.1016/j.anclin.2016.01.004

49. Bobb B, Smith TJ. When should epidural or intrathecal opioid infusions and pumps be considered for pain management? In: Goldstein N, ed. *Evidence-Based Practice in Palliative Medicine*. Philadelphia, PA: Elsevier; 2012:93–98.

50. Aslakson R, Brookman J, Smith TJ. When should nerve blocks be used for pain management? In: Goldstein N, ed. *Evidence-Based Practice in Palliative Medicine*. Philadelphia, PA: Elsevier; 2012:99–102.

51. Roeland EJ, LeBlanc TW. Palliative chemotherapy: oxymoron or misunderstanding? *BMC Palliat Care*. 2016;15(1):33. doi:10.1186/s12904-016-0109-4

52. Lutz S, Berk L, Chang E, et al. Palliative radiotherapy for bone metastases: an ASTRO evidence-based guideline. *Int J Radiat Oncol Biol Phys*. 2011;79(4):965–976. doi:10.1016/j.ijrobp.2010.11.026

53. Varma S, Friedman DL, Stavas MJ. The role of radiation therapy in palliative care of children with advanced cancer: Clinical outcomes and patterns of care. *Pediatr Blood Cancer*. 2017;64(5):e26359. doi:10.1002/pbc.26359

54. Eaton LH, Brant JM, Mcleod K, Yeh C. Nonpharmacologic pain interventions: a review of evidence-based practices for reducing chronic cancer pain. 2017;21:54–79. doi:10.1188/17.CJON.S3.54-70

55. Running A, Seright T. Integrative oncology: Managing cancer pain with complementary and alternative therapies. *Curr Pain Headache Rep*. 2012;16(4):325–331. doi:10.1007/s11916-012-0275-x

Drug-Related Endocrine System Disruption and Management in Palliative Cancer Care

14

Ashley Anderson and Jaydira Del Rivero

INTRODUCTION

Pain is considered a major public health topic estimated to cost society more than $500 billion annually, and as many as 39 million people in the United States have persistent pain (1). The National Institute of Health (NIH) reported that approximately 200 million prescriptions for opioids were distributed in 2013. Prescriptions for opioids have increased by over 50% in the last 10 years. Nearly all patients requiring chronic opioid therapy develop side effects, most commonly affecting the central nervous and gastrointestinal systems (2,3).

Moreover, long-term opioid use has a negative impact on the endocrine system leading to a decrease in the maintenance of homeostasis for the secretion of hormones in the body. When focusing on patients with existing endocrine disorders, long-term opioid use could exacerbate their already present problems and conditions. Common conditions that are associated with long-term opioid use in the endocrine system are opioid-induced androgen deficiency (OPIAD) and opioid-induced endocrinopathy (OIE). In this chapter, we describe the effects of opioids on the endocrine system during palliative cancer care.

OPIAD AND OIE

Opioids have been used as medicines and analgesics for both oncological and palliative purposes for many years. However, their effects on the endocrine system have not been widely discussed or researched in the medical field. Systematic studies have provided new and needed knowledge regarding the effects of opioids on the endocrine system. Despite such findings, signs of opioid endocrinopathy are often unreported, not monitored clinically, and thus are undermanaged. As a result, long-acting opioids use for the treatment of chronic pain can result in OPIAD or OIE, which in turn contribute to infertility, decreased libido, and sexual functioning, and can also be associated with osteopenia and osteoporosis. Specific evidence for these effects are noted in brief in the following text.

Results Reported in Studies

- A case-control study conducted by Rajagopal and colleagues compared sexual desire, anxiety, depression, fatigue, and general functioning in 20 male cancer survivors, who were prescribed opioids chronically, with 20 matched controls. The opioid group had significantly greater depression, fatigue, and sexual dysfunction (4). These findings indicate the need to monitor mood, sexual and general functioning of cancer survivors being treated in an ongoing manner with opioids.

- In another study by Abs and colleagues (5), libdo and impotency and a series of endocrine test levels (including serum testosterone, serum luteinizing hormone [LH] levels, free androgen, serum follicle-stimulating hormone [FSH], peak cortisol) were compared in 73 patients (29 men and 44 women; mean age, 49.2 +/− 11.7 yr) receiving opioids intrathecally for nonmalignant pain with a control group of 20 patients with chronic pain but who were not receiving opioid treatment. Libido, serum testosterone, free androgen, serum LH, and peak cortisol were significantly lower in the group receiving opioids than in the control group. Findings support the need to monitor all patients receiving intrathecal opioids.

Opioid Dose Effects and Monitoring Needs

There are limited data regarding the negative effects of long-term use of opioids and of opioid dosages on the endocrine system, but there is evidence of hypogonadal suppression when opioid dosages range from 100 to 200 mg of oral morphine equivalents daily; however, lower doses may create the same effects.

- It is important to understand the physiologic impact of chronic opioid administration and monitor patients accordingly. If symptoms of endocrine dysfunction are recognized during chronic opioid therapy, appropriate evaluation, treatment, and follow-up should be instituted (6).
- The possibility that opioids could be adding to the symptom burden by inducing hypogonadism makes it a relevant clinical issue (7).
- The problem of hypogonadism may be less relevant for patients in active cancer treatment or in the advanced stage of disease (8).

Pathophysiology and the Effects of Opioids on the Hypothalamic-Pituitary-Gonadal Axis

The *hypothalamic-pituitary-gonadal axis* controls the production and excretion of sex hormones in both males and females.

- The primary sex hormones are testosterone and estrogen, which are controlled by the secretion of GnRH from the hypothalamus.

GnRH stimulates the pituitary gland allowing for the release of LH and FSH, which then stimulate the gonads (testes and ovaries) to secrete the primary growth hormones testosterone and estrogen. These are vital for normal sexual, reproductive behavior in males and females.

- The hypothalamic-pituitary-gonadal axis can also be affected by external influences.
  - Opioids have been recognized to have an influence on this system.
    - *Long-term* use of opioids, whether for medicinal or other purposes, can risk analgesic or addiction effects.

○ Patients taking opioids for *short-term* treatment are not at the same level of risk as patients on long-term treatment for OPIAD. "Evidence suggests that opioids, both endogenous and exogenous, can bind to opioid receptors primarily in the hypothalamus, but potentially also in the pituitary and the testis, to modulate gonadal function" (9).

Opioids may decrease the release of GnRH and subsequently LH and FSH, and thereby decrease the available levels of testosterone and estrogen. A decrease in primary hormone levels leads to hypogonadism. Patients treated with opioids for 1 or more months can have abnormally low dehydroepiandrosterone sulphate (DHEAS) levels. DHEAS is secreted by the adrenal glands and aids in the production of certain hormones such as testosterone and estrogen (10,11). All patients receiving long-term opioid treatment should be monitored for hypogonadism and the DHEAS laboratory test in combination with a clinical interview with a focus on relevant symptoms can help to confirm this condition.

Symptoms of Hypogonadism in Males and Females

The symptoms that can be anticipated and monitored:

- Loss of libido
- Infertility
- Erectile dysfunction
- Depression
- Anxiety
- Decreased muscle mass and strength
- Weight gain
- Fatigue or tiredness
- Amenorrhea
- Irregular menses
- Galactorrhea
- Hot flashes/ night sweats
- Osteoporosis
- Anemia
- Cortisol deficiency

Hypogonadism—A Side Effect of Chemotherapy in Cancer Patients

- According to McWilliams et al., for many patients who are on long-term opioid protocols and are also undergoing chemotherapy, there may be a multifactorial etiology (7).
- Chemotherapy is known to be toxic to the testes and ovaries in patients and can cause hypogonadism.
- In conjunction with the long-term use of opioids it is hard to determine what in fact is causing the hypogonadism is those patients when reviewing systematic studies of OPIAD and OIE.

Severity and Onset of Symptoms of OPIAD and OIE in Patients

- Choice of opioids and dosage can impact severity and onset of symptoms.
- OPIAD and OIE symptoms may exacerbate pain in patients.
  - Pain management is necessary for quality of life.
  - Nonopioid pain management options should be considered based on severity.
    - Physical exercise
    - Cognitive therapies
    - Physiotherapy
    - Adjuvant drugs (e.g., antidepressants or anticonvulsants)
    - Invasive techniques (such as kyphoplasty or nerve blocks)
  - Chronic opioid treatment with well-defined goals should be considered when nonopioid pain management options have failed (12).

In palliative or end-of-life care, however, taking away overall pain despite the negative symptoms may be the preferred choice due to the patients' (and their families') desire to be pain free during their last days. Patients who are receiving hospice or end-of-life care and their families should be educated on the potential side effects of chronic opioid use and as well as on the positive effects of opioids. "In contrast, in patients in the final stages of cancer, the most important aim of palliative and supportive care is to maintain as long as possible the best possible mobility and overall quality of life" (8).

Laboratory Evaluation

The Endocrine Society Guidelines recommend measuring testosterone levels in patients requiring long-term opioid therapy based on several studies that have reported androgen deficiency in males with cancer treated with opioids (13–15).

- *Screening* for gonadal dysfunction should be considered in all male patients with symptoms of:
  - Fatigue
  - Depressed mood
  - Poor appetite
  - Insomnia
  - Anxiety
  - Decreased libido
- Differences in laboratory assays; diurnal (16), genetic (17), and age variation (18); and the effect of inflammation on total testosterone can make laboratory evaluation for hypogonadism in cancer patients challenging.
- *Laboratory assessment* can be complex and may include total testosterone, free testosterone, LH, FSH,), sex hormone binding globulin (SHBG), DHEAS, and estradiol. It may also require specific evaluation of the pituitary-adrenal function (9).

The levels should be measured early in the morning since testosterone reaches a maximum level at 8 a.m. and the level decreases by 70% at 8 p.m. (19). The measurement should be repeated in the morning to confirm testosterone deficiency (20). Because of cost or availability constraints, total testosterone level may be the most practical way to screen cancer patients with symptoms of hypogonadism; however, free testosterone or bioavailable testosterone levels should be measured when low normal total testosterone levels are found on initial testing. Consultation with an endocrinologist may be necessary to confirm the diagnosis.

The endocrine system in women can also be affected by opioids associated with hypopituitarism and secondary hypogonadism and, hence, low levels of total testosterone, free testosterone, androstenedione, DHEAS levels (21,22). While women receiving chronic opioids may also develop similar symptoms related to testosterone deficiency, there are no guidelines for the assessment and treatment of opioid-related androgen deficiency in women (23).

Management Options

- Low testosterone levels in chronic pain patients can be managed with testosterone replacement to counteract the negative side effects of long-term opioid therapy.
  - Libido, mood, muscle mass, and erectile dysfunction can be improved with hormone therapy.
  - Low testosterone can be supplemented by various routes: oral and buccal tablets, subcutaneous pellets, transdermal patches and gels, and intramuscular injections (20).
    - The oral formulation may cause liver toxicity and is best avoided (24), and buccal tablets can cause changes in taste (25).
    - Testosterone intramuscular injections are inexpensive and safe. It is injected every 2 weeks resulting in rapid rise to supraphysiological levels of testosterone in 48 hr with a gradual decline (26).
    - Testosterone patches and gels have the advantage of achieving stable serum concentrations of testosterone and are easy to administer.
    - Patients using gels must wash their hands well after use, since there is a risk of transferring the hormone to children or females (27).

Risks associated with testosterone replacement therapy for both men and women for treatment of opioid-related endocrinopathy need to be communicated to patients and closely monitored:

- Sleep disordered breathing
- Lipid abnormalities
- Hypercalcemia
- Polycythemia

The Endocrine Society guidelines recommend against testosterone replacement in patients with breast or prostate cancer. Other contraindications include hematocrit greater than 50%, untreated severe obstructive sleep apnea, uncontrolled heart failure, an acute coronary event in the previous 6 months, and severe lower urinary tract symptoms. Because of the litany of potential side effects from hormonal supplementation, clinicians should monitor the outcomes of treatment over time (20,28).

CONCLUSION

OPIAD and OIE are poorly understood and are often overlooked by clinicians. Moreover, recognizing endocrine dysfunction in men and women can be a diagnostic challenge. Clinicians should be aware that chronic use of opioids can lead to hypogonadism causing significant morbidity. Hypogonadism is common in patients with cancer but most of the symptoms of this condition are treatable. Testosterone replacement can improve the signs and symptoms related to androgen deficiency such as erectile and sexual dysfunction, decreased libido, mood disturbances, hot flashes, and irregular menses and can improve muscle strength, bone health, and quality of life. However, more formal recommendations and guidelines by a dedicated pain management and endocrine task force are warranted to better optimize clinical outcomes and safety.

REFERENCES

1. Kennedy J, Roll JM, Schraudner T, et al. Prevalence of persistent pain in the U.S. adult population: new data from the 2010 national health interview survey. *J Pain*. 2014;15(10):979–984. doi:10.1016/j.jpain.2014.05.009
2. Bawor M, Dennis BB, Samaan MC, et al. Methadone induces testosterone suppression in patients with opioid addiction. *Sci Rep*. 2014;4:6189. doi:10.1038/srep06189
3. Kumar L, Barker C, Emmanuel A. Opioid-induced constipation: pathophysiology, clinical consequences, and management. *Gastroenterol Res Pract*. 2014;2014:1–6. doi:10.1155/2014/141737
4. Rajagopal A, Vassilopoulou-Sellin R, Palmer JL, et al. Symptomatic hypogonadism in male survivors of cancer with chronic exposure to opioids. *Cancer*. 2004;100(4):851–858. doi:10.1002/cncr.20028
5. Abs R, Verhelst J, Maeyaert J, et al. Endocrine consequences of long-term intrathecal administration of opioids. *J Clin Endocrinol Metab*. 2000;85(6):2215–2222. doi:10.1210/jcem.85.6.6615
6. Elliott JA, Horton E, Fibuch EE. The endocrine effects of long-term oral opioid therapy: a case report and review of the literature. *J Opioid Manag*. 2011;7(2):145–154. doi:10.5055/jom.2011.0057
7. McWilliams K, Simmons C, Laird BJ, Fallon MT. A systematic review of opioid effects on the hypogonadal axis of cancer patients. *Support Care Cancer*. 2014;22(6):1699–1704. doi:10.1007/s00520-014-2195-2
8. Buss T, Leppert W. Opioid-induced endocrinopathy in cancer patients: an underestimated clinical problem. *Adv Ther*. 2014;31(2):153–167. doi:10.1007/s12325-014-0096-x
9. Katz N, Mazer NA. The impact of opioids on the endocrine system. *Clin J Pain*. 2009;25(2):170–175. doi:10.1097/AJP.0b013e3181850df6
10. Colameco S, Coren JS, Ciervo CA. Continuous opioid treatment for chronic noncancer pain: a time for moderation in prescribing. *Postgrad Med*. 2009;121(4):61–66. doi:10.3810/pgm.2009.07.2032
11. Colameco S, Coren JS. Opioid-induced endocrinopathy. *J Am Osteopath Assoc*. 2009;109(1):20–25. doi: 10.7556/jaoa.2009.109.1.20
12. Carmona-Bayonas A, Jiménez-Fonseca P, Castañón E, et al. Chronic opioid therapy in long-term cancer survivors. *Clin Transl Oncol*. 2017;19(2):236–250. doi:10.1007/s12094-016-1529-6

13. Rajagopal A, Vassilopoulou-Sellin R, Palmer JL, et al. Hypogonadism and sexual dysfunction in male cancer survivors receiving chronic opioid therapy. *J Pain Symptom Manage.* 2003;26(5):1055–1061. doi:10.1016/S0885-3924(03)00331-2

14. Araujo AB, Esche GR, Kupelian V, et al. Prevalence of symptomatic androgen deficiency in men. *J Clin Endocrinol Metab.* 2007;92(11):4241–4247. doi:10.1210/jc.2007-1245

15. Skipworth RJ, Moses AGW, Sangster K, et al. Interaction of gonadal status with systemic inflammation and opioid use in determining nutritional status and prognosis in advanced pancreatic cancer. *Support Care Cancer.* 2011;19(3):391–401. doi:10.1007/s00520-010-0832-y

16. Panizzon MS, Hauger R, Jacobson KC, et al. Genetic and environmental influences of daily and intra-individual variation in testosterone levels in middle-aged men. *Psychoneuroendocrinology.* 2013;38(10):2163–2172. doi:10.1016/j.psyneuen.2013.04.003

17. Travison TG, Zhuang WV, Lunetta KL, et al. The heritability of circulating testosterone, oestradiol, oestrone and sex hormone binding globulin concentrations in men: the Framingham Heart Study. *Clin Endocrinol (Oxf).* 2014;80(2):277–282. doi:10.1111/cen.12260

18. Brambilla DJ, Matsumoto AM, Araujo AB, McKinlay JB. The effect of diurnal variation on clinical measurement of serum testosterone and other sex hormone levels in men. *J Clin Endocrinol Metab.* 2009;94(3):907–913. doi:10.1210/jc.2008-1902

19. Bremner WJ, Vitiello MV, Prinz PN. Loss of circadian rhythmicity in blood testosterone levels with aging in normal men. *J Clin Endocrinol Metab.* 1983;56(6):1278–1281. doi:10.1210/jcem-56-6-1278

20. Bhasin S, Cunningham GR, Hayes FJ, et al. Testosterone therapy in men with androgen deficiency syndromes: an Endocrine Society clinical practice guideline. *J Clin Endocrinol Metab.* 2010;95(6):2536–2559. doi:10.1210/jc.2009-2354

21. Miller KK. Androgen deficiency in women. *J Clin Endocrinol Metab.* 2001;86(6):2395–2401. doi:10.1210/jc.86.6.2395

22. Miller KK, Sesmilo G,Schiller A, et al. Androgen deficiency in women with hypopituitarism. *J Clin Endocrinol Metab.* 2001;86(2):561–567. doi:10.1210/jc.86.2.561

23. Daniell HW. Opioid endocrinopathy in women consuming prescribed sustained-action opioids for control of nonmalignant pain. *J Pain.* 2008;9(1):28–36. doi:10.1016/j.jpain.2007.08.005

24. Westaby D, Paradinas FJ, Ogle SJ, et al. Liver damage from long-term methyltestosterone. *Lancet.* 1977;2(8032):262–263. doi:10.1016/S0140-6736(77)90949-7

25. Dinsmore WW, Wyllie MG. The long-term efficacy and safety of a testosterone mucoadhesive buccal tablet in testosterone-deficient men. *BJU Int.* 2012;110(2):162–169. doi:10.1111/j.1464-410X.2011.10837.x

26. Giagulli VA, Triggiani V, Corona G, et al. Evidence-based medicine update on testosterone replacement therapy (TRT) in male hypogonadism: focus on new formulations. *Curr Pharm Des.* 2011;17(15):1500–1511. doi:10.2174/138161211796197160

27. Dobs AS, Meikle W, Arver S, et al. Pharmacokinetics, efficacy, and safety of a permeation-enhanced testosterone transdermal system in comparison with bi-weekly injections of testosterone enanthate for the treatment of hypogonadal men. *J Clin Endocrinol Metab.* 1999;84(10):3469–3478. doi:10.1210/jc.84.10.3469

28. Gudin JA, Laitman A, Nalamachu S. Opioid Related Endocrinopathy. *Pain Med.* 2015;16 Suppl 1:S9–S15. doi:10.1111/pme.12926

Psychosocial and Spiritual Distress in the Advanced Adult and Pediatric Cancer Patient

15

Laura Hofmann, Rita A. Manfredi, Robert M. Kaiser, Najmeh Jafari, and Christina M. Puchalski

INTRODUCTION

Nonphysical causes of suffering, which are less frequently studied than physical causes, may go unnoticed and contribute greatly to the distress of the patient (1). Illness is a complex interplay of biology, cognition, behavioral and emotional responses, social factors, and the patient's religiosity and/or spirituality (2). Spirituality plays an important role in patients' lives and has been incorporated into the traditional biopsychosocial model, currently known as the "biopsychosocial spiritual" model. To highlight this, the 2009 National Consensus Conference for Spiritual Care in Palliative Care describes the following three tenets to address suffering and distress: (a) address all aspects of the patient's and family's suffering; (b) discover what the patient may need spiritually; and (3) respect the struggles and beliefs of the patient and family (3).

DEFINITIONS

- **Spirituality** is a "dynamic and intrinsic aspect of humanity through which persons seek ultimate meaning, purpose, and transcendence, and experience relationship to self, family, others, community, society, nature, and the significant or sacred. Spirituality is expressed through beliefs, values, traditions, and practices" (4).
- **Religiosity** and spirituality, though often considered synonymous, have important distinctions that may need to be addressed separately when caring for a patient (5).
- **Religion** is an organized belief system that offers an approach for thinking about life, death, suffering, and universal questions by using texts, rituals, and practices shared by a community (6).
- Psychosocial distress is discomfort related to a patient's cognition, behavior, emotions, and social interactions and includes unhealthy thought patterns, emotional dysregulation, diagnosable psychiatric conditions (e.g., depression, suicidality), interpersonal conflict, and social upheaval.
- **Spiritual distress** is difficulty in finding purpose, meaning, or connection with others, God, or another transcendent belief (Table 15.1).
- **Religious struggle** includes envisioning God as a punishing entity, ascribing a demonic cause to illness, questioning God's powers, and feeling religious discontent (7,8).

195

Table 15.1 Presentations of Spiritual Distress

Lack of meaning and purpose	Fear
Despair	Concerns one won't be remembered
Hopelessness	Anger at God/others
Guilt/shame	Feeling out of control
Sense of abandonment by God/others	Problems with trust
Existential suffering	Grief/loss
Concerns about reconciliation	Lack of love or connection to God/others
Loneliness	

Many clinicians acknowledge that patients with robust psychological and emotional health, social support, and spiritual or religious beliefs who are undergoing a complicated treatment regimen tend to cope better. Patients with psychosocial difficulties have more problems during treatment. Similarly, spiritual support and distress have effects on treatment outcomes (Table 15.2).

PREVALENCE OF DISTRESS

* Psychosocial distress and spiritual distress are common. In a recent systematic review study, the point prevalence of spiritual distress within

Table 15.2 Spiritual Support and Spiritual Distress

Support	Distress
Spiritual support in advanced cancer correlates with improved quality of life (9,10).	Spiritual distress is significantly associated with poor emotional well-being, general distress, and depression (10).
Majority of advanced cancer patients report their religious/spiritual needs were largely unmet by their care team; 60% report adequate support from their religious community (9).	Spiritual distress is associated with worse physical pain, depression, anxiety, well-being, and financial distress (FD) (11).
Highly religious patients pursue more aggressive treatments at end-of-life; this risk decreases five-fold when spiritual support is provided by non-pastoral members of the medical team resulting in greater acceptance of hospice (12).	Negative spiritual/religious coping was associated with an increased risk for suicidal ideation (13).

an inpatient setting ranged from 16% to 63%, and 96% of patients had experienced spiritual pain at some point in their lives(14). In a study of 113 cancer patients in an acute palliative care unit, 44% of them reported spiritual distress during the initial chaplain visit, and patients with spiritual distress were more likely to be younger, to have pain, and to have depression (15). In a study from Israel, 23% of cancer patients in an outpatient setting reported spiritual distress, and the main parameters for spiritual distress included "not feeling peaceful," "feeling unable to accept that this is happening," and "perceived severity of one's illness (16)." In a sample of 300 adult cancer patients in India, 76.3% of the participants found their illness unfair, and 83.3% kept wondering why the illness had happened to them (17). Evidence shows that 73% of cancer patients express at least one spiritual need, and up to 44% of cancer patients in palliative care report a significant level of spiritual distress (18).

- Distress may vary with the time-point in the illness trajectory, the location of care, and with the underlying cancer type (Table 15.3) (8,19–23).
- Psychosocial distress may vary in different patient populations. For example, a literature review on health-related quality of life of Black survivors of breast cancer less than 55 years old, found that these women had a greater fear of dying, unmet supportive care needs, financial distress, and lower physical/functional and well-being (24).
- In outpatient congestive heart failure (CHF) patients with diabetes and inpatient oncology patients, younger age and less attendance at religious worship services were associated with higher negative religious coping (8).

Table 15.3 Rates of Distress in Different Patient Populations	
Population	**Rate**
Psychosocial distress	
Oncology patients undergoing treatment	24.5%
Oncology patients receiving some form of palliative care	59.3%
Cancer survivors in the general community	16.5%
Oncology patients in an outpatient clinic	41.6%
Oncology patients on inpatient oncology unit	63.5%
Patients with all types of cancer	35.1%
Patients with lung cancer	43.3%
Patients with gynecologic cancer	29.6%
Spiritual distress	
Advanced cancer patients with spiritual pain	44%
Outpatient diabetic, CHF, and inpatient oncology patients with any religious struggle (of note, CHF rates were greatest, followed by oncology and then diabetic rates)	48%

(continued)

Table 15.3 Rates of Distress in Different Patient Populations (*continued*)

Population	Rate
Outpatient diabetic, CHF, and inpatient oncology patients with moderate to high negative religious struggle	15%

Source: From Fitchett G, Murphy PE, Kim J. Religious struggle: prevalence, correlates and mental health risks in diabetic, congestive heart failure, and oncology patients. *Int J Psychiatry Med.* 2004;34(2):179–196; Gao W, Bennett MI, Stark D, et al. Psychological distress in cancer from survivorship to end of life care: Prevalance, associated factors and clinical implications. *Eur J Cancer.* 2010;46(11):2036–2044; Delgado-Guay MO, Hui D, Parsons HA, et al. Spirituality, religiosity, and spiritual pain in advanced cancer patients. *J Pain Symptom Manage.* 2011;41(6):986–994; Bauwens S, Baillon C, Distelmans W, Theuns P. Sytematic screening for distress in oncology practice using the Distress Barometer: the impact on referrals to psychosocial care. *Psychooncology.* 2014;23(7):804–811; Clark PG, Rochon E, Brethwaite D, Edmiston KK. Screening for psychological and physical distress in a cancer inpatient treatment setting: a pilot study. *Psychooncology.* 2011;20(6):664–668; Zabora J, Brintzenhofeszoc K, Curbow B, et al. The prevalence of psychological distress by cancer site. *Psycho-Oncology.* 2001;10(1):19–28.

MAKING THE CASE FOR ADDRESSING SPIRITUALITY IN CLINICAL CARE

- The psychological and spiritual impact of illness is influenced by the patient's resources and his or her relationship with the healthcare team. It is also affected by the degree of disability, severity of symptoms, intensity of treatment, and the adverse side effects of treatment. Symptom burden, treatment side effects, and disability related to cancer may cause significant psychosocial and spiritual distress (25). Financial stability may be jeopardized, and roles in relationships may change drastically. Prior sources of fulfillment, such as work, may be beyond an oncology patient's abilities. Patients may begin to question purpose and meaning.

- Confronting mortality may raise troubling questions about what happens after death, how a deity could allow death and suffering, and if the patient has made a mark in life and will be missed (25).

- Distress rates may be highest in lung cancer due to the possible association of lung cancer and personal behavior (i.e., history of smoking). This could lead to a sense of personal responsibility for the effect of the disease on oneself and one's family and impact the way people accept their illness (23).

- Cancers of the brain and pancreas, which have had a poor prognosis despite treatment, correlate with relatively high patient distress including psychosocial and spiritual distress (23).

- The meaning of life may change as people encounter illness, either in themselves, their loved ones, or their patients, or face the prospect of dying. Exploring deep questions about meaning and purpose can profoundly affect patients and can be transforming in a positive way (toward spiritual growth). Patients may also not be able to move through the suffering and questioning, which could lead to spiritual distress (26). Some people find meaning in suffering in terms of self-improvement or a trigger for enlightenment. In a study in Australia, cancer patients defined their illness as a "spiritual journey" that had direct positive consequences on their personal development and the meaning they are making out of life (27). In another study in Iran, Muslim cancer patients described suffering as delightful pain that turned toward a feeling of rebirth and spiritual growth (28).

- Therefore, in addressing spiritual issues with patients, it is also important to look for signs of spiritual well-being, which can be defined as the ability to experience and integrate meaning and purpose in life through connectedness with self, others, art, music, literature, nature, and/or a power greater than oneself that can be strengthened (29).

- Spiritual well-being can occur through a dynamic and interactive growth process that leads to a realization of the ultimate purpose and meaning of life (30).

CLINICAL CHARACTERISTICS

- The presenting symptoms of distress may be depression, anxiety, social, interpersonal, or financial concerns, a lack of meaning or purpose, hopelessness, despair, concern about being remembered after death, feelings of guilt or shame, anger toward and feelings of abandonment by God or others, and feelings of disconnection and impotence. If patients do not voice these concerns, they may be subsequently detected during routine screening. However, patients may not endorse these problems explicitly, and providers should have a high level of suspicion, especially if other symptoms or behaviors seem to signal distress.

  - **Physical pain** may be a presenting symptom of psychosocial or spiritual distress and may warrant screening for such distress. Cancer patients with high levels of pain are more likely to develop depression, anxiety, and mood disturbance (31). Severe pain may be a marker for socioeconomic disadvantage, which was the most important predictor of disabling pain in a probability sample of telephone interviews of the general population (32). Pain that does not respond to pharmacologic treatment may be a result of or be exacerbated by underlying spiritual pain (20). Spiritual or existential distress may be expressed as increased pain or pain not improving with medications. Spiritual intervention may be as effective as medication in pain management (37). Thus, addressing only physical pain will not adequately assess for spiritual or psychosocial pain.

  - Depression may be an indicator of psychosocial and spiritual difficulties. Depression can be a marker for social isolation. Increased rates of depression are found in patients who practice behavioral disengagement or self-imposed isolation (33). In older hospitalized patients, depression rates are higher and quality of life lower in those with more negative religious coping (33). Also, spiritual pain can worsen emotional symptoms (20). Spiritual or existential distress may also be incorrectly diagnosed as depression. Anger and diminished self-esteem may also be spiritually related (National Cancer Institute, Cancer Care for Whole Person). It is critical to always assess for spiritual or existential distress. The treatments for spiritual distress are different from the treatment for clinical depression. Also, patients may be dually diagnosed with depression and spiritual or existential distress. Treatment may include antidepressants, referral to a board certified chaplain and spiritually directed counseling, meaning-oriented therapy (34), art or music therapy (35,36).

- A **desire for death** should trigger a detailed evaluation, since it correlates with pain severity and effect on function, perceived low levels of social support, and depression (38). Spiritual or existential distress is the most prevalent reason for physician assisted suicide (PAS) and should be evaluated when a patient expresses a desire to die or a request for PAS (39).

- **Behaviors that interfere with care** can signify psychosocial or spiritual distress. Patients may refuse care based on a spiritual or religious belief (25). Nonadherence to a treatment plan is more common in patients with distress and, especially, in those with depression (40). Family and caregiver distress may manifest as disruptive behaviors, including the following: being unavailable, not obeying visiting hours, criticizing staff, delaying treatments, speaking for the patient, dividing the team, demanding information repetition, and counseling the patient to disregard medical advice (25).

ASSESSMENT

- Every patient evaluation should include a psychiatric, social, and spiritual history; screening for distress should take place at every visit and especially during periods of vulnerability (Table 15.4) (41). The social history is where social and spiritual distress as well as resources of strength are addressed. The checklist in the following text identifies a complete social history that also includes a spiritual history:

Table 15.4 Periods of Increased Vulnerability/Risk for Distress		
Initial evaluation/ treatment	**During treatment**	**After treatment**
Finding a suspicious symptom	Complications	Transition to survivorship
During diagnostic workup	Change in treatment plan	Follow-up and surveillance
Receiving a diagnosis	Hospital admission	Recurrence/ progression
Awaiting treatment	Hospital discharge	End of life
	End of treatment Treatment failure	Learning of familial/ genetic cancer risk
Source: From www.nccn.org, 2018.		

Social and Spiritual History Checklist*

☐ Living situation (alone or with others and type of home; e.g., house, apartment, assisted living, shelter)
☐ Significant relationships
☐ Occupation
☐ Sexual activity
☐ Tobacco use
☐ Alcohol use
☐ Recreational drugs use
☐ Diet
☐ Exercise
☐ Hobbies, interests
☐ Spiritual history

*From George Washington University School of Medicine.

- In psychosocial assessment, a brief screening tool for distress may be used (25). This is efficient and more sensitive in identifying distress than a provider's impression alone (21). Several screening tools exist including the National Comprehensive Cancer Network (NCCN) Distress Thermometer (42).
- Some patient characteristics are associated with an increased risk of distress (Table 15.5).
- **Spiritual History**
  - Useful spiritual history-taking tools include FICA (Table 15.7), HOPE, SPIRIT, and Open Invite (43). The FICA tool has been validated for cancer patients (44). A quality improvement project encouraged

Table 15.5 Factors Associated With an Increased Risk of Moderate or Severe Distress

Psychiatric	Social	Miscellaneous
History of psychiatric disorder	Communication barriers	Uncontrolled symptoms
History of substance abuse	Financial problems	Severe comorbid illness
History of depression	Living alone	Younger age
Cognitive impairment	Family/caregiver conflicts	Female sex
History of physical abuse	Inadequate social support	
History of sexual abuse	Limited access to medical care	
	Having young/dependent children	

Source: From www.nccn.org, 2018.

clinicians to use the FICA tool to establish a trusting patient–clinician relationship, to allow patients to share spiritual concerns, and to make referrals to chaplains, as needed. Subsequent to the interventions, the number of completed FICA histories and chaplain consults doubled as an indicator of quality improvement in a palliative care setting (45).

- Expressions of spiritual distress that may arise during the spiritual history are seen in Table 15.6.
- Once the assessment of distress, as well as resources of strength, are made and the exam is completed, a whole person assessment and treatment plan is completed, which includes all four domains of the biopsychosocial and spiritual model of palliative care—physical, emotional, social, and spiritual.

Table 15.6 Spiritual Distress

Diagnoses (primary)	Key feature from history	Example statements
Existential	Lack of meaning / questions meaning about own existence / concern about afterlife / questions the meaning of suffering / seeks spiritual assistance	"My life is meaningless." "I feel useless."
Abandonment by God or others	Lack of love, loneliness / not being remembered / no sense of relatedness	"God has abandoned me." "No one comes by anymore."
Anger at God or others	Displaces anger toward religious representatives / inability to forgive	"Why would God take my child... it's not fair."
Concerns about relationship with deity	Closeness to God / deepening relationship	"I want to have a deeper relationship with God."
Conflicted or challenged belief systems	Verbalizes inner conflicts or questions about beliefs or faith / conflicts between religious beliefs and recommended treatments / questions moral or ethical implications of therapeutic regimen / expresses concern with life/death and/or belief system	"I am not sure if God is with me anymore."

(continued)

Table 15.6 Spiritual Distress (*continued*)

Diagnoses (primary)	Key feature from history	Example statements
Despair/ hopelessness	Hopelessness about future health, life / despair as absolute hopelessness, no hope for value in life	"Life is being cut short." "There is nothing left for me to live for."
Grief/loss	Grief is the feeling and process associated with a loss of person, health, etc.	"I miss my loved one so much." "I wish I could run again."
Guilt/shame	Guilt is feeling that the person has done something wrong or evil; shame is a feeling that the person is bad or evil	"I do not deserve to die pain free."
Reconciliation	Need for forgiveness and/ or reconciliation of self or others	"I need to be forgiven for what I did." "I would like my wife to forgive me."
Isolation	From religious community or other	"Since moving to assisted living I am not able to go to my church anymore."

Source: Puchalski C, Ferrell B, Virani R, et al. Improving the quality of spiritual care as a dimension of palliative care: the report of the consensus conference. *J Palliat Med.* 2009;12(10):885–904. doi:10.1089/jpm.2009.0142

TREATMENT

Evaluation and treatment should be undertaken by all members of the interdisciplinary team. The interdisciplinary team should include a trained chaplain. Chaplains are trained to address spiritual and existential issues and are the experts in spiritual and existential distress. They work with all patients, religious, nonreligious, secular humanist, and so on. Any team member can perform a screening. The clinician will then review the screening with the patient and ask further questions. Psychosocial and spiritual histories are taken by clinicians, usually physicians, advanced practice nurses, and physician assistants, who then develop treatment and care plans. In the absence of distress, this process should be repeated at appropriate intervals. If distress is identified, an assessment should be performed by an appropriate interdisciplinary

Table 15.7 FICA Spiritual History Tool	
Item	**Possible questions**
Faith and belief	"Do you consider yourself spiritual or religious?" or "Is spirituality something important to you" or "Do you have spiritual beliefs that help you cope with stress/difficult times?" (Contextualize to reason for visit if it is not the routine history.) If the patient responds "No," the healthcare provider might ask, "What gives your life meaning?" Sometimes patients respond with answers such as family, career, or nature.
Importance	"What importance does your spirituality have in your life? Has your spirituality influenced how you take care of yourself, your health? Does your spirituality influence you in your healthcare decision making (e.g., advance directives, treatment etc.)?
Community	"Are you part of a spiritual community?" Communities such as churches, temples, and mosques, a group of like-minded friends, family, or yoga, can serve as strong support systems for some patients. Can explore further: "Is this of support to you and how? Is there a group of people you really love or who are important to you?"
Address in care	"How would you like me, your healthcare provider, to address these issues in your healthcare?" (With the newer models including diagnosis of spiritual distress, this also refers to the "Assessment and Plan" of patient spiritual distress or issues within a treatment or care plan.)

Source: From Puchalski C, Romer AL. Taking a spiritual history allows clinicians to understand patients more fully. J Palliat Med. 2000;3(1): 129–137. doi:10.1089/jpm.2000.3.129

team member. The interdisciplinary team should develop a treatment plan, which should be updated on a regular basis. This process is visualized in Figure 15.1.

Psychosocial interventions often involve caregivers and should be introduced shortly after cancer diagnosis to normalize their inclusion (46).

- For patients with psychosocial comorbidities, the NCCN provides detailed treatment algorithms (41).
- Patients with spiritual or existential distress should be treated by all clinicians on the team with compassionate presence and deep listening (3). Referral to trained healthcare chaplains should be considered for patients with moderate to severe distress, or with distress that does not resolve with initial support and attentive listening from the clinicians.

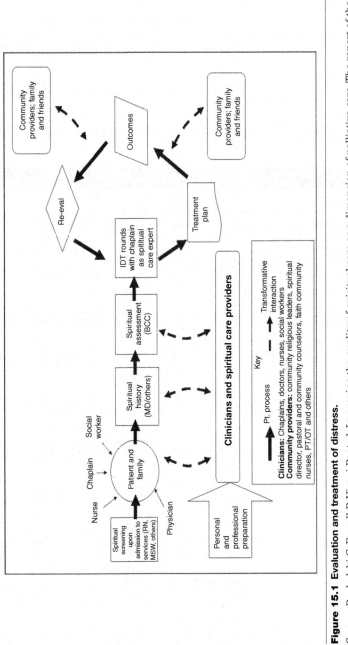

Figure 15.1 Evaluation and treatment of distress.

Source: Puchalski C, Ferrell B, Virani R, et al. Improving the quality of spiritual care as a dimension of palliative care: The report of the consensus conference. *J Palliat Med.* 2009;12(10):885–904. doi:10.1089/jpm.2009.0142

Physical symptoms (i.e., pain) must be addressed as part of any psychosocial-spiritual intervention (i.e., treat pain) (25).

- Psychiatric disorders may warrant pharmacotherapy to alleviate psychiatric symptoms, reduce associated physical symptoms, improve the ability to adhere to the treatment plan (25) and decrease a desire for death (38). Table 15.8 is an example of a Biopsychosocial–Spiritual Treatment Plan

Special Considerations

- While all caregivers are at risk of psychosocial distress, some populations have been shown to experience certain symptoms or disorders at greater rates (Table 15.9) (47–50).

Table 15.8 Case Example With Assessment and Treatment Plan

Ms. G is a 65-year-old female with metastatic lung cancer admitted to the inpatient hospice unit for control of chest wall pain. Although she reports her mood is good and denies depression and anxiety, she is tearful during the visit and expresses interest in voluntary cessation of eating and drinking to hasten her death. She identifies as a Catholic but has not been particularly observant prior to her diagnosis. She finds meaning in family and nature, and used to meditate, but cannot do that now. She does not want to share her distress with her family for fear of upsetting them.

Domain	Issue	Treatment
Physical	Less than optimal control of chest wall pain	Employ adequate pain medication regimen
Emotional/ psychological	Fear of loss of control Inability to care for self	Refer to counselor for exploration of issues about loss of control. Consider pastoral counselor in outpatient setting as spiritual distress also present
Social	Difficulty accepting dependence on others	Counseling with social worker; discuss support services available
Spiritual	Conflict with spiritual beliefs Unable to utilize her spiritual practices (e.g., meditation) Despair Isolation from family and church community	Refer to trained chaplain for spiritual counseling, continued presence and deep listening by clinicians on team

Table 15.9 Common Caregiver Issues

Issue	Caregiver population particularly at risk
Depression	Caring for a patient diagnosed with late stage cancer Adult caregivers of ill parents Those working or actively looking for work
Life disruption	Caring for a patient with high symptom burden
Feeling abandoned by family/friends	Women Adult caregivers of ill parents Non-spouse caregivers
Spiritual distress	Spouse caregivers Caregivers of family members or friend

Source: From Delgado-Guay MO, Parsons HA, Hui D, et al. Spirituality, religiosity, and spiritual pain among caregivers of patients with advanced cancer. *Am J Hosp Palliat Care*. 2013;30(5):455–461. doi:10.1177/1049909112458030; Given B, Wyatt G, Given C, et al. Burden and depression among caregivers of patients with cancer at the end of life. *Oncol Nurs Forum*. 2004;31(6):1105–1117. doi:10.1188/04.ONF.1105-1117; Kim Y, Spillers RL, Hall DL. Quality of life of family caregivers 5 years after a relative's cancer diagnosis: follow-up of the national quality of life survey for caregivers. *Psycho-Oncology*. 2012;21(3):273–281. doi:10.1002/pon.1888; Sun V, Kim JY, Irish TL, et al. Palliative care and spiritual well-being in lung cancer patients and family caregivers. *Psycho-Oncology*. 2015;25:1448–1455. doi:10.1002/pon.3987

- 98% of caregivers identify as religious or spiritual and 58% have reported spiritual pain. These caregivers had higher levels of anxiety, depression, denial, behavioral disengagement, dysfunctional coping strategies, and poor quality of life (47).
- Children in the home of adult patients may require additional considerations based on developmental stage. In particular, their comfort level and understanding is important to consider if a patient may die at home.
- Professional providers may experience distressful symptoms including fear, loneliness, abandonment, loss of faith, loss of meaning in life (especially as the time to engage in valued activities is limited by caregiving responsibilities), and guilt for not being able to cure or be ever-available for the patient. It is essential that providers practice self-care to ensure personal mental and physical health, remain effective and present for the patient, and model healthy behaviors for caregivers. Debriefing with colleagues, self-reflection, talking with a trusted mentor, or accessing more formal mental health services are all strategies to ensure well-being in a palliative provider.
- Providers should be cognizant of the views of major religions and philosophies on death and dying (Tables 15.10 and 15.11) (51). Keep in mind that each patient is an individual, and beliefs may vary from those listed in Tables 15.10 and 15.11, and there is great variation in practices and philosophies among the branches of major religions.

Table 15.10 Key Religious Beliefs Toward Illness and End of Life

Religion/ belief	Key beliefs and possible practices
Buddhism	Harming or taking the life of any living creature is against the first precept of Buddhism; euthanasia is not supported but the natural dying process is supported without requiring aggressive interventions that would simply prolong the dying process. Dying is an accepted part of life and a transition in the reincarnation process. Meditation is felt to promote healing in all life phases, including at the end of life. The Western concept that brain death signifies death may not be accepted and Buddhists may not support organ donation; some, however, may consider organ donation a compassionate act. Practices may also include divination, recitation of mantras and sutras, and the use of amulets and exocrcism.
Christianity	Patients may view suffering as a punishment for sins; enduring suffering may bring one closer to Christ by offering understanding of His suffering; however, doctrine advises a patient be made comfortable; it is permissible to forego extraordinary measures to prolong life if poor chance of benefit. Patients may pray for a miracle cure but can be advised to also prepare for death if a cure is not achieved. All healing comes from God. Death is a passage to another life. Euthanasia and assisted suicide are unacceptable, but medicines may be used to ensure end-of-life comfort and dignity as long as their purpose is not to hasten death (Double Effect Principle); organ donation is permissible. Practices include attending church, prayer, and reading the Bible, and receiving sacraments including Holy Communion; for Catholics this may also include Confession, and Anointing of the Sick (this requires presence of the priest but there are blessings [viaticum] that can be done by laity).
Hinduism	Dying is a natural step in the continual cycle of the reincarnation process, which is organized by karma and the rules of moral evaluation. A supreme being exists in the universe and in individual souls and is the ultimate end of all. Spiritual progression can lead to Moksha (liberation from reincarnation), so death is considered a step taking one closer to this goal. Practices include meditation and yoga.

(continued)

Table 15.10 Key Religious Beliefs Toward Illness and End of Life (*continued*)

Religion/ belief	Key beliefs and possible practices
Islam	One should surrender to Allah's will; Allah offers forgiveness and redemption when a person repents; this can occur until death. Clergy, chaplains, and family should remind the dying person of this possibility up to the moment of death. Modesty may cause female patients to prefer female providers. The male head of the family is expected to make serious healthcare decisions. Life exists after death and death is simply a link to the afterlife. Suicide and assisted suicide are not permissible. Practices include the Sahadah, a set of prayers important before death that attest to faith in Allah as the one God; closing the eyes and reciting blessings for the deceased; funerals are felt to be of benefit to the deceased and the family.
Judaism	Daily life is dictated by religious law, including dietary practice and keeping the Sabbath; a rabbi may help interpret these laws; different branches of Judaism may differ in interpretation of these laws; it is important to ask a patient about his or her religious observances. Orthodox women may refuse to be touched by a male healthcare provider. The body is entrusted to the individual by God and should be respected; physicians are God's agents and when individuals are ill, they must consult a doctor. Family and community are important; visiting the sick is an important duty and can promote healing. Hope in the face of illness must be preserved, but the focus of hope can change with time. The tzidduk hadin, a prayer asking for god's forgiveness and accepting his judgment, should be said by or for the patient close to death. Palliative care is acceptable, but hastening death is not; however, foregoing life-sustaining therapies in the face of incurable illness may be acceptable. The body of the deceased should be washed by the Jewish Burial Society; the body should be accompanied overnight and the attendee repeat prayers; the burial should occur within 3 days. Orthodox adherents do not permit organ donation. Mourning begins with the 7-day period of Shiva when family greets mourners at the home and lasts for 11 months; on the anniversary of a death, close family members recite the Kaddish.

Source: From Puchalski CM, O'Donnell E. Religious and spiritual beliefs in end of life care: how major religions view death and dying. *Tech Reg Anesth Pain Manag.* 2005;9(3);114–121. doi:10.1053/j.trap.2005.06.003

Table 15.11 Key Beliefs of Nonreligious Frameworks

Humanism—a way of life centered on human interests or values; *especially* a philosophy that usually rejects supernaturalism and stresses an individual's dignity and worth and capacity for self-realization through reason. British Humanism Society has resources for funerals for atheists, agnostics, humanists, and others who do not belong to a religion. These include rites, ethnographic records, and other secular rituals (52).

CLINICAL PEARLS

- Spiritual and psychosocial distress are common and underdiagnosed. Distress has negative effects on outcomes.
- Pain symptoms must be treated adequately to minimize their effects on distress.
- Pharmacological treatment may be needed for psychiatric disorders.
- Caregivers and providers are at risk for distress, and impairments associated with distress may affect patient treatment. Distress management should encompass the entire care team.
- Children related to the patient may require special assistance to prevent and manage distress.
- Providers should routinely screen for psychosocial and spiritual distress through spiritual history and screening; introducing these evaluations early normalizes the inclusion of distress treatment in a cancer care plan.
- America Ethical Union: Culture is a moral faith that respects the dignity and worth of all life (53).
- Appropriate specialists in the interdisciplinary team should address psychosocial and spiritual distress. Trained chaplains should be members of all healthcare teams and are the specialists for spiritual issues.
- All team-members should address psychosocial and spiritual distress and attend to the suffering of patients.
- The NCCN provides detailed treatment algorithms for those with particular underlying problems (e.g., history of abuse, bipolar disorder, cognitive impairment).

REFERENCES

1. Abraham A, Kutner JS, Beaty B. Suffering at the end of life in the setting of low physical symptom distress. *J Palliat Med*. 2006;9(3):658–665. doi:10.1089/jpm.2006.9.658
2. Berger AM, Shuster JL, Von Roenn JH. *Principles and Practice of Palliative Care and Supportive Oncology*. Philadelphia, PA: Lippincott Williams & Wilkins; 2007.
3. Puchalski C, Ferrell B, Virani R, et al. Improving the quality of spiritual care as a dimension of palliative care: The report of the consensus conference. *J Palliat Med*. 2009;12(10):885–904. doi:10.1089/jpm.2009.0142
4. Puchalski CM, Vitillo R, Hull SK, Reller N. Improving the spiritual dimension of whole person care: Reaching national and international consensus. *J Palliat Med*. 2014;17(6):642–656. doi:10.1089/jpm.2014.9427

5. Doherty WJ. Morality and spirituality in therapy. In: Walsh F, eds. *Spiritual Resources in Family Therapy*. New York, NY: Guilford Publications; 1999:179–192.

6. Sulmasy D. Spiritual issues in the care of dying patients, "…It's Okay Between Me and God". *JAMA*, 2006;1385–1392.

7. Pargament K, Koenig H, Tarakeshwar M, Hahn J. Religious struggle as a predictor of mortality among medically ill elderly patients: a 2-year longitudinal study. *Arch Intern Med*, 2001;1881–1885.

8. Fitchett G, Murphy PE, Kim J. Religious struggle: prevalence, correlates and mental health risks in diabetic, congestive heart failure, and oncology patients. *Int J Psychiatry Med*, 2004;34(2):179–196.

9. Balboni TA, Vanderwerker LC, Block SD, et al. Religiousness and spiritual support among advanced cancer patients and associations with end-of-life treatment preferences and quality of life. *J Clin Oncol*. 2007;25(5):555–560. doi:10.1200/jco.2006.07.9046

10. Salsman JM, Pustejovsky JE, Jim HS, et al. A meta-analytic approach to examining the correlation between religion/spirituality and mental health in cancer. *Cancer*. 2015;121:3769–3778. doi:10.1002/cncr.29350

11. Delgado-Guay MO, Chisholm G, Williams J, et al. Frequency, intensity, and correlates of spiritual pain in advanced cancer patients assessed in a supportive/palliative care clinic. *Palliat Support Care*. 2016;14(4):341–348. doi:10.1017/S147895151500108X

12. Balboni TA, Paulk ME, Balboni MJ, et al. Provision of spiritual care to patients with advanced cancer: Associations with medical care and quality of life near death. *J Clin Oncol*. 2010;28(3):445–452. doi:10.1200/JCO.2009.24.8005

13. Trevino KM, Balboni M, Zollfrank A, et al. Negative religious coping as a correlate of suicidal ideation in patients with advanced cancer. *Psycho-Oncology*. 2014;23(8):936–945. doi:10.1002/pon.3505

14. des Ordons AR, Sinuff T, Stelfox HT, et al. Spiritual distress within inpatient settings–A scoping review of patient and family experiences. *J Pain Symptom Manage*. 2018;56:122–145. doi:10.1016/j.jpainsymman.2018.03.009

15. Hui D, de la Cruz M, Thorney S, et al. The frequency and correlates of spiritual distress among patients with advanced cancer admitted to an acute palliative care unit. *Am J Hosp Palliat Care*. 2011;28(4):264–270. doi:10.1177/1049909110385917

16. Schultz M, Meged-Book T, Mashiach T, Bar-Sela G. Distinguishing between spiritual distress, general distress, spiritual well-being, and spiritual pain among cancer patients during oncology treatment. *J Pain Symptom Manage*. 2017;54(1):66–73. doi:10.1016/j.jpainsymman.2017.03.018

17. Bhatnagar S, Gielen J, Satija A, et al. Signs of spiritual distress and its implications for practice in indian palliative care. *Indian J Palliat Care*. 2017;23(3):306. doi:10.4103/IJPC.IJPC_24_17

18. Astrow AB, Wexler A, Texeira K, et al. Is failure to meet spiritual needs associated with cancer patients' perceptions of quality of care and their satisfaction with care? *J Clin Oncol*. 2007;25(36):5753–5757. doi:10.1200/JCO.2007.12.4362

19. Gao W, Bennett MI, Stark D, et al. Psychological distress in cancer from survivorship to end of life care: prevlance, associated factors and clinical implications. *Eur J Cancer*, 2010;46(11):2036–2044. doi:10.1016/j.ejca.2010.03.033

20. Delgado-Guay MO, Hui D, Parsons HA, et al. Spirituality, religiosity, and spiritual pain in advanced cancer patients. *J Pain Symptom Manage*. 2011;41(6):986–994. doi:10.1016/j.jpainsymman.2010.09.017

21. Bauwens S, Baillon C, Distelmans W, Theuns P. Systematic screening for distress in oncology practice using the Distress Barometer: the impact on referrals to psychosocial care. *Psycho-oncology*, 2014;23(7):804–811. doi:10.1002/pon.3484

22. Clark PG, Rochon E, Brethwaite D, Edmiston KK. Screening for psychological and physical distress in a cancer inpatient treatment setting: a pilot study. *Psychooncology*, 2011;20(6):664–668. doi:10.1002/pon.1908

23. Zabora J, Brintzenhofeszoc K, Curbow B, et al. The prevalence of psychological distress by cancer site. *Psycho-Oncology*. 2001;10(1):19–28. doi:10.1002/1099-1611(200101/02)10:1<19::AID-PON501>3.0.CO;2-6

24. Samuel CA, Pinheiro LC, Reeder-Hayes KE. To be young, Black, and living with breast cancer: a systematic review of health-related quality of life in yong Black breast cancer survivors. *Breast Cancer Res Treat*, 2016;160(1):1-15.

25. Berger AM, Shuster JL, Von Roenn JH. *Principles and Practice of Palliative Care and Supportive Oncology.* 4th ed. Philadelphia, PA: Lippincott Williams & Wilkins; 2013.

26. Peteet JR, Balboni MJ. Spirituality and religion in oncology. *CA Cancer J Clin.* 2013;63(4):280–289. doi:10.3322/caac.21187

27. McGrath P. Reflections on serious illness as spiritual journey by survivors of haematological malignancies. *Eur J Cancer Care.* 2004;13(3):227–237. doi:10.1111/j.1365-2354.2004.00457.x

28. Farsi Z. The meaning of disease and spiritual responses to stressors in adults with acute leukemia undergoing hematopoietic stem cell transplantation. *J Nurs Res.* 2015:1. doi:10.1097/jnr.0000000000000088

29. North American Nursing Diagnosis Association. *NANDA International Nursing Diagnoses: Definitions and Classification.* Hoboken, NJ: Wiley-Blackwell; 2012.

30. Hungelmann J, Kenkel-Rossi E, Klassen L, Stollenwerk R. Focus on spiritual well-being: Harmonious interconnectedness of mind-body-spirit—Use of the JAREL spiritual well-being scale: assessment of spiritual well-being is essential to the health of individuals. *Geriatr Nurs.* 1996;17(6):262–266. doi:10.1016/S0197-4572(96)80238-2

31. Spiegel D, Sands S, Koopman C. Pain and depression in patients with cancer. *Cancer,* 1994;74(9):2570–2578.

32. Portenoy RK, Bruera E. *Issues in Palliative Care Research.* New York, NY: Oxford University Press, USA; 2003.

33. Koenig HG, George LK, Hays JC, et al. The relationship between religious activities and blood pressure in older adults. *Int J Psychiatry Med.* 1998;28(2):189–213. doi:10.2190/75JM-J234-5JKN-4DQD

34. Breitbart W, Rosenfeld B, Pessin H, et al. Meaning-centered group psychotherapy: an effective intervention for improving psychological well-being in patients with advanced cancer. *J Clin Oncol.* 2015;33(7):749–754. doi:10.1200/JCO.2014.57.2198

35. Masko MK. Music therapy and spiritual care in end-of-life: A qualitative inquiry into ethics and training issues identified by chaplains and music therapists. *J Music Ther.* 2016;53(4):309–335. doi:10.1093/jmt/thw009

36. Slayton SC, D'Archer J, Kaplan F. Outcome studies on the efficacy of art therapy: a review of findings. *Art Ther.* 2010;27(3):108–118. doi:10.1080/07421656.2010.10129660

37. McGrath P. Creating a language for 'spiritual pain' through research: a beginning. *Support Care Cancer.* 2002;10(8):637–646. doi:10.1007/s00520-002-0360-5

38. O'Mahony S, Goulet J, Kornblith A, et al. Desire for hastened death, cancer pain and depression: Report of a longitudinal observational study. *J Pain Symptom Manage.* 2005;29(5):446–457. doi:10.1016/j.jpainsymman.2004.08.010

39. Radbruch L, Leget C, Bahr P, et al. Euthanasia and physician-assisted suicide: a white paper from the european association for palliative care. *Palliat Med.* 2016;30(2):104–116. doi:10.1177/0269216315616524

40. DiMatteo MR, Lepper HS, Croghan TW. Depression is a risk factor for noncompliance with medical treatment. *Arch Intern Med,* 2000;160(4):2101–2107.

41. https://www.nccn.org/professionals/physician_gls/pdf/distress.pdf

42. National Comprehensive Cancer Network. *NCCN distress thermometer for patients;* 2015. https://www.nccn.org/professionals/physician_gls/pdf/distress.pdf

43. Saguil A, Phelps K. The spiritual assessment. *Am Fam Physician,* 2012;86(6):546–550.

44. Puchalski C, Romer AL. Taking a spiritual history allows clinicians to understand patients more fully. *J Palliat Med.* 2000;3(1):129–137. doi:10.1089/jpm.2000.3.129

45. Gomez-Castillo BJ, Hirsch R, Groninger H, et al. Increasing the number of outpatients receiving spiritual assessment: A pain and palliative care service quality improvement project. *J Pain Symptom Manage.* 2015;50(5):724–729. doi:10.1016/j.jpainsymman.2015.05.012

46. Fawzy FI, Fawzy NW, Arndt LA, Pasnau RO. Critical review of psychosocial interventions in cancer care. *Arch Gen Psychiatry.* 1995;52(2):100–113. doi:10.1001/archpsyc.1995.03950140018003

47. Delgado-Guay MO, Parsons HA, Hui D, et al. Spirituality, religiosity, and spiritual pain among caregivers of patients with advanced cancer. *Am J Hosp Palliat Care.* 2013;30(5):455–461. doi:10.1177/1049909112458030

48. Given B, Wyatt G, Given C, et al. Burden and depression among caregivers of patients with cancer at the end of life. *Oncol Nurs Forum*. 2004;31(6):1105–1117. doi:10.1188/04. ONF.1105-1117

49. Kim Y, Spillers RL, Hall DL. Quality of life of family caregivers 5 years after a relative's cancer diagnosis: follow-up of the national quality of life survey for caregivers. *Psycho-Oncology*. 2012;21(3):273–281. doi:10.1002/pon.1888

50. Sun V, Kim JY, Irish TL, et al. Palliative care and spiritual well-being in lung cancer patients and family caregivers. *Psycho-Oncology*. 2015;25:1448–1455. doi:10.1002/pon.3987

51. Puchalski CM, O'Donnell E. Religious and spiritual beliefs in end of life care: how major religions view death and dying. *Tech Reg Anesth Pain Manag*. 2005;9(3);114–121. doi:10.1053/j.trap.2005.06.003

52. Engelke M. The coffin question: death and materiality in humanist funerals. *Material Religion*. 2015;11(1):26–48. doi:10.2752/205393215x14259900061553

53. Ippei S. Secularism in america: a brief history of non-religion movement. *Social Sciences*. 2007;29:97–106.

Supportive Oncology and Quality of Life Considerations for Patients, Families, and Caregivers

III

Intimacy, Sexuality, and Fertility Issues Associated With Cancer Treatment 16

Tara Berman

INTRODUCTION

Despite treatment advances in the world of oncology, problems with sexuality, intimacy, and fertility persist for many women and men treated for cancer. Life expectancy of cancer patients, both young and old, has significantly increased due to advances in treatments of malignant diseases. Consequently, medical attention has expanded its focus to improving the quality of life of patients who have undergone cancer treatment. Treatment decisions made at diagnosis significantly impact interpersonal relationships and reproductive capacity of survivors (1). Fertility represents one of the greatest concerns of cancer survivors of childbearing age (2). Most young survivors are interested in having children, according to studies, even if they were childless at the time of their cancer diagnosis (2).

Sexual function and feeling healthy enough to be a parent represent two of the strongest predictors of emotional well-being in cancer survivors, and parenthood can represent a return to normalcy, contributing happiness and life-fulfillment (3). Often, cancer survivors fear that their disease or treatment history may adversely affect offspring conceived posttreatment, contributing risk for congenital anomalies, impaired growth and development, or even for malignancy (3). Concerns about the risks of cancer recurrence, infertility, miscarriage, and achieving a successful pregnancy outcome are also prevalent.

The ability to preserve fertility depends on several variables: age, type of cancer, and types of treatment (4). Pregnancy does not appear to increase the risk of recurrence of cancer (5). The American Society of Clinical Oncologists (ASCO) recommends that (a) oncologists address the possibility of infertility with patients in their reproductive years and that (b) fertility preservation should be considered as early as possible during treatment.

PREVALENCE

Despite these concerns, only about 50% of female cancer survivors surveyed in California and Sweden recalled receiving reproductive health counseling (6,7); the proportion is higher in male cancer survivors (7). According to another study, survivors, however, do desire counseling about reproductive loss and the option to try to preserve fertility before treatment, even if chemotherapy precludes them from having children after treatment (8). Patient education regarding future reproductive function is thus an important component of the care of individuals with cancer.

The Childhood Cancer Survivor Study (CCSS) represents the largest database on the risk of infertility in cancer survivors. CCSS is a cohort of several thousand 5-year cancer survivors, from 26 Canadian and United States institutions, who were younger than 21 years at the time of diagnosis (between January 1, 1970 and December 21, 1986) and who had an eligible malignancy: leukemia, central nervous system (CNS) cancer, Hodgkin lymphoma, non-Hodgkin lymphoma, Wilms' tumor, neuroblastoma, soft-tissue sarcoma, or bone tumors. Major findings included a lower relative risk (RR) of pregnancy among female survivors compared to female siblings (RR 0.81, 95% CI 0.73–0.90).

CAUSES

Cancer treatment may affect reproductive health in many ways. Not all patients encounter fertility problems after treatment but determining who will be affected is challenging. Factors affecting fertility include the type of surgery performed, the type and dose of chemotherapy received, the dose of radiation delivery, and the area of the body irradiated. Temporary or permanent fertility problems may result.

For women, cytoxic damage from chemotherapy and/or radiation to ovarian stromal cells and germ cells appears to be progressive and irreversible, and chemotherapy occasionally exerts detrimental and often unavoidable effects on ovarian function, resulting in female sterility. Unlike men, female patients are most susceptible to gonadal toxicants because they are born with an irreplaceable supply of germ cells in their ovaries. Male fertility, however, is affected by various cancer treatments, as described in the following text.

For women and/or girls:

- Treatment may require surgical removal of cancerous reproductive organs (e.g., hysterectomy, oophorectomy).
- Pelvic radiation and certain chemotherapy drugs may destroy oocytes in the ovary, causing primary ovarian insufficiency (POI), making it more difficult or impossible to become pregnant. (See chemotherapy drugs stratified by risk, Table 16.1.) POI is synonymous with premature menopause: amenorrhea, that is, loss of menstrual periods, due to lack of ovarian function, before the age of 40 (9).
- Low ovarian reserve can be entangled with loss of ovarian function in POI, although these are two separate entities requiring different management (9).
- The risk of developing ovarian failure is higher in older patients, presumably due to a lower ovarian reserve (10). Conversely, studies show younger patients may expect recovery of ovarian function in 30% of the cases at 6 to 48 months after therapy for various cancers (10).
- Pelvic radiation may cause changes in the female anatomy that precludes the possibility of maintaining pregnancy. As a result of uterine radiation, for example, an embryo may not be able to implant, or the uterus may not be able to expand to hold a growing fetus. This can result in complications during pregnancy such as miscarriage, preterm (early) birth, or low birth weight babies.

- Radiation to or surgery in certain areas of the brain may reduce development of pituitary gland hormones that stimulate the ovaries each month, disrupting the monthly menstrual cycle and interfering with ovulation.
  - Poor prognostic fertility factors, including data from the CCSS study (11), include:
    - Hypothalamic/pituitary radiation dose ≥30 Gy
    - Ovarian/uterine radiation dose >5 Gy
    - Exposure to alkylating agents >4,000 mg/m^2 (12)
    - Treatment with lomustine or cyclophosphamide
  - In addition, female survivors possessed a higher risk of nonsurgical premature menopause than siblings (8 %vs. 0.9%; RR 13.21, 95% CI 3.26–53.51) (11). Risk factors include:

Table 16.1 Cancer Therapy and Risk of Infertility for Women	
Risk level	**Treatments**
High	• Whole abdominal or pelvic radiation doses >6 Gy in adult women • TBI • Cranial/brain irradiation >40 Gy • CMF, CEF, or CAF x 6 cycles in women >40 years • Total cyclophosphadmide 5 g/m^2 in women >40 years • Total cyclophosphadmidey >7.5 g/m^2 <20 years • Alkylating chemotherapy (e.g., cyclophosphamide, busulfan, melaphan) conditioning for transplant • Any alkylating agent (e.g., cyclophosphamide, ifosfamide, busulfan, BCNU [carmustine], CCNU [lomustine]) + TBI or pelvic radiation • Protocols containing procarbazine: MOPP, MVPP, COPP, ChlVPP, ChlVPP/EVA, BEACOPP, MOPP/ABVD, COPP/ABVD
Intermediate	• Abdominal/pelvic radiation • CMF, CEF, or CAF x 6 cycles in women 30–40 years • Spinal radiation doses >25 Gy CMF, CEF, or CAF x 6 cycles in women 30–40 years • Bevacizumab (Avastin) • Protocols containing cisplatin • FOLFOX4 • Total cyclophos-phamide 5 g /m^2 in women age 30–40 years
Low	• CMF, CEF, or CAF x 6 cycles in women <30 years • Nonalkylating chemotherapy: ABVD • Anthracycline + cytarabine
No Risk	• Radioactive iodine • MF • Multi-agent therapies using vincristine

(continued)

Table 16.1 Cancer Therapy and Risk of Infertility for Women *(continued)*

Risk level	Treatments
Unknown Risk	• Monoclonal antibodies (e.g., cetuximab [Eributx]) • Tyrosine kinase inhibitors (e.g., erlotinib [Tarceva], imatinib [Gleevec])

ABVD, adriamycin/bleomycin/vinblastine/ dacarbazinel; AC, adriamycin/cyclophosphamidel; BEACOPP, bleomycin/etoposide/adriamycin/cyclophosphamide/oncovin/procarbazine/prednisonel; CAF, cyclophosphamide/adriamycin (doxorubicin)/ fluorouracil; CEF, cyclophosphamide/epirubicin/fluorouracil; ChlVPP, chlorambucil/vinblastine/procarbazine/prednisolonel; CHOP, cyclophosphamide/hydroxydaunomycin/oncovin/prednisonel; CMF, cyclophosphamide/methotrexate/fluorouracil; COP, cyclophosphamide/oncovin/ prednisonel; COPP, cyclophosphamide/oncovin/procarbazine/prednisonel; EVA, etoposide/vinblastine/adriamycinl; MOPP, mechlorethamine/oncovin (vincristine)/procarbazine/prednisonel; MVPP, mechlorethamine/vinblastine/procarbazine/prednisolonel; MF, methotrexate/5-fluorouracil; TBI, total body irradiation.

Source: From SaveMyFertility, Northwestern University, Chicago, Illinois, 2018. https://www.savemyfertility.org/pocket-guides/providers/fertility-preservation-women-diagnosed-cancer

- ○ Attained age
- ○ Exposure to increasing doses of radiation to the ovaries (highest risk with ≥1,000 cGy)
- ○ Exposure to alkylating agents, and increased risk with exposure to increasing quantities of alkylating agents
- ○ Exposure to both alkylating agents and abdominopelvic radiation, with a cumulative risk of nonsurgical premature menopause approaching 30%
- For men and/or boys:
  - ▪ Surgery of reproductive structures affected by cancer may result in erectile dysfunction or retrograde ejaculation, leading to the inability to release sperm naturally into the vagina (3).
  - ▪ Testicular radiation and certain chemotherapy drugs can impair healthy sperm production. Recovery is possible following treatment after several months to years. (See chemotherapy drugs stratified by risk, Table 16.2.)
  - ▪ Radiation or surgery to certain brain areas may reduce pituitary gland hormones production, negatively impacting the hormones that stimulate sperm production (3).
  - ▪ In the CCSS, male cancer survivors were overall less likely to father a pregnancy than siblings (HR 0.56, 95% CI -0.49 to 0.63) (13). Poor prognostic factors include (13):
    - ○ Radiation dose >7.5 Gy to the testes

Table 16.2 Cancer Therapy and Risk of Infertility for Men

Risk level	Treatments
High	• Total body irradiation (TBI) • Testicular radiation dose >2.5 Gy in men • Testicular radiation dose >6 Gy in boys • Cranial radiation >40 Gy • Protocols containing procarbazine: COPP, MOPP, MVPP, ChlVPP, ChlVPP/EVA, MOPP/ABVD, COPP/ABVD • Alkylating chemotherapy for transplant conditioning (cyclophosphamide, busulfan, melphalan) • Any alkylating agent (e.g., procarbazine, nitrogen mustard, cyclophosphamide) + TBI, pelvic radiation, or testicular radiation • Total cyclophosphamide >5 g/m² • Surgical removal of one or both testicles or the pituitary gland
Intermediate	• Testicular radiation dose 1–6 Gy (due to scatter from abdominal/pelvic radiation) • BEP x 2–4 cycles • Cumulative cisplatin dose >400 mg/m² • Cumulative carboplatin dose ≥ 2 g/m² • Hormone treatments (prostate cancer) • Surgical procedures within in the pelvis (prostate, bladder, lower large intestine, rectum) • CHOP/COP
Low	• Testicular radiation dose 0.2−0.7 Gy • Non-alkylating agents: ABVD, multiagent therapies for leukemia • Anthracycline + cytarabine • Bevazicumab (Avastin)
No Risk	• Radioactive iodine • MF • Multi-agent therapies using vincristine
Unknown Risk	• Monoclonal antibodies (e.g., cetuximab [Eributx]) • Tyrosine kinase inhibitors (e.g., erlotinib [Tarceva], imatinib [Gleevec])

ABVD, adriamycin/bleomycin/vinblastine/ dacarbazinel; ChlVPP, chlorambucil/vinblastine/procarbazine/prednisolonel; CHOP, cyclophosphamide/hydroxydaunomycin/oncovin/prednisonel; COP, cyclophosphamide/oncovin/ prednisonel; COPP, cyclophosphamide/ oncovin/procarbazine/prednisonel; EVA, etoposide/vinblastine/ adriamycinl; MOPP, mechlorethamine/oncovin (vincristine)/procarbazine/ prednisonel; MVPP, mechlorethamine/vinblastine/procarbazine/ prednisolonel; MF, methotrexate/5-fluorouracil; TBI, total body irradiation.

Source: From SaveMyFertility, Northwestern University, Chicago, Illinois, 2018. https://www.savemyfertility.org/pocket-guides/providers/fertility -preservation-women-diagnosed-cancer

- ○ Higher cumulative alkylating agent dose score
- ○ Treatment with cyclophosphamide or procarbazine

ASSESSMENT

After treatment, there are several ways to analyze fertility. For men, at-home semen analysis kits can be sent in to a lab to ascertain the structure and function of the sperm. For women, a comprehensive appointment with a reproductive physician specialist to review medical history and perform a thorough physical exam should be scheduled. Certain tests will be ordered or performed, such as ovarian function tests to evaluate hormone levels, including day 3 follicle stimulating hormone (FSH) and estradiol (measuring estrogen), along with inhibin B levels and transvaginal ultrasound (to confirm ovulation occurred). Luteal phase testing will involve evaluating progesterone levels, as well as levels of other hormones, along with a possible endometrial biopsy. Additional hormone level tests include prolactin, free T3, total and free testosterone, dehydroepiandrosterone sulfate (DHEAS), and androstenedione.

PHYSICAL PSYCHOSOCIAL SPIRITUAL DIMENSIONS OF THE ISSUE OR SYMPTOM

Infertility can be associated with psychological strain, which can be both a contributing factor and, more often, a consequence of the disorder (14). Stress prevalence can be as high as 80% in married women with infertility, according to one study (15). The primary negative emotional response to infertility manifests as either anxiety (a sense of threat, tension, worry), or depression (a sense of loss, sadness, lack of contro) (16).

NONPHARMACOLOGICAL TREATMENT INCLUDING COMPLEMENTARY ALTERNATIVE MEDICINE (CAM)

Several strategies exist to cope with the stress related to infertility, including yoga, mindfulness meditation, relaxation response testing, group therapy, exercise, or starting a new hobby. Based on recommendations from *RESOLVE: The National Infertility Association*, steps to focus attention on mind and body can bring a calmer perspective and stress relief to patients' lives. Such recommendations include: acknowledging feelings; sharing questions and fears; allowing oneself to cry and feel anger; grieving; keeping a journal; staying connected to family and friends; communicating with one's partner; establishing intimacy in both sensual and nonsexual ways; researching infertility treatments; finding ways to reduce stress as described earlier; practicing deep breathing; and maintaining a healthy lifestyle with a low-sugar diet and adequate sleep.

Several supplements have been reported to have a positive fertility effect in men, although more research is needed before clinical recommendations can be considered. A meta-analysis of randomized controlled trials with supplements effective for treating male fertility in men without cancer resulted in the following supplements having a positive fertility effect: aescin, coenzyme Q $_{10}$, glutathione, Korean red ginseng, L-carnitine, nigella sativa, omega-3, selenium, combination of zinc and folate, and the Menevit antioxidant (17). Acupuncture and acupuncture-like therapies, including electroacupuncture (EA) and transcutaneous electrical acupoint stimulation (TEAS), have become popular worldwide for treating infertility, although no randomized controlled trials have been conducted to prove their efficacy, as of yet.

PHARMACOLOGICAL TREATMENT

Fertility Preservation

For men, fertility preservation involves collecting and freezing semen prior to beginning cancer therapy. The sperm can later be thawed and used to fertilize eggs of a partner when choosing to start a family. For pre-pubertal boys, testicular tissue banking may be an option, but should be done under the guidance of an institutional review board, as outcomes of this procedure are still uncertain (18). Fertility preservation for women involves collecting eggs (oocytes) prior to beginning cancer treatment, a procedure performed by a reproductive endocrinologist (19). First, medication will be administered to stimulate the ovaries so that multiple eggs will mature. Next, the woman undergoes egg retrieval during an office visit. The eggs can either be cryopreserved as unfertilized oocytes or fertilized with sperm to create embryos (in vitro fertilization), which are monitored for several days before being cryopreserved. After any number of years, the cryopreserved embryos can later be thawed and transferred into that woman's uterus or into the uterus of another woman, a "gestational carrier" (19). Cryopreserved oocytes can be thawed to later be fertilized with sperm in vitro. For pre-pubertal girls, ovarian tissue banking is available, although more research is needed to ascertain the success of this treatment (19).

ASCO has just released new fertility guidelines for 2018, summarized in Table 16.3 (20). More investigational options for fertility preservation may become available or more established with time.

RECOMMENDATIONS

Table 16.3 2018 ASCO Fertility Guidelines Summarized	
Target audience	**Recommendations summarized from ASCO guidelines**
Health care providers (HCPs)	• Cancer patients are interested in discussing fertility preservation. HCPs caring for adult and pediatric cancer patients should address the possibility of infertility as early as possible before treatment starts. • Refer patients interested in fertility preservation and those who are ambivalent to reproductive specialists. • Fertility preservation approaches should be discussed as early as possible, before starting treatment. The discussion can reduce future stress and improve quality of life. Another discussion/referral may be necessary upon follow-up for completion of therapy and/or if pregnancy is being considered. Document discussions in the medical record.

(continued)

Table 16.3 2018 ASCO Fertility Guidelines Summarized (*continued*)

Target audience	Recommendations summarized from ASCO guidelines	
Health care roviders (HCPs) (cont.)	• Discuss infertility as potential risk of therapy. Discussion should take place as soon as possible once a cancer diagnosis is made and can occur simultaneously with staging and formulation of a treatment plan. There are benefits for patients in discussing fertility information with providers at every step of the cancer journey. • Encourage patients to participate in registries and clinical studies, as available, to further define the safety and efficacy of these interventions and strategies. • Refer patients to psychosocial providers when distressed about potential infertility.	
Adult men	**Sperm cryopreservation**	• Effective • HCPs should discuss sperm banking with postpubertal males receiving cancer treatment
	Hormonal gonadoprotection	• Not successful in fertility preservation • Not recommended
	Other methods to preserve male fertility	• Testicular tissue cryopreservation and reimplantation or grafting of human testicular tissue should be performed only as part of clinical trials or experimental protocols
	Post-chemotherapy	• Potentially higher risk of genetic damage in sperm collected after initiation of therapy • Sperm should be collected before initiation of treatment because the quality of the sample and sperm DNA integrity may be compromised after a single treatment • Although sperm counts and quality of sperm may be diminished even before initiation of therapy, and even if there may be a need to initiate chemotherapy quickly, these concerns should not dissuade patients from banking sperm • Intracytoplasmic sperm injection allows the future use of a very limited amount of sperm; thus, even in these compromised scenarios, fertility may still be preserved.

(*continued*)

Table 16.3 2018 ASCO Fertility Guidelines Summarized (*continued*)		
Target audience	**Recommendations summarized from ASCO guidelines**	
Adult women	**Embryo cryopreservation**	• Established fertility preservation method • Routinely used for storing surplus embryos after in vitro fertilization.
	Cryopreservation of unfertilized oocytes	• Well-suited to women without a male partner, who do not wish to use donor sperm, or have religious or ethical objections to embryo freezing • Performed in centers with necessary expertise • Concern in estrogen-sensitive breast and gynecologic malignancies with increased estrogen levels either from ovarian stimulation regimens or future pregnancy for cancer recurrence • Aromatase inhibitor (AI)-based stimulation protocols ameliorate this concern—no increased cancer recurrence risk from AI-supplemented ovarian stimulation and subsequent pregnancy
	Ovarian suppression	• Conflicting evidence to recommend GnRHa and other means of ovarian suppression for fertility preservation • GnRHa may be offered to patients in the hope of reducing likelihood of chemotherapy-induced ovarian insufficiency when proven fertility preservation methods are not feasible or in the setting of young women with breast cancer • GnRHa should not be used in place of proven fertility methods
	Ovarian tissue cryopreservation and transplantation	• Does not require ovarian stimulation • Can be performed immediately • Does not require sexual maturity; may be the only method available in children • May also restore global ovarian function

(*continued*)

Table 16.3 2018 ASCO Fertility Guidelines Summarized (*continued*)		
Target audience	**Recommendations summarized from ASCO guidelines**	
		• Further investigation needed to confirm safety in leukemia patients • Remains experimental in the United States
Children	**Special consideration**	• Suggest established methods of fertility preservation (e.g., semen or oocyte cryopreservation) for postpubertal children, with patient assent and parent/guardian consent

Source: Adapted from ASCO: The American Society of Clinical Oncology (ASCO) recently published new guidelines for fertility preservation for adults, adolescents, and children with cancer; Oktay K, Harvey BE, Partridge AH, et al. Fertility Preservation in Patients With Cancer: ASCO Clinical Practice Guideline Update. *J Clin Oncol.* 2018;36:1994–2001. doi:10.1200/JCO.2018.78.1914

SEXUAL HEALTH: SEXUALITY AND INTIMACY

Sexuality is one of the first elements of daily living disrupted by a cancer diagnosis, and the phenomenon of sexual dysfunction following treatment for cancer has been well documented (21). Sexual health represents a vital aspect of life and an area of concern patients consistently identify after cancer treatment (22). Cancer diagnosis and/or its treatments can abruptly change one's expression and experience of sexual and emotional closeness (23).

Discussing sexual health should become a routine part of conversations with patients before, during, and especially after cancer treatment. Despite the importance of sexual health to women and men surviving cancer, this issue often remains unaddressed (24).

Sexuality

In order for providers to begin assessing sexuality in patients, it is important to understand what sexuality encompasses. Sexuality is a broad term encompassing social, emotional, and physical components (25). "It is genetically endowed, phenotypically embodied, hormonally nurtured; it is not age related, but matured by experience," as Mary Hughes eloquently explains in a palliative care text (26). Sexuality includes affection, sexual orientation, sexual activity, eroticism, reproduction, intimacy, gender roles, and encompasses feelings of trust (26). The human sexual response cycle has four cycles, any of which could be affected by physiologic or emotional sequelae of cancer diagnosis or treatment (27). Libido, the desire for sexual activity, precedes the first phase, sexual excitement. This is where the penis stiffens and engorges in men, and when vaginal secretions start to occur in women for lubrication. The vagina will enlarge in depth and width and the clitoris also enlarges during this time, and arousal will continue into the plateau phase for men and women (26). Sexual intercourse peaks in orgasm, the height of sexual pleasure and release of sexual tension. Muscular spasms of the penis emit semen into the vagina, and rhythmic contractions of the vagina can help propel semen in through the cervix into the uterus up to the fallopian tube, where fertilization may occur. During the final resolution phase, the genitals return to their normal, non-excited state. A refractory period follows, when the genitals are resistant to sexual stimulation. Certain medications or medical conditions like cancer can extend this refractory phase in men (26).

Clinical Assessment of Sexuality

A survey of approximately 26,000 men and women between the ages of 40 and 80 spanning 29 countries pointed out that physicians do not make it a common practice to discuss sexuality and intimacy; this was a global phenomenon (28). Within the United States alone, only 14% of patients reported physicians inquiring about their sexual issues within a time span of 3 years. This reticence may be explained by an assumption on the part of clinicians (explicit or presumed) that patients will bring up sexual concerns to them without first being asked. Unfortunately, it is unrealistic to expect patients to bring up a potentially sensitive issue. In one study involving 878 women diagnosed with a gynecologic malignancy, only 3% brought sexual concerns to providers spontaneously; in contrast, 16% did so only when asked directly (29).

Sexual Health Discussion Guidelines

To help clinicians incorporate questions about sexual health in their routine review of systems both during and after active treatment, a patient-centric communication strategy can be effective (30). One approach to introducing sexual health discussions is the PLISSIT model: "Permission, Limited Information, Specific Suggestions, and Intensive Therapy (Table 16.4) (31)." Park et al. propose the 5 As—Ask, Advise, Assess, Assist, Arrange—which is a separate framework that builds on PLISSIT and is designed to aid clinicians in communicating with cancer survivors (32). Open and closed questions should be used, with sensitivity shown to the patient, as he or she describes sexuality-related issues.

Intimacy

Clinicians should recognize that sexual activity is not synonymous with intimacy. Intimacy is a term often used as a euphemism for sexual function, when more appropriately, it describes a sharing of identity, mutual acceptance, closeness, and reciprocated rapport, more closely linked to communication than sexual function (33). In a recent study by Perz et al. involving over 40 patients, their partners, and clinicians, clinicians tended to emphasize their queries on the ability of their patients

Table 16.4 Permission, Limited Information, Specific Suggestions, and Intensive Therapy (PLISSIT) Model for Sexual Conversations. Open-Ended Questions to be Used to Start Discussions at Each Step Are Included, Followed by Closed-Ended Questions That May Help During the Conversation

Permission	• Invite patient to enter into a discussion about sexual health • "I'd like to review how you are doing as it relates to both sexuality and intimacy. Would that be okay?" • "Are you (and your partner) having problems with being intimate?
Limited Information	• Normalize that issues related to sexual health are common • "Some patients complain that sex and intimacy are different now. In fact, it is pretty common. How has your experience been?" • "A common complaint is pain during intercourse. Is this something that is happening with you?"
Specific Suggestions	• Offer advice that can be actionable and easy to incorporate if possible. • "If you have trouble with vaginal dryness, it may help to use a lubricant before and during sex."
Intensive Therapy	• If one is not comfortable with issues brought up or does not know what to advise, offer expert consultation locally (if possible) or refer to educational resources. • "It sounds like you might benefit from seeing an expert in sexual health. Can I suggest a referral?"

Source: Adapted from Annon JS. Behavioral Treatment of Sexual Problems: Brief Therapy. New York, NY: Harper & Row, 1976;45.

to perform sexually, but patients and their partners cautioned that the inability to perform should not be presumed to mean there was a lack of intimacy (34). Intimacy is valued by patients, and alternative means of expressing intimacy could be highly satisfying, despite being unable or uninterested in having penile-vaginal intercourse (the "coital imperative") (24). Another study found that many patients searched for practical strategies and emotional support about how to come to terms with their altered sense of sexual or intimate self, yet assumed if the topic was not raised by health professionals caring for them, these issues must not be important (35). Even partaking in such a study about palliative care and sexuality in and of itself had therapeutic and emotionally cathartic patient outcomes.

A number of validated questionnaires exist for sexual health, as given in Table 16.5.

Table 16.5 Examples of Validated Questionnaires for Sexual Health

Measure	Construction	Comment
Female Sexual Function Index (36)	19 items; domains tested (desire, arousal, lubrication, orgasm, pain, satisfaction) are summed to a total score	Recall period is 4 weeks, thus may be less useful in those who are not sexually active
Female Sexual Distress Scale-Revised (37)	13 items; quantifies the personal distress caused by any sexual complaint	Recall period on revised scale is 7 days
Body Image Scale (38)	10 items; evaluates appearance and any changes as a result of disease or treatment	Recall period is past 7 days
Dyadic Adjustment Scale (39)	32 items; evaluates adjustment, consensus, satisfaction, cohesion, and affectional expression	No set recall period
Personal Assessment of Intimacy in Relationships	36 items; assesses five types of intimacy—emotional, social, sexual, intellectual, and recreational	Describes both perceived and expected levels of intimacy within a relationship

Sexual Dysfunction

Sexual dysfunction is when one or more aspects of the sexual response cycle fail to function properly (33). Up to 90% of sexual dysfunction cases contain a psychological component while 75% have clear physiologic sources, with obvious significant overlap (26). In the realm of oncology, mainly physiologic causes affect sexual dysfunction (26). The *DSM-5* outlines sexual disorders (Table 16.6), which is just one category of causes of sexual dysfunction, in addition to psychosocial/interpersonal stressors, medical illness, depressive illness, and medication.

Chemotherapy often causes fatigue associated with loss of desire and decreased frequency of intercourse for most women (40). The effect of chemotherapy on gonadal function causing menopause can also lead to decreased sexual stimulation, sexual energy, and erotic pleasure (41). Chemotherapy-related neuropathies not only affect the hands and feet, but also the clitoris, which can decrease sexual arousal and women's sexual pleasure (41). In women, pelvic radiation can cause neurovascular damage resulting in delayed arousal and orgasm and vaginal changes that can lead to vaginal stenosis and fibrosis.

Management

Arguably, the most important factor in treating sexual problems is to ask about them (26). Beyond pharmacologic interventions, both dilators to

Table 16.6 Sexual Dysfunction According to *DSM-5* Summarized

Types of sexual dysfunction	Description
Female Dysfunctions	
Female sexual interest/arousal disorder	An absence or significant reduction in sexual fantasies or thoughts, desire, or receptivity to sexual activity at any time during the sexual encounter.
Female orgasmic disorder	Marked delay in, infrequency of, or absence of orgasm or reduced intensity of orgasmic sensations.
Genito-pelvic pain/penetration disorder	Persistent or recurrent difficulties with one (or more) of the following: vaginal penetration during intercourse, marked vulvovaginal or pelvic pain during vaginal intercourse or penetration attempts; marked fear or anxiety about vulvovaginal or pelvic pain in anticipation of, during, or as a result of vaginal penetration; marked tensing or tightening of the pelvic floor muscles during attempted vaginal penetration.
Male dysfunctions	
Erectile disorder	Marked difficulty in obtaining or maintaining an erection during sexual activity or marked decrease in erectile rigidity.
Male hypoactive sexual desire	Persistently or recurrent deficient (or absent) sexual/erotic thoughts or fantasies and desire for sexual activity.
Premature (early) ejaculation	A persistent or recurrent pattern of ejaculation occurring during partnered sexual activity within approximately 1 minute following vaginal penetration and before the individual wishes it.
Delayed ejaculation	Marked delay in, infrequency of, or absence of ejaculation.
Other dysfunctions	
Substance/ medication-induced sexual dysfunction	A clinically significant disturbance in sexual function that developed during or soon after substance intoxication or withdrawal after exposure to a medication.
Other specified and unspecified sexual dysfunctions	Symptoms characteristic of a sexual dysfunction that cause clinically significant distress but do not meet full criteria for any of the disorders in the sexual dysfunctions diagnostic class.

treat vaginismus or genito-pelvic pain/penetration syndrome and liberal use of lubrication can aid penetrative intercourse (24). Vaginal moisturizers and suppositories for vaginal dryness can be prescribed, including polycarbophilic ones like Replens or vaginal pH-balanced gels (e.g., RepHresh), although the data on their efficacy are limited (24). Beyond vaginal moisturizers, vaginal suppositories that contain vitamin A or E can also be used, with limited available data about treatment efficacy. Vaginal estrogen can be prescribed as a cream, ring, or table to effectively treat vaginal dryness (42). Further recommendations for women and men can be found in Table 16.7.

Recent studies have noted the success of brief psychosexual interventions and of addressing the informational needs of cancer patients

Table 16.7 Treatment of Sexual Dysfunction	
Treatment	**Example**
Psychosexual therapy	Sex therapists, marital counselors, or psychotherapists to address poor body image, guilt, fear, anxiety, or past sexual trauma, for example
Behavioral treatments	Various techniques, including insights into harmful behaviors in the relationship or techniques such as self-stimulation for arousal/orgasm problems
Mechanical aids	Vacuum devices for men or women (Eros for women), penile implants or bands to maintain erection, or vaginal dilators
Medication	For hormone deficiency: hormone shots, pills, or creams. For men: sildenafil (Viagra®) or tadalafil (Cialis®), for example, to increase penile blood flow to help improve sexual function. Take medications for symptoms control, for example, for pain, nausea, fatigue, if relevant.
Integrative medical treatments	Acupuncture or supplements, including yohimbine or L-arginine to improve genital blood flow.
Education and communication	Education about sex and sexual behaviors and responses to help overcome one's anxieties about sexual function.
Physical therapy	Pelvic floor exercises with a specially-trained physical therapist
Water-soluble or silicon vaginal lubricants and moisturizers	K-Y, Astroglide, or other lubricants for sexual activity. Replens or other vaginal moisturizers for female health and comfort.
Erotica	Videos, magazines, books, music, websites to help stimulate sexual arousal

(26). An effective method of treating sexual difficulties in cancer patients would be through the coordinated provision of information, support, and symptom management at one site, for example, in a sexual health program. The resources to develop such a program are not always available, but medical professionals can identify local practitioners with expertise in the treatment of sexual and fertility concerns—both physical and psychological—and may provide their patients with a referral list of such practitioners, making help with these problems more accessible as needs arise. Figure 16.1 explains how to build a successful referral network. Overall, by legitimizing the topics of sexuality and intimacy, and addressing fertility concerns early on in treatment visits, providers can help provide a comprehensive modicum of support for their patients.

The oncologist and healthcare team should build a referral network of specialists for the treatment of sexual dysfunction. The type of referral will depend on the patient's presenting problem.

A comprehensive referral network should include:

• A mental health professional to provide sex therapy and sexual counseling
• An endocrinologist to treat hormone excess production or deficiency, which may lead to diabetes, thyroid disease, or menopause
• A urologist to treat male and female urinary tract problems, and provide medical treatment for loss of sexual desire and erectile dysfunction.
• A gynecologist to assess and treat pain with sexual activity and to advise women making decisions about hormone replacement therapy after cancer treatment
• A sperm bank to store semen samples from men before starting cancer treatment.
• An infertility clinic offering in vitro fertilization and successful donor gamete programs, with staff familiar with cancer-related infertility in men and women
• A genetics clinic to counsel survivors regarding their concerns about birth defects or offspring cancer risks.

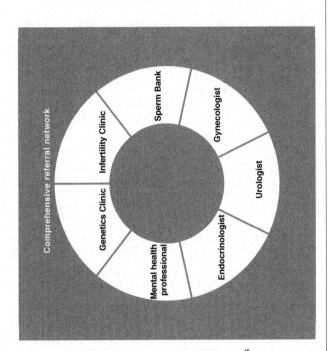

Figure 16.1 Building blocks of a successful referral network.

Source: Adapted from Richards TA, Bertolotti PA, Doss D, et al. Sexual dysfunction in multiple myeloma: survivorship care plan of the International Myeloma Foundation Nurse Leadership Board. *Clin J Oncol Nurs.* 2011;15 Suppl:53–65. doi:10.1188/11.CJON.S1.53-65

REFERENCES

1. Thaler-DeMers D. Intimacy issues: sexuality, ferility, and relationships. *Semin Oncol Nurs*. 2001;17:255–262. doi:10.1053/sonu.2001.27919
2. Schover LR. Sexuality and fertility after cancer. *Hematology Am Soc Hematol Educ Program*. 2005;2005:523–527. doi:10.1182/asheducation-2005.1.523
3. Cardonick, EH. Overview of infertility and pregnancy outcome in cancer survivors. *UpToDate*.Literature review current through October 2018.2018.https://www.uptodate.com/contents/overview-of-infertility-and-pregnancy-outcome-in-cancer-survivors
4. Moody LE, Beckie T, Long C, et al. Assessing readiness for death in hospice elders and older adults. *Hosp J*. 2000;15:49–65. doi:10.1300/J011v15n02_04
5. Fossa SD, Dahl AA. Fertility and sexuality in young cancer survivors who have adult-onset malignancies. *Hematol Oncol Clin North Am*. 2008;22:291–303, vii. doi:10.1016/j.hoc.2008.01.002
6. Niemasik EE, Letourneau J, Dohan D, et al. Patient perceptions of reproductive health counseling at the time of cancer diagnosis: a qualitative study of female California cancer survivors. *J Cancer Surviv*. 2012;6:324–332, doi:10.1007/s11764-012-0227-9
7. Armuand GM, Rodriguez-Wallberg KA, Wettergren L, et al. Sex differences in fertility-related information received by young adult cancer survivors. *J Clin Oncol*. 2012;30:2147–2153. doi:10.1200/JCO.2011.40.6470
8. Letourneau JM, Ebbel EE, Katz PP, et al. Pretreatment fertility counseling and fertility preservation improve quality of life in reproductive age women with cancer. *Cancer*. 2012;118:1710–1717. doi:10.1002/cncr.26459
9. Webber L, Davies M, Anderson R, et al. ESHRE Guideline: management of women with premature ovarian insufficiency. *Hum Reprod*. 2016;31(5):929–937. doi:10.1093/humrep/dew027
10. Imai A, Ichigo S, Matsunami K, et al. Ovarian function following targeted anti-angiogenic therapy with bevacizumab. *Mol Clin Oncol*. 2017;6:807–810. doi:10.3892/mco.2017.1237
11. Green DM, Kawashima T, Stovall M, et al. Fertility of female survivors of childhood cancer: a report from the childhood cancer survivor study. *J Clin Oncol*. 2009;27:2677–2685. doi:10.1200/JCO.2008.20.1541
12. Kelly JC. No "Safe" Dose for Avoiding Sperm Damage with Alkylating Agents. 2014 Annual Meeting of the American Society of Clinical Oncology (ASCO). Medscape; 2014.
13. Green DM, Kawashima T, Stovall M, et al. Fertility of male survivors of childhood cancer: a report from the Childhood Cancer Survivor Study. *J Clin Oncol*. 2010;28:332–339. doi:10.1200/JCO.2009.24.9037
14. Greil AL. Infertility and psychological distress: a critical review of the literature. *Soc Sci Med*. 1997;45:1679–1704. doi:10.1016/S0277-9536(97)00102-0
15. Patel A, Sharma PSVN, Narayan P, et al. Prevalence and predictors of infertility-specific stress in women diagnosed with primary infertility: a clinic-based study. *J Hum Reprod Sci*. 2016;9:28–34. doi:10.4103/0974-1208.178630
16. Matthiesen SM, Frederiksen Y, Ingerslev HJ, Zachariae R. Stress, distress and outcome of assisted reproductive technology (ART): a meta-analysis. *Hum Reprod*. 2011;26:2763–2776, doi:10.1093/humrep/der246
17. Yao DF, Mills JN. Male infertility: lifestyle factors and holistic, complementary, and alternative therapies. *Asian J Androl*. 2016;18:410–418. doi:10.4103/1008-682X.175779
18. Hussein AA, Tran ND, Smith JF. Fertility preservation for boys and adolescents facing sterilizing medical therapy. *Transl Androl Urol*. 2014;3:382–390. doi:10.3978/j.issn.2223-4683.2014.11.06
19. National Comprehensive Cancer Network (NCCN): Patient and Caregiver Resources. "Cancer and Fertility." 2018. https://www.nccn.org/patients/resources/life_with_cancer/fertility.aspx
20. Oktay K, Harvey BE, Partridge AH, et al. Fertility Preservation in Patients With Cancer: ASCO Clinical Practice Guideline Update. *J Clin Oncol*. 2018;36:1994–2001. doi:10.1200/JCO.2018.78.1914

21. PDQ Supportive and Palliative Care Editorial Board. Sexuality and Reproductive Issues (PDQ®): Health Professional Version. In: *PDQ Cancer Information Summaries [Internet]*. Bethesda, MD: National Cancer Institute (US); 2002. https://www.ncbi.nlm.nih.gov/books/NBK65975

22. Bruner DW, Boyd CP. Assessing women's sexuality after cancer therapy: checking assumptions with the focus group technique. *Cancer Nurs.* 1999;22:438–447. doi:10.1097/00002820-199912000-00007

23. Lee JJ. Sexual dysfunction after hematopoietic stem cell transplantation. *Oncol Nurs Forum.* 2011;38:409–412. doi:10.1188/11.ONF.409-412

24. Dizon DS, Suzin D, McIlvenna S. Sexual health as a survivorship issue for female cancer survivors. *Oncologist.* 2014;19:202–210. doi:10.1634/theoncologist.2013-0302

25. Southard NZ, Keller J. The importance of assessing sexuality: a patient perspective. *Clin J Oncol Nurs.* 2009;13:213–217. doi:10.1188/09.CJON.213-217

26. Hughes MK. *Disorders of Sexuality and Reproduction.* Philadelphia, PA: Lippincott Williams & Wilkins; 2013.

27. Masters WH, Johnson V. *Human Sexual Response.* 1st ed. Boston, MA: Little Brown; 1966.

28. Montejo-Gonzalez AL, Llorca G, Izquierdo JA, et al. SSRI-induced sexual dysfunction: fluoxetine, paroxetine, sertraline, and fluvoxamine in a prospective, multicenter, and descriptive clinical study of 344 patients. *J Sex Marital Ther.* 1997;23:176–194. doi:10.1080/00926239708403923

29. Bachmann GA, Leiblum SR, Grill J. Brief sexual inquiry in gynecologic practice. *Obstet Gynecol.* 1989;73:425–427.

30. Parish SJ, Rubio-Aurioles E. Education in sexual medicine: proceedings from the international consultation in sexual medicine, 2009. *J Sex Med.* 2010;7:3305–3314. doi:10.1111/j.1743-6109.2010.02026.x

31. Annon JS. *Behavioral Treatment of Sexual Problems: Brief Therapy.* Vol. 45. New York, NY: Harper & Row; 1976.

32. Park ER, Norris RL, Bober SL. Sexual health communication during cancer care: barriers and recommendations. *Cancer J.* 2009;15:74–77. doi:10.1097/PPO.0b013e31819587dc

33. Lemieux L, Kaiser S, Pereira J, Meadows LM. Sexuality in palliative care: patient perspectives. *Palliat Med.* 2004;18:630–637. doi:10.1191/0269216304pm941oa

34. Perz J, Ussher JM, Gilbert E. Constructions of sex and intimacy after cancer: Q methodology study of people with cancer, their partners, and health professionals. *BMC Cancer.* 2013;13:270. doi:10.1186/1471-2407-13-270

35. Redelman MJ. Is there a place for sexuality in the holistic care of patients in the palliative care phase of life? *Am J Hosp Palliat Care.* 2008;25:366–371. doi:10.1177/1049909108318569

36. Baser RE, Li Y, Carter J. Psychometric validation of the Female Sexual Function Index (FSFI) in cancer survivors. *Cancer.* 2012;118:4606–4618. doi:10.1002/cncr.26739

37. Derogatis L, Clayton A, Lewis-D'Agostino D, et al. Validation of the female sexual distress scale-revised for assessing distress in women with hypoactive sexual desire disorder. *J Sex Med.* 2008;5:357–364. doi:10.1111/j.1743-6109.2007.00672.x

38. Hopwood P, Fletcher I, Lee A, Al Ghazal S. A body image scale for use with cancer patients. *Eur J Cancer.* 2001;37:189–197. doi:10.1016/S0959-8049(00)00353-1

39. Spanier GB. The measurement of marital quality. *J Sex Marital Ther.* 1979;5:288–300. doi:10.1080/00926237908403734

40. Hughes AL, Hughes MK. Adaptive evolution in the rat olfactory receptor gene family. *J Mol Evol.* 1993;36:249–254. doi:10.1007/BF00160480

41. Hughes MK. Alterations of sexual function in women with cancer. *Semin Oncol Nurs.* 2008;24:91–101. doi:10.1016/j.soncn.2008.02.003

42. Frechette D, Paquet L, Verma S, et al. The impact of endocrine therapy on sexual dysfunction in postmenopausal women with early stage breast cancer: encouraging results from a prospective study. *Breast Cancer Res Treat.* 2013;141:111–117. doi:10.1007/s10549-013-2659-y

Caregiver and Family Grief and Bereavement (Including Anticipatory and Complicated)

Rachel Ombres, Karen Baker, and Lori Wiener

INTRODUCTION

Upon a patient's death, the focus of caregiving changes to attending to the grief of the patient's family and friends. Grief manifests in innumerable ways depending on several factors, including one's culture, religion, and personality, but is a universal stressor. As a clinician encountering grief, it is important to familiarize oneself with the family's background in order to contextualize their experience. However, regardless of the inherent variability of grief's manifestations, there are trends one can anticipate. In this chapter, we examine the constitution of normal as well as complicated grief. Grieving is not intrinsically pathological, but identifying characteristics of complicated grief, which can be associated with increased rates of depression and even mortality, is essential to provide appropriate care for those experiencing it.

NORMAL GRIEF

Grief: The emotional, cognitive behavioral response to loss of attachment; what we feel.

    Bereavement: The state of loss resulting from experiencing a death; what happens to you.

    Mourning: The process of adaptation that may also include established rituals or social spiritual passages to follow.

Grief During Chronic Illness

Grief is a reaction to the experience of a loss. Loss can manifest in several ways. Therefore, one can imagine that for many people caring for someone with a serious illness, grieving can begin long before that person dies. For example, a woman whose husband has advanced Parkinson's disease and dementia may grieve the loss of his typical companionship. The patient himself may grieve the loss of his function and independence.

- Be aware of these emotions in order to help patient and family cope with illness and the losses it brings.
- Empathically recognize the loss to provide comfort and a sense of communion between clinician and patient.
- Seek opportunity to direct care in a way that addresses the loss. In the example given earlier, depending on the goals of the patient's care, recognizing that the loss of independence is particularly troubling may lead a clinician to prioritize care that aims to maximize or preserve function, instead of recommending treatments that may further deteriorate it.

Anticipatory Grief

As end of life draws near there may be an emergence of anticipatory grief, a pre-death contemplation. What will the future be like in the absence of this person? These thoughts may not be expressed, but may present as anxiety. Prevalence of pre-death symptoms in care givers can be as high as 38% (1). Families that acted in preparation of death were less likely to suffer depression or complicated grief (2).

Emergent Grief

The way in which a person will ultimately experience grief and progress through bereavement may begin immediately upon the notification of a loved one's death. Studies have shown that the way in which a person discovers that a loved one has died can contribute to the grieving experience and can be associated with the development of complicated grief. Therefore, training in death notification communication is essential for clinicians.

Techniques for notifying family of a patient's death:

- Preparation
  - Choose who should deliver the news
    - A person with sufficient time available to support the family after the discussion
    - A person well informed about the medical details and other relevant circumstances relating to the illness or injury
    - Notably, this ideal notifier is not always the attending physician. However, in cases of unexpected deaths, it is recommend that the attending physician be present during news delivery
  - Confirm the details of the case prior to conversing with family
    - Review the chart for medical details related to the death
    - Discuss the case with the nurse; often he or she may know more about the family's dynamics and how to prepare for the conversation
    - Determine the patient's and/or family's faith and if chaplain accompaniment is appropriate
    - Notify the attending physician
  - Find a quiet, private location
    - Avoid telephone notification if possible, especially if death is unexpected. See following text.
- Meeting with family/loved ones
  - Consider having a nurse or chaplain accompany you during the notification conversation
  - Introduce yourself and your relationship to the deceased and ask that all others present do the same if possible
  - Take a comfortable position in the room, inviting those present to sit if possible
- Language
  - Refer to the deceased by his or her name

- Offer a preparatory statement, such as "I am afraid I am here to discuss some difficult news" if the death was not imminently expected
- Use direct, unambiguous terminology to avoid misunderstanding, specifically using the words "died" or "dead"
- Express condolence with words ("I'm very sorry for your loss") and nonverbal gestures (e.g., hand holding) if appropriate and accepted
- Explain the circumstances of the death in nonmedical terms if requested. Know that many questions will arise in the following hours to days
- Be prepared for the following general questions, often encountered during death notifications:
  - Did he suffer?
  - Why did he die?
  - Was this preventable?
  - What do we do now?
- Follow-up
  - Ensure notification of the deceased's primary care physician
  - Sign a condolence card for the bereaved family
  - Consider attending the memorial service
  - Consider referral to supportive bereavement service agency

Techniques for Death Notification by Telephone

It is highly recommended that when delivering news of a person's death, communication should occur in person. This allows for more precise communication, more meaningful expressions of support and empathy, and it also enables clinicians to assess and ensure the safety of the bereaved during a vulnerable moment.

However, many times it is not possible to meet with families in person. During these circumstances, telephone notification should include the following unique steps, in addition to those outlined in the "Emergent Grief" secton :

- During your preparation for the call, ensure you know your hospital's policy about how long after death a body can remain in a room. Some families may want to travel to visit with the deceased prior to its transport to the morgue.
- Upon calling, ensure you are speaking with the deceased patient's emergency contact. Do not deliver news of death to a minor.
- Introduce yourself, where you are calling from, who you are calling to discuss.
- If you are unfamiliar with the person with whom you are speaking, take a moment to assess their understanding of the patient's illness.
- If the person is alone, consider delaying the news of death until they can come to the hospital or find a companion.
- Offer a preparatory statement before proceeding with more information, for example: "I am calling with what I am afraid is some difficult news."
- Allow for silence.

In addition to answering questions, if they arise, and offering words of condolence as you would in an in-person setting, be sure to also address arrangements for family to visit with the body of the deceased. If anyone plans to come to the hospital to view the body:

- Advise safe travel with companions.
- Notify the nurse manager or other unit personnel in order to arrange for someone to greet the family in the hospital lobby or parking area upon their arrival. Family should not enter the room alone and should be escorted.
- Inform the chaplain of the family's planned arrival.
- Visit with the family at the bedside upon their arrival.

The Normal Bereavement Course

There is no designated time frame for grieving to begin or end. It is a dynamic process, with initial recognition and reaction to the anticipated loss or at the actual time of death. There is then a phase of the lived experience of the loss, change in normalcy or routine that may be quite different without their loved one. Physical influences of grief have been described as feeling like they are in a fog, changes in sleep patterns, lacking energy. There is eventual release of or adaptation to the loss, ideally with eventual clarity of meaning and purpose in this new reality and future focused.

COMPLICATED GRIEF

Complicated grief is a pathological outcome from loss with a more extreme psychosocial, spiritual, or physical impact with a prevalence rate of 7% (3). The symptoms of grief distress can be recurring, persistent sorrow and often a preoccupation with the individual who died, or prolonged feelings of apathy or guilt. Complicated grief can develop into Posttraumatic Stress Disorder (PTSD), depression, Generalized Anxiety Disorder, or substance abuse. Those at high risk for complicated grief are those with a strong, unilaterally dependent relationship to the deceased, young age at the time of the death, poor social support, if the death was traumatic or violent, if they feel disenfranchised, or have an existing comorbid psychiatric diagnoses. Prevention is based on early assessment and recognition of poor coping or poor adjustment to the loss, encouraging counseling, connecting with others, group bereavement support, mind-body programs.

Death of a Child

From the moment a child is born, babies invite us into a mutually loving relationship that evolves with each developmental milestone as parents anticipate and plan for their child's future (4). Grief begins when parents realize that their hopes and dreams for their child's future need to be radically altered and occurs repeatedly as they witness their child's physical changes (hair loss, weight loss or gain, loss of limb, reduced energy, and quality of life), withdrawal from social activities (school, sports), and the emotional consequences associated with progressive illness such as pain, anxiety, and sadness.

- Regardless of the length of illness or cause of death, parents rarely feel prepared for their child to die.
- The special bond between the parent and child is threatened and grief often feels unbearable.
- The intensity of grief ebbs and flows, dependent on individual factors, family dynamics, cultural factors, the quality of the parent–child relationship, and the nature of the child's illness and death.

Normative and Adaptive Responses in Children

- Grief can present with a range of "normal" reactions (anxiety, sense of emptiness, sleep disturbances, withdrawal, frequent crying, yearning), consequently psychological morbidity should not be judged within the first year after the death of a child. Assessment of the acuity of grief is important.
- Most families can restore a potentially satisfying and meaningful life (5).

Clinical Presentations of Grief (4)

- *Anticipatory*—experiencing many of the same symptoms of grief while the child is alive as those experienced after the death. When excessive, parents risk not being emotionally present while the child is alive.
- *Acute*—intense grieving that occurs in the early aftermath of death. A parent may experience flashbacks of their child and events that took place at the time of death, listlessness, heightened startled reactions, nightmares, poor appetite, disinterest in previous activities or relationships, and transient thoughts of suicide (6).
- *Integrated*—grief no longer as disabling or preoccupying and becomes more integrated into day to day functioning (6). Acute grief reactivates on certain holidays, important family celebration days, and anniversaries (day and month of death).
- *Prolonged*—grief that does not dissipate with time and persists for years (7,8). Prolonged Grief Disorder includes symptoms such as difficulty accepting the loss, feeling shocked, bitter, distrustful, avoidance of reminders of the child, unending waves of acutely painful emotions that persist for more than 6 months post death (8).

Factors That Contribute to Positive Adaptation

- Clear and positive communication with the child's medical providers; sense of being part of the team
- Communication with the ill child (9)
- Strong family relationship (10)
- Faith and strong faith community
- Ability to find meaning (11)

Families at Risk of Difficult Bereavement Adaptation

- Pre-death suffering (12)
- Family dysfunction, including stressed family relationships

- Conflict with the ill child
- Conflict with the surviving child(ren)
- Prior psychiatric difficulties
- Substance use
- Poor social support
- Illness of other family members
- Financial crises

The Dying Child's Experience of Grief

- Talking about death is one of the most difficult and compassionate conversations a parent can have with the child.
- Providing honest information in age-appropriate words is helpful.
- Allowing the child to talk about worries and fears can reduce anxiety and emotional isolation at a time when closeness is most needed. It also enables families to talk about memories, express love, and say good-bye. Younger children can communicate their thoughts, hopes, and anxieties through play and art. Children's books have the potential to facilitate communication about death for children living with a serious illness and for children coping with the death of a loved one (13).
- Encouraging the child to express end-of-life preferences (including people they want near them and where they want to die) informally or with age appropriate advance care planning documents can be useful to the child, family, and medical providers.
- Discussing the family's religious or spiritual beliefs about death and what happens after death can be reassuring.
- Reassuring the child that he or she will not be alone is essential.
- Reminding the child that he or she will forever be loved and remembered is comforting.
- Giving the child time to create legacies (art, photographs, letters) or to give away belongings can be healing for the child and the family and friends after the child's death.

Grief and Bereavement Presenting as an Existential Distress

The spiritual diagnosis of grief and bereavement may stem from a shaken faith, feelings of resentment, estrangement, guilt, or loneliness.

The clinical assessment can uncover these through three areas of inquiry.

1. What gives you purpose and meaning?
2. Do you have a community that you are regularly involved with?
3. Are you embraced in a caring relationship?

Spiritual treatment may include:
- Spiritual care and counseling
- Connection with others
- Story creation

- Engaging in support groups
- Practice of meditation
- Receive Reiki, or other energy medicine modalities
- See a music therapist or seek out healing music, such as laments, chants, or vocalization

Grief Resources

Apps: Flutter helps teens deal with death
       Grief Support (apple)
       Cope with bereavement hypnosis (blackberry, android)
       Lilies; grief support for young people

Web: Griefnet.org
       Compassionate friends
       Mygrief.com
       Grieving.com
       MyGriefAngels.com

Blog: whatsyourgrief.com
       Refuge in grief; unexpected death
       Grieving Dads project

PEARLS

- Awareness of our own mortality
- Acknowledge the grief you assess, anticipate and teach what is expected and reframe as a normal response, meet the grieving patient or family where they are.
- It's okay not to be okay stoicism or masking feelings from patients and their families can come across as impersonal. Shedding a tear is real human connection as long as the focus is the patient and family not yourself.
- The best therapeutic intervention is your presence, no words need to be spoken; listen, avoid using clichés.
- Grief can challenge your own beliefs or re-emerge past personal experiences, allow time for processing and debriefing with a trusted mentor. If not addressed, accumulative grief can lead to work dissatisfaction, compassion fatigue, and burn out.
- Allow yourself work-life balance.
- Rituals of mourning can help as a collective team such as an annual memorial service, healing art and music, sending cards to families, and holding debriefing sessions.

REFERENCES

1. Coelho A, de Brito M, Barbosa A. Caregiver anticipatory grief: phenomenology, assessment and clinical interventions. *Curr Opin Support Palliat Care.* 2018;12(1):52–57. doi:10.1097/SPC.0000000000000321
2. Mori M, Yoshida S, Shiozaki M, et al. What I did for my loved one is more important than whether We talked about death: A nationwide survey of bereaved family members. *J Palliat Med.* 2018;21:335–341. doi:10.1089/jpm.2017.0267
3. Simon N. Treating complicated grief. *JAMA.* 2013;10(4):416–423. doi:10.1001/jama.2013.8614

4. Wiener L, Gerhardt CA. Family bereavement care after the death of a child. *Bereavement care for families.* New York, NY: Routledge; 2014.

5. Bonanno GA, Moskowitz JT, Papa A, Folkman S. Resilience to loss in bereaved spouses, bereaved parents, and bereaved gay men. *J Pers Soc Psychol.* 2005;88(5):827–843. doi:10.1037/0022-3514.88.5.827

6. Zisook S, Shear K. Grief and bereavement: What psychiatrists need to know. *World Psychiatry.* 2009;8(2):67–74. doi:10.1002/j.2051-5545.2009.tb00217.x

7. Lichtenthal WG, Cruess DG, Prigerson HG. A case for establishing complicated grief as a distinct mental disorder in *DSM-V. Clin Psychol Rev.* 2004;24:637–662. doi:10.1016/j.cpr.2004.07.002

8. Prigerson HG, Vanderwerker LC, Maciejewski PK. A case for inclusion of prolonged grief disorder in *DSM-V.* In: Stroebe MS, Hansson RO, Schut H, Stroebe W, eds. *Intervention.* Washington, DC: American Psychological Association; 2008:165–186.

9. Kreicbergs U, Valdimarsdóttir U, Onelöv E, et al. Talking about death with children who have severe malignant disease. *N Engl J Med.* 2004;351(1):175–186. doi:10.1056/NEJMoa040366

10. Kreicbergs UC, Lannen P, Onelov E, Wolfe J. Parental grief after losing a child to cancer: impact of professional and social support on long-term outcomes. *J Clin Oncol.* 2007;25(22):3307–3312. doi:10.1200/JCO.2006.10.0743

11. Kubler-Ross E, Kessler D. *On grief and grieving.* New York, NY: Scribner Press; 2005.

12. Jalmsell L, Kreicbergs U, Onelöv E, et al. (2010). Anxiety is contagious—symptoms of anxiety in the terminally ill child affect long-term psychological well-being in bereaved parents. *Pediatr Blood Cancer.* 2010;54:751–757. doi:10.1002/pbc.22418

13. Arruda-Colli M, Weaver M, Wiener L. Communication about dying, death, and bereavement: a systematic review of children's literature. *J Palliat Med.* 2017;20(5):548–559. doi:10.1089/jpm.2016.0494

Running a Family Meeting With the Palliative Care Team 18

Juanita L. Smith, Margaret M. Mahon, and Shana S. Jacobs

INTRODUCTION

Though many find achieving a successful family meeting challenging, it is a skill set that any provider may acquire. Understanding the elements of and common hurdles encountered in these meetings can improve a clinician's comfort with the process, and add to the patient's quality of care. Family meetings conducted with open communication, empathy, and consistency of information increase trust in the medical teams that are involved, and can improve family satisfaction (1). In addition, involving palliative care team members in family meetings is often key to a good outcome; participation in family meetings is one of the core "procedures" that a palliative team performs.

DEFINITION OF A FAMILY MEETING

Dimensions of a family meeting include time and attention dedicated to the exchange of information and ideas among the patient's care teams, the patient, and family members. A meeting may be formal or informal; both offer value. The meeting may focus on updates on the patient's condition, address family concerns, and/or involve specific care decisions that need to be made. Almost inevitably, psychological, interpersonal, and/or spiritual issues will affect the content and process of the meeting. Cognizance of this allows modification of content and process to meet the needs of the participants (Table 18.1).

PLANNING FOR A FAMILY MEETING

Who should participate? Participants in an informal meeting are typically those who are in the patient's room at the time of a provider's visit, or the patient and those who accompany the patient to an out-patient visit. Participants in a formal family meeting are more carefully planned.

Formal Family Meeting Participants: Who Should Be Invited?

- Patient
- Family or other close people, even if they disagree. (Ask the patient.)
- Physician and/or other clinicians from the primary team (the attending, if in a teaching hospital, trainees involved in the patient's care, nurse practitioners [NPs], others)
- Consulting physicians relevant to the discussion
- Members of the palliative care team (physician, NP, RN)

Table 18.1 Characteristics of Formal and Informal Family Meetings

Meetings structure	Characteristics
Formal	• Typically involve multiple medical teams • Scheduled • Interdisciplinary (multiple specialists, multiple caregiver roles) • Updates on patient's condition, often when things have not improved as hoped, or when the patient's condition has declined • Often involve breaking bad news • Often occur when a discussion about change in goals of care is warranted
Informal	• Typically short; often spontaneous • Likely occur multiple times during a hospital stay • 1:1 with patient and provider, or patient/family and provider • Provide brief status updates • Ensure patient/family understanding of patient's condition • May occur on morning rounds or during a routine daily visit • Discussion of more routine tests and procedures • Can contribute to getting to know patient/family, building trust, clarifying, and providing support

• Patient's social worker and/or other psychosocial team members
• Pastoral care/chaplain and/or patient's spiritual leader

Other attendees, depending on the purpose of the meeting, might include a representative from pharmacy, legal, the ethics committee, administration, or others.

It might be appropriate for students or trainees without a long-term relationship with the patient to participate in the meeting. If, however, there are too many white coats in the room or if the family seems overwhelmed by the number of participants, students should be asked to leave.

Should the Patient Participate?

Yes, whenever possible, the patient should participate in the meeting. A seriously ill patient may have an array of difficult treatment options to consider. Identifying the patient's goals (in the context of what is physiologically possible) may help alleviate uncertainty and moral distress among family members and even among caregivers. Using the patient's values as a guide, clinicians can more confidently recommend treatments that align with both sound medical practice and the patient's wishes. Ultimately, the patient can choose how much involvement he or she has in the process. If a surrogate is needed to assist with decision making, the patient's goals and values should still undergird decision making, hopefully also alleviating any decision-making burden for a surrogate.

Who Should Lead the Meeting?

The primary physician, who often has the most trusted relationship with the patient, generally leads the meeting, although other clinicians who know the patient well (NP, social worker, chaplain) may also play this role. If the focus is medical decision making, often the physician or another provider will take the lead. A palliative care specialist can assist and help navigate complicated family dynamics or guide complex decision making.

Where Is the Meeting Held?

A good meeting space should be able to offer privacy, provide enough seating for everyone to sit comfortably, and be clean. Ideally, the meeting should be held in a place where interruptions are minimal. The meeting leader should be able to see everyone in the room, to monitor how things progress during the meeting. If difficult topics are on the agenda, have tissues available.

Structuring the Meeting

1. Planning for the meeting
   Before starting a family meeting, the healthcare team should meet to lay some groundwork. Issues to discuss ahead of time:

   - *What are the expectations for the meeting?* This should be agreed upon among healthcare providers, perhaps in a pre-meeting. Examples of meeting expectations might be: the family will understand that the patient is very sick and unlikely to survive; the patient will understand his treatment options, change in code status, and so on.

   - *Is there a consensus on the patient's condition and the best next steps?* If there is not a clear next step for this patient clinically, is there a consensus on the options? For example, due to the progressive cancer, the patient may choose to go home with hospice or to remain in the hospital. The patient may choose comfort care only or might consider a clinical trial or palliative chemo. Are there options that are no longer available for this patient? Specifying options that are not available is at least as important as identifying valid disease focused therapies.

   - *Who is leading the family meeting?* This also should be discussed in the pre-meeting. The leader could be the primary provider for the patient, the attending individual on the specialist service (e.g., intensivist, cardiologist), or sometimes a member of the palliative care team. If the focus is not related to a specific medical treatment, a chaplain, social worker, or other team member might lead the meeting. The meeting's leader will start the meeting, set the agenda and tone, elicit the thoughts and concerns of the patient and family, and seek the input of the other staff and family in attendance.

Box 18.1 Helpful Sentences for Family Meetings

- Is everyone present who should be present?
- What is your understanding of your son's condition?
- What would your brother tell us if he were sitting with us?
- Did your mother ever say anything to you about what she would want in this circumstance?
- What kind of person is your husband? What were his beliefs about medical care?
- We should never ask you what *you* want us to do. We should only ask you what you believe your cousin would want.
- So I just want to make sure we have the same understanding. Our plan is. . . .

---

2. During the meeting (2–4) (Box 18.1)
   - *Always start with introductions*, making sure that the patient and family hear the name and role of every healthcare giver present, even students, or other observers.

   - *State the purpose of the meeting*, for example: "We are here to talk about what is happening with your cancer, and what our next steps might be." Keep it simple.

   - *Start with the patient and family's voice.* First, elicit their understanding of the patient's condition. This provides a basis for giving information based on what they already know. It also allows clarification of any misunderstandings that might shape patient or family responses or decision making. Further, if the patient or family talk first, they are more likely to hear what the team then says, rather than being focused on trying to remember their agenda.

   - *Tell the information.* Describe the patient's condition as clearly and with as little medical jargon as possible. Always start with the big picture before asking sub-specialists to focus on individual problems or organs.

   - *Identify decisions to be made, and ask specific questions.* That is, saying, "What do you want us to do?" begs for a similarly big answer, such as, "Everything." Explain options in the context of *this* particular patient and the likelihood of various treatments that can help toward achievement of the goals of care. For example, if a patient is dying of progressive cancer with lung metastases, CPR is not going to reverse the dying process, so patients and families should not be asked "If your heart stops, do you want us to do CPR?" Rather, the question should be structured with a limited number of feasible answers, such as "She is unlikely to survive CPR, and if she does, she will likely spend the end of her life in the ICU. Because she told us this is not how she would want to live, we recommend *not* doing CPR. What do you think?"

- *Give space for emotions.*
- *Summarize and next steps.* Ensure that the patient and family understand and agree with the medical team's perception of what was discussed at the meeting. Review what decisions have been made, what a short-term plan for care is, and allow for final questions. Make a plan for next steps, ensuring the patient and family never feel abandoned.

When Meeting Plans Go Awry

Many of the challenges of family meetings can be obviated by preplanning, especially identifying who will lead the meeting, and what outcome the primary team wants (e.g., a specific decision will be made, the family will understand the patient's condition). Still, there will be times when the best laid plans are abandoned because of unexpected dynamics. Flexibility is essential for successful family meetings (5).

- *When one person dominates the meeting.* There may be one person who commandeers the meeting, who talks a lot, and who listens little. This may be a provider who keeps talking, even saying the same thing repeatedly. This may reflect that provider's discomfort with silence. A family member might dominate the family meeting by talking about his own life challenges, repeatedly. A strong leader can bring things back to the patient-centered focus.
  - *"Mr. Washington, it sounds like you've really struggled with your own health. Does that help you to know what your sister would want?"*
  - *"As Dr. Adams has said, understanding your brother's course of treatment is very important. What would your brother say about what is happening today?"*

  Acknowledging the other's agenda, while bringing the focus back to the patient, and to the meeting's goal can be difficult, especially if discussions veer counter to the planned agenda. Gritti (6) suggests repeating and rephrasing as a means to keep the focus on those things the family needs to understand.

- *An apparent change in meeting goals . . . during the meeting.* Often, the goal of a family meeting, agreed in the pre-meeting, is to discuss a transition in the goals of care to a focus on comfort. If a provider unexpectedly introduces the possibility of more disease-focused therapies, it may not be possible to accomplish the meeting's goal. That is, if the plan was to inform the patient and/or family that further disease-focused treatments were not available, and there is a surprise announcement of more chemotherapy or more surgery for which the patient and/or family have been hoping, the planned goal of the meeting may not be achievable. Often, however, the language, is:
  - *"If your wife [gets stronger, gains weight, does well off the ventilator], then this other therapy might be available."*

  At that point, the meeting goal may be changed to "hope for the best and plan for the worst."

  - *"We will still work to get your wife off the ventilator, but at the same time, we will not escalate her level of care. If her heart stops, we still will accept that as her natural death, and not attempt resuscitation."*

- *A new voice enters the conversations.* There are times when a consensus about goals of care seems to have been established, but then a new perspective arrives. This may be a family member who has been estranged or otherwise out of touch, or a family member from a great geographic distance. Distance often breeds lack of understanding of the reality of the patient's condition. It may take time and consistency to get the sister-from California (or New York, or Florida, or Texas) current in her understanding of the patient's condition, and thus able to participate in decision making. Keeping the focus on the *patient's* preferences may unburden this relative whose responses are often mediated by guilt (7).

- *Nothing versus everything.* Far too often, in family meetings and other discussions, a patient is told, "We've done everything. There is nothing else we can do." There is *never* nothing else we can do. If this phrase comes up in a meeting, it is an opportunity to change the framework. "Dr. Jefferson is right. All treatments for the heart disease have been offered. We still have many options for your care. We will always be able to manage your symptoms with the goal of having you live as well as possible for as long as possible."

When the Patient Is a Child

Involving children in treatment discussions and family meetings makes some clinicians uncomfortable. Many children, however, can and should be included in hearing news about their illness and in making decisions about their care. There is no set age at which a child should be included in care decisions. Rather, the decision to involve a child depends on what is being discussed, the child's state of wellness (i.e., whether the child is too ill to participate), the child's preferences for inclusion, and the family's comfort with having the child present.

Children are capable of being involved in hearing bad news about their health and making and understanding important medical decisions. Bluebond-Langner (8) found that dying children know that they are dying, whether or not they have been told. Hinds and colleagues found that even children as young as 10 years old understood end of life decisions being made about them (9). Teens often seek to participate in advance care planning, and doing so does not cause them considerable stress or depression (10–12).

Perhaps the best way to determine if a child should be involved in a treatment discussion is to ask the child and family how they would like the child to be involved, whether the child would prefer to be part of the family meeting directly, or would prefer to be told the information later on. Again, the *child* should be included in this decision, not just the parents deciding for the child. Some children, especially younger children, may be intimidated by a large meeting with multiple medical staff and may prefer to discuss news and medical decisions with their parents, possibly including clinical staff they feel most comfortable with. Other children, especially older teens, may prefer to be involved directly.

For children too young or too cognitively impaired to be involved in decision making or even discussions, families are put in the position of making decisions in the best interest of children who have never have had the ability to articulate their own thoughts or preferences. Parents, however, generally know their children, even nonverbal children, extremely well. Most parents of ill children seek to be "good parents" (13,14), which they defined in a number of ways including "making sure that my child feels loved," "focusing on my child's health," "making informed medical care decisions," and "advocating for my child with medical staff." Clinicians should empower parents to be "good parents" to their ill children and to trust their instincts about their child's wishes and needs.

Very rarely, parents are unable to act in the best interests of their children. This may be because the pain of the child's possible death, or the perceived burden of making a decision that "caused" death (as opposed to allowing it) is perceived as imposing too great of a burden. In this case, multiple family meetings, and targeted parental support may help the parents to act in the child's best interest. In those cases in which this does not happen, the involvement of the ethics committee may provide additional support and guidance.

A Review of Surrogacy

The patient is the decision maker about her care. Even if the patient is unable to participate, her preferences should still guide decision making.

- *What is a surrogate?* "Surrogate" comes from the Latin, meaning, "to stand in the shoes of"." The surrogate is not the decision maker, per se, but rather is the patient's voice in decision making.
- *Surrogate responsibilities.* The role of a surrogate is to represent the *patient's* preferences in decision making, if the patient is unable, or chooses not to participate in decision making. The role of the surrogate is not to make decisions for the patient, but rather to be the patient's voice, indicating the patient's preferences. Ensuring that the surrogate understands the *patient's* preferences can unburden the surrogate (15) and perhaps alleviate tension arising from disagreements among family members.

One of the greatest difficulties in decision making, especially when the patient is unable to participate, is when family members insist on something that does not meet the patient's goals, or is physiologically not possible. When there is such a disagreement, the first inclination is often to ask, "Who is the power of attorney (POA)?"

- *What is a Power of Attorney?* Someone with PoA has legal authority to represent another person's interests in legal or financial affairs. *Power of attorney for healthcare* is a separate document, or a separate section of the same document in which a person (in this case, the patient) designates another (often called *the agent)* to make decisions on behalf of the patient. The PoA-HC is entrusted to make decisions that represent the patient's preferences.

  When a decision is needed about a patient's care, and the patient is unable to participate, the first step is often to look to the PoA for decision making. It is often possible to avoid recourse to legal considerations with a well-structured family meeting. Convening those involved in the patient's life (family, close friends) is an optimal setting for a discussion about the patient's preferences. Having a family meeting is often a way to avoid legal recourse while keeping the focus on the patient's preferences.

- *What if there is no surrogate or PoA?* If a patient has not appointed someone to act as the surrogate decision maker, either informally (e.g., written designation or during a discussion with a healthcare provider) or legally (through a PoA document), there is an order for who is the presumed decision maker for a patient who cannot speak for himself.

The typical legal order of surrogacy for decision making for an adult is typically as follows, but can vary by state:

1. Legal guardian
2. Spouse/partner
3. Adult children acting together; no priority by age
4. The patient's parent (the parents do not have to agree)
5. A sibling of the patient (no requirement for agreement)
6. A close friend

In the situation of surrogacy, health caregivers have a central role to ensure that the right thing happens. That is, by asking the right question, ("What would your father tell us if he were able to talk with us?") rather than keeping the focus on the surrogate providers ("What do you want us to do?"), and others can help the surrogate to be the voice of the patient.

CONCLUSION

A family meeting is an ideal mechanism for sharing information among providers and patients and families. A well-constructed family meeting takes planning, knowledge, and skills. Involving clinicians from a range of disciplines (physicians, nurses, social workers, chaplains, and others) is likely to improve the content and process of the meeting. The focus should always be on the patient's preferences in the context of what is physiologically beneficial. Family meetings can help patients and families adapt to the sometimes burdensome realities of a member's illness. Discussions that allow for understanding and even planning for the end of a patient's life may lead to decreased depression and complicated grief in surviving family members (16). While primary teams may be very good at leading family meetings, involvement of the palliative care team may facilitate understanding and help patients to achieve their goals of care (17).

REFERENCES

1. Wood GJ, Chaitin E, Arnold RM. Communication in the ICU: Holding a family meeting. *Up To Date.* 2017. https://www.uptodate.com/contents/communication-in-the-icu -holding-a-family-meeting
2. Baile WF, Buckman R, Lenzi R, et al. SPIKES. A six-step protocol for delivering bad news: application to the patient with cancer. *Oncologist.* 2000;5(4):302–311. doi:10.1634/ theoncologist.5-4-302

3. Feudtner C. Collaborative communication in pediatric palliative care: a foundation for problem-solving and decision-making. *Pediatr Clin North Am.* 2007;54(5):583–607. doi:10.1016/j.pcl.2007.07.008

4. Levetown M. Communicating with children and families: from everyday interactions to skill in conveying distressing information. American Academy of Pediatrics Committee on Bioethics. *Pediatrics.* 2008;121(5):e1441–e1460. doi:10.1542/peds.2008-0565

5. Weissman DE, Quill T, Arnold RM. Fast Facts and Concepts #222. Preparing for the family meeting. 2015. https://www.mypcnow.org/blank-qrd7h

6. Gritti P. The family meetings in oncology: some practical guidelines. *Front Psychol.* 2015;5:1552. doi:10.3389/fpsyg.2014.01552

7. Ambuel B, Weissman DE. Fast Facts & Concepts #16. Moderating an end-of-life family conference. 2015. https://www.mypcnow.org/blank-qy84d

8. Bluebond-Langner M. *The Private Worlds of Dying Children.* Princeton, NJ: Princeton University Press; 1978.

9. Hinds PS, Drew D, Oakes LL, et al. End-of-Life care preferences of pediatric patients with cancer. *J Clin Oncol.* 2005;23:9146–9154. doi:10.1200/JCO.2005.10.538

10. Bluebond-Langner M, Belasco JB, DeMesquita Wander M. I want to live, until I don't want to live anymore: Involving children with life-threatening and life-shortening illnesses in decision making about care and treatment. *Nurs Clin North Am.* 2010;45:29–43. doi:10.1016/j.cnur.2010.03.004

11. Jacobs S, Perez J, Cheng YI, et al. Teen end of life preferences and congruence with their parents' perceptions: results of a survey of teens with cancer. *Pediatr Blood Cancer.* 2015;62(4):710–714. doi:10.1002/pbc.25358

12. Lyon ME, Jacobs S, Briggs L, et al. Family-centered advance care planning for teens with cancer. *JAMA Pediatr.* 2013;167(5):460–467. doi:10.1001/jamapediatrics.2013.943

13. Feudtner C, Walter JK, Faerber JA, et al. Good-parent beliefs of parents of seriously ill children. *JAMA Pediatr.* 2015;169(1):39–47. doi:10.1001/jamapediatrics.2014.2341

14. Hinds PS, Oakes LL, Hicks J, et al. "Trying to be a good parent" as defined by interviews with parents who made phase I, terminal care, and resuscitation decisions for their children. *J Clin Oncol.* 2009;27:5979–5985. doi:10.1200/JCO.2008.20.0204

15. Weissman DE, Quill T, Arnold RM. Fast Facts and Concepts #226. Helping surrogates make decisions. 2015. https://www.mypcnow.org/blank-fpu2r

16. Yamaguchi T, Maeda I, Hatano Y, et al. Effects of end-of-life discussions on the mental health of bereaved family members and quality of patient death and care. *J Pain Symptom Manage.* 2017;54:17–26. doi:10.1016/j.jpainsymman.2017.03.008

17. Carson SS, Cox CE, Wallenstein S, et al. Effect of Palliative Care-Led meetings for families of patients with chronic critical illness. A randomized clinical trial. *JAMA.* 2016;316:51–62. doi:10.1001/jama.2016.8474

Caring for the Family Caregiver of Cancer Patients 19

Lori Wiener, Margaret Bevans, Amy M. Garee,
and Allison J. Applebaum

INTRODUCTION

Caregivers of patients with chronic, acute, or life-limiting illness have been described as "isolated, invisible, and in need" (1). This chapter provides an overview of the experience of caregivers, and interventions that can be implemented at various points throughout the trajectory of the illness.

WHAT AND WHO IS A CAREGIVER?

The National Cancer Institute defines a "caregiver" as a family member or friend who helps a loved one manage cancer treatment in ways ranging from day-to-day activities of daily living to healthcare needs at home (2). The terms "informal caregiver," "unpaid caregiver," and "family caregiver" are often used interchangeably to refer to unpaid assistance to an adult or child with functional and/or cognitive limitations.

- Caregivers are diverse in terms of age, gender, socioeconomic status, and race/ethnicity.
- They may be family members, friends, health professionals, or members of the clergy.
- Caregivers may give care at home or in a hospital or other healthcare setting. The care they provide extends from diagnosis, treatment, through survivorship and end of life.
- They may provide physical, social, emotional, financial, spiritual, and logistical support.
- Caregivers bring a set of predisposing factors (genetic, attitudinal, personality, and environmental) that impact or hinder their resilience as caregivers.

Approximately 2.8 million Americans provide unpaid care to an adult family member or friend diagnosed with cancer (3). Being a caregiver is demanding, as it is associated with persistent emotional, mental, and physical needs. When the caregiver reports poor health, the patient is negatively affected (4).

PSYCHOSOCIAL CHALLENGES OF CAREGIVING

An increasing number of papers, in both the lay and professional literature, have documented the physical, social, and psychological impact of family caregiving for cancer patients (5–9). Caregivers are often called upon to understand complex medication regimens, contact 'hard to reach' medical providers, navigate a difficult health and legal system, advocate for services, negotiate with insurance companies, and/or manage the household, finances, and children (10). In addition, worrying about the future and the emotional strain of renegotiating roles within the relationship to the patient and the family can be burdensome, frustrating, and exhausting.

Caregiving can also give one a sense of meaning and pride. These positive feelings can help provide the strength and endurance to continue in the role and to adapt to their loved one's changing needs. In addition, the experiences, skills, and internal resources that caregivers bring into their role may enhance their emotional well-being (11).

ASSESSING CAREGIVER BURDEN

The needs of caregivers are often overlooked by healthcare providers, friends, and family members in the face of the complex needs of the person with cancer (12–14). At the time of diagnosis or early in the cancer trajectory, it is critical to acknowledge the primary caregiver(s) and complete an initial assessment (8) that includes:

- Willingness to care for the patient and availability (e.g., proximity to the patient)
- Ability to provide care
  - General health
  - Physical health and mobility
  - Emotional health and stability (e.g., mental health history including depression or anxiety)
  - Cognitive skills
  - Competing demands
- Knowledge and skill related to the patient's needs

Providers should repeat these assessments of the caregiver at critical points along the cancer trajectory to assess distress that might suggest a change in their burden and ability to cope with the role as caregiver. Well-established questionnaires can provide valid and reliable estimates of the caregiver strain and burden (Table 19.1). Challenges and risk factors that can lead to increased distress might include:

- Role recognition, role shifts (roles that the caregiver enjoys and those that are problematic)
- Increased patient needs (e.g., expanding required skills) or change in patient acuity (e.g., end of life)
- Caregiver poor health and psychosocial needs (e.g., emotional distress of the caregiver)
- Outside demands (e.g., employment, financial stresses)
- Isolation or loneliness in being disconnected from support network/ activities

Table 19.1 Screening of Caregiver Distress and Quality of Life		
Caregiver Self-Assessment	American Psychological Association: www.apa.org/pi/about/publications/caregivers/practice-settings/assessment/tools/self-assessment.aspx	18-item measure of caregiver stress
CareGiver Oncology Quality of Life Questionnaire (CarGOQoL)	Karine Baumstarck and Pascal Auquier: eprovide.mapi-trust.org	
Distress Thermometer	National Comprehensive Cancer Network: www.nccn.org/about/permissions/thermometer.aspx	Single-item global distress scale with 36 common problems
PROMIS Global Health	Health Measures: www.healthmeasures.net	10 item measure of physical and mental health
PROMIS, Patient-Reported Outcomes Measurement Information System.		

Importantly, assessment of psychosocial needs of caregivers needs to continue following the death of the patient, as the loss of the positives and benefits of the caregiving role is mourned along with the loss of the loved one (15).

EDUCATION FOR ONCOLOGY PROVIDERS

To infuse a systematic, formal assessment of caregivers of cancer patients into practice, education needs to be considered for all oncology providers (16). The Caregiver Advise, Record, Enable (CARE) Act is one major step in advancing the care of caregivers and holding hospitals and providers accountable. This legislation requires a hospital to have the patient designate a family caregiver at the time of admission. The hospital is then required to take reasonable steps to communicate with the caregiver regarding discharge plans and to educate the caregiver regarding the skills needed to care for the patient (states.aarp.org/tag/care-act).

INTERVENTIONS

Although most research on caregiver interventions finds them effective, very few interventions have been implemented in practice because they were not initially designed for the realities and cost restrictions of the practice setting (8). Categories of interventions that might benefit caregivers are vast with those often recommended for practice (www.ons.org/practice-resources/pep/caregiver-strain-and-burden) including cognitive behavioral therapy (CBT) or elements of CBT, psycho-education, or general supportive care.

Cognitive Behavioral Therapy

CBT is a psychotherapy that addresses the problem of how unhelpful thoughts and behaviors can lead to distress. The basis of CBT is that thoughts—not situations—cause emotional experiences. CBT therefore is particularly appropriate in the setting of cancer, where the situations are so frequently challenging.

- CBT has the most empirical support for ameliorating anxiety and depression in individuals in the general population. CBT, delivered in its traditional format among caregivers, however, appears to be less robust. A recent meta-analysis of interventions for caregivers that included one or more elements of CBT (17) found a small, statistically significant effect of CBTs but this effect disappeared when randomized controlled trials were evaluated alone.
- CBTs tailored to the unique needs of caregivers will likely be more efficacious. Studies have already shown that a CBT intervention for insomnia among caregivers (CAregiver Sleep Intervention [CASI]; Carter (2006), which incorporates stimulus control, relaxation therapies, cognitive therapy, and sleep hygiene (all of which have been found to be effective in the treatment of insomnia and other sleep disorders) led to improvements in sleep quality and depressive symptoms.

Psychoeducation

The information needs of caregivers are great (18–20). Psychoeducation is an evidence-based therapeutic intervention that provides information and support to better understand and cope with illness. A large number of psychoeducational interventions have been designed to provide caregivers with various types of information.

- Psychoeducational interventions have been shown to have a positive impact on caregivers' knowledge and/or ability to provide care (e.g., 21–27). Several have also been shown to have significant and positive changes on psychological correlates of burden (23,28).
- The majority of studies of psychoeducation have targeted caregivers of patients who were recently diagnosed with cancer, or who are at early stages of their disease (e.g., 22,24,28–31). Fewer have been specifically developed for caregivers of advanced or palliative care patients (26,27,32).
- Importantly, studies have shown that psychoeducation can be particularly effective when delivered to both patients and caregivers (21,24,26,30–32).

Supportive Therapy

Caregivers have great need for emotional support (e.g., 33,34) and hence, the majority of psychosocial interventions for caregivers includes some element of support. Interventions that are purely supportive in nature, however, are less efficacious at impacting psychological correlates of burden (e.g., emotional well-being, anxiety, depression; 35–38) than other, more targeted therapies.

Problem Solving/Skills Building Interventions

Caregivers are often unprepared to provide the care needed by the patient (e.g., 39,40), and such skill deficits contribute to the psychological burden they experience (41). Enhancing caregivers' ability—and confidence in their ability—to provide care may attenuate burden (42).

- Problem-solving and skill-building interventions aim to develop caregivers' repertoire of caregiving skills, including the ability to assess and manage patients' symptoms. Caregivers are taught how to quickly identify solutions to caregiving problems that arise, and how to enhance their coping with cancer caregiving in general (43–53).

- Problem solving therapies have significant and positive effects on psychological correlates of burden and problem-solving skills for caregivers. (45,48,50,51). Caregivers also report positive effects among the patients for whom they are providing care, including decreased depressive symptomatology (48,51) and attitudes toward treatment and coping (50).

- A recent study of an early palliative care intervention (ENABLE [Educate, Nurture, Advise Before Life Ends]) that addressed caregivers' unique self-care needs and assisted them with problem solving, communication, decision making, and advance care planning found that training in these areas led to lower depressive symptoms (54).

- Pediatric cancer caregivers' emotional well-being is important not only in itself, but because of its close relationship with the child's adjustment at diagnosis and during treatment (55). The Problem-Solving Skills Training (PSST) program has been established as an effective intervention for enhancing problem-solving skills and decreasing depression and anxiety in parents of children newly diagnosed with cancer (46). Following PSST, caregivers' mood improved and depressive and posttraumatic stress symptoms decreased over time (56).

- A second evidence-based approach uses cognitive behavioral and family therapy approaches within a medical trauma framework to reduce or prevent posttraumatic stress symptoms and enhance family functioning. This intervention, the Surviving Cancer Competently Intervention Program (SCCIP), has two versions. The first version of SCCIP was adapted for use with families at diagnosis in a three-session format that incorporated video discussions and was directed toward caregivers. The second version is delivered in a one-day, multiple-family intervention format (57).

Family/Couples Therapy

As cancer is a disease affecting the family, interventions that address family functioning show effects on caregiver burden (58–68).

- Couples therapy interventions have positive and significant outcomes for caregivers and patients, including improvements in relationship quality and functioning (60,63,66), communication (64,65), and sexual satisfaction (61) for both partners, as well as improvements in physical functioning (65) and psychological functioning (e.g., depression, anxiety, posttraumatic growth) in patients (60,61,64,66) and caregivers (60,61,64,66).

- Family-based interventions have also shown improvements in psychological functioning in patients and caregivers. For example, Kissane et al.'s (59) study of Family Focused Grief Therapy found that the intervention (which involved four to eight family sessions delivered from palliative care through bereavement care phases) led to significant reductions in distress and depressive symptomatology for those family members identified at baseline as having the greatest amount of distress, depression, and social adjustment problems.

- Delivery of care to families can be challenging. To address this fact, the FOCUS intervention (58) included three sessions conducted in the home and two follow-up phone calls, which focused on the following five components: family involvement, optimistic attitude, coping effectiveness, uncertainty education, and symptom management. The intervention led to significant decrease in negative appraisals of caregiving for caregivers and decreased hopelessness and negative appraisals of illness in patients.

Self-Care

Self-care activities are those that are performed daily to maintain and promote health and prevent disease (69). As noted throughout this chapter, when taking care of loved ones with cancer, caregivers have needs that are largely unmet and often overlooked (12). "Putting on one's own oxygen mask before helping another person with theirs" is analogous to the context of practicing good self-care. In providing care to oneself first, we are able to more effectively help others.

Studies have shown that caregivers for a loved one with an illness report high levels of caregiving stress, poor self-rated health, worse physical function, symptoms, and depressed mood (70,71). As more care is being provided in the outpatient setting, it is imperative that caregivers become capable self-care agents and invest time caring for themselves at home (72).

Examples of self-care activities are provided in Box 19.1. Resources for caregivers are provided in Table 19.2.

Box 19.1 General Self-Care

General Self-Care

- Invest in yourself. You are as important as those you care for.
- Get a massage or some other type of body work.
- Attend to your own healthcare needs (e.g., attend own physician appointments).
- Eat healthy meals.
- Learn and use stress-reduction techniques (e.g., meditation, prayer, yoga, Tai Chi).
- Caregiving is hard work so take respite breaks whenever possible.

(continued)

Box 19.1 General Self-Care (*continued*)

Cognitive/Internal Self-Care

- Embrace your caregiving choice.
- Focus on the things you can control.
- Learn to set boundaries. Only say yes to what you have the energy to do.
- Find what rejuvenates you, such as a walk in nature, time with a good friend, a cup of tea, or a fitness activity.
- Take time off without feeling guilty.
- Identify and acknowledge your feelings; you have a right to *all* of them.
- Change any negative ways you view situations.
- Set goals in small, manageable time increments.
- Celebrate the small victories and applaud your own efforts.

Physical Self-Care

- Set personal health goals.
- Get proper rest and nutrition.
- Exercise regularly, if only for 10 minutes at a time.
- Participate in pleasant, nurturing activities, such as reading a good book, taking a warm bath.
- Listen to soothing music.
- Journal about your caregiving journey.

Social Support

- Get connected
- Seek and accept the support of others.
- Seek supportive counseling when you need it, or talk to a trusted counselor, friend, or pastor.
- Attend caregiver meetings that are available on-line or in person.
- Build a support team to assist in meeting the patient's needs.
- Suggest specific things people can do to help you.
- Find services that include pet sitting, bookkeeping, transportation, shopping, cooking, and personal care to assist with certain tasks.

Future Directions

- Retaining caregivers in in-person support is challenging due to the temporal and financial demands of caregiving. The literature suggests that interventions that are time-limited (between 1 and 12 sessions) and

Table 19.2 Resources for Caregivers	
AARP/ New State Law to Help Family Caregivers	www.aarp.org/politics-society/advocacy/caregiving-advocacy/info-2014/aarp-creates-model-state-bill.html
The National Cancer Institute. Resources for Caregivers	www.caregiver.org/taking-care-you-self-care-family-caregivers
LIVESTRONG. For Caregivers	www.livestrong.org/we-can-help/caregiver-support
National Alliance for Caregiving and the Cancer Support Community	www.caregiver.org/taking-care-you-self-care-family-caregivers
The National Cancer Institute. Resources for Caregivers	https://www.cancer.gov/about-cancer/coping/caregiver-support
Navigate Cancer Foundation	www.navigatecancerfoundation.org
Oncology Nursing Society. Caregiver Strain and Burden	www.ons.org/practice-resources/pep/caregiver-strain-and-burden

allow for the possibility of sessions conducted via telehealth modalities (e.g., Internet, Skype) appear to be the most feasible and acceptable.

- While individually delivered therapies attend to the temporal demands faced by caregivers, the group setting has the benefit of providing social support, even when support is not the focus of the intervention.
- Caregivers of patients with advanced cancer at end-of-life are particularly in need of support. Interventions that attend to existential distress and death anxiety (e.g., Meaning-Centered Psychotherapy) (73) show promise in assisting caregivers at this particularly difficult moment in the care trajectory.

SUMMARY

The multidimensional burden that results from providing care to a patient with cancer is significant. It is critically important to assess the primary caregiver's needs early and consistently throughout the cancer trajectory. Fortunately, a growing number of psychosocial interventions have been developed specifically to address the psychosocial burden on caregivers. However, as each caregiver and care situation is unique, interventions need to be tailored depending on the patient's medical condition, emotional and physical needs, and required medical/nursing tasks. Interventions must also always address the caregiver's own problems, strengths, and resources. The provision of such support to caregivers in a timely fashion has the potential to buffer distress throughout the caregiving trajectory, and to foster a sense of benefit finding and growth in both the caregiver and the patient.

REFERENCES

1. Applebaum A. Isolated, invisible, and in-need: there should be no "I" in caregiver. *Palliat Support Care*. 2015;13(3):415–416. doi:10.1017/S1478951515000413
2. National Cancer Institute. 2017. https://www.cancer.gov/about-cancer/coping/family-friends/family-caregivers-pdq
3. National Alliance for Caregiving. Caregiving in the U.S. 2016. https://www.caregiving.org/wp-content/uploads/2016/06/CancerCaregivingReport_FINAL_June-17-2016.pdf
4. Litzelman K, Kent EE, Mollica M, Rowland JH. How Does Caregiver Well-Being Relate to Perceived Quality of Care in Patients With Cancer? Exploring Associations and Pathways. *J Clin Oncol*. 2016;34(29):3554–3561. doi:10.1200/JCO.2016.67.3434
5. Carter PA, Acton GJ. Personality and coping: predictors of depression and sleep problems among caregivers of individuals who have cancer. *J Gerontol Nurs*. 2006;32(2):45–53. doi:10.3928/0098-9134-20060201-11
6. Gilbar O, Ben-Zur H. *Cancer and the Family Caregiver: Distress and Coping*. Springfield, IL: Charles C Thomas Publisher; 2002.
7. Kent EE, Rowland JH, Northouse L, et al. Caring for caregivers and patients: research and clinical priorities for informal cancer caregiving. *Cancer*. 2016;122(13):1987–1995. doi:10.1002/cncr.29939
8. Northouse L, Williams A, Given B, McCorkle R. Psychosocial care for family caregivers of patients with cancer. *J Clin Oncol*. 2012;30(11):1227–1234. doi:10.1200/JCO.2011.39.5798
9. Stenberg U, Ruland CM, Miaskowski C. Review of the literature on the effects of caring for a patient with cancer. *Psychooncology*. 2010;19(10):1013–1025. doi:10.1002/pon.1670
10. Kim Y, Baker F, Spillers RL, Wellisch DK. Psychological adjustment of cancer caregivers with multiple roles. *Psycho-Oncology*. 2006;15:795–804. doi:10.1002/pon.1013
11. Litzelman K, Tesauro G, Ferrer R. Internal resources among informal caregivers: trajectories and associations with well-being. *Qual Life Res*. 2017;26:3239–3250. doi:10.1007/s11136-017-1647-9
12. Harding R, List S, Epiphaniou E, Jones H. How can informal caregivers in cancer and palliative care be supported? An updated systematic literature review of interventions and their effectiveness. *Palliat Med*. 2012;26(1):7–22. doi:10.1177/0269216311409613
13. O'Mara A. Who's taking care of the caregiver? *J Clin Oncol*. 2005;23(28):6820–6821. doi:10.1200/JCO.2005.96.008
14. Varner A. Caregivers of cancer patients. In: Christ G, Messner C, Behar L, eds. *Handbook of Oncology Social Work*. New York, NY: Oxford University Press; 2015:385–390.
15. Boerner K, Schulz R, Horowitz A. Positive aspects of caregiving and adaptation to bereavement. *Psychol Aging*. 2004;19:668–675. doi:10.1037/0882-7974.19.4.668
16. Ferrell B, Hanson J, Grant M. An overview and evaluation of the oncology family caregiver project: improving quality of life and quality of care for oncology family caregivers. *Psycho-Oncology*. 2013;22(7):1645–1652. doi:10.1002/pon.3198
17. O'Toole MS, Zachariae R, Renna ME, et al. Cognitive behavioral therapies for informal caregivers of patients with cancer and cancer survivors: a systematic review and meta-analysis. *Psycho-Oncology*. 2017;26:428–437. doi:10.1002/pon.4144
18. Aoun SM, Kristjanson LJ, Currow DC, et al. Caregiving for the terminally ill: at what cost? *Palliat Med*. 2005;19:551–555. doi:10.1191/0269216305pm1053oa
19. Adams E, Boulton M, Watson E. The information needs of partners and family members of cancer patients: a systematic literature review. *Patient Educ Couns*. 2009;77:179–186. doi:10.1016/j.pec.2009.03.027
20. Gansler T, Kepner J, Willacy E, et al. Evolving information priorities of hematologic cancer survivors, caregivers, and other relatives. *J Cancer Educ*. 2010;25:302–311. doi:10.1007/s13187-009-0034-9
21. Ferrell B, Grant M, Chan J, et al. The impact of cancer pain education on family caregivers of elderly patients. *Oncol Nurs Forum*. 1995;22:1211–1218.
22. Grahn G, Danielson M. Coping with the cancer experience. II. Evaluating an education and support programme for cancer patients and their significant others. *Eur J Cancer Care*. 1996;5:182–187. doi:10.1111/j.1365-2354.1996.tb00231.x

23. Horowitz S, Passik SD, Malkin MG. In sickness and in health: A group intervention for spouses caring for patients with brain tumors. *J Psychosoc Oncol*. 1996;14:43–56. doi:10.1300/J077v14n02_03

24. Derdiarian AK. Effects of information on recently diagnosed cancer patients' and spouses' satisfaction with care. *Cancer Nurs*. 1989;12:285–292. doi:10.1097/00002820-198910000-00004

25. Pasacreta JV, Barg F, Nuamah I, McCorkle R. Participant characteristics before and 4 months after attendance at a family caregiver cancer education program. *Cancer Nurs*. 2000;23(4):295–303. doi:10.1097/00002820-200008000-00007

26. Keefe F, Ahles T, Sutton L, et al. Partner-guided cancer pain management at the end of life: a preliminary study. *J Pain Symptom Manage*. 2005;29:263–272. doi:10.1016/j. jpainsymman.2004.06.014

27. Hudson P, Quinn K, Kristjanson L, et al. Evaluation of a psycho-educational group programme for family caregivers in home-based palliative care. *Palliat Med*. 2008;22:270–280. doi:10.1177/0269216307088187

28. Bultz BD, Speca M, Brasher PM, et al. A randomized controlled trial of a brief psycho-educational support group for partners of early stage breast cancer patients. *Psycho-Oncology*. 2000;9:303–313. doi:10.1002/1099-1611(200007/08)9:4<303::AID-PON462> 3.0.CO;2-M

29. Manne S, Babb J, Pinover W, et al. Psychoeducational group intervention for wives of men with prostate cancer. *Psycho-Oncology*. 2004;13:37–46. doi:10.1002/pon.724

30. Cartledge Hoff A, Haaga DG. Effects of an education program on radiation oncology patients and families. *J Psychosoc Oncol*. 2005;23:61–79. doi:10.1300/J077v23n04_04

31. Budin WC, Hoskins CN, Haber J, et al. Breast cancer: education, counseling and adjustment among patients and partners: a randomized clinical trial. *Nurs Res*. 2008;57:199–213. doi:10.1097/01.NNR.0000319496.67369.37

32. Hudson P, Aranda S, Hayman-White K. A psycho-educational intervention for family caregivers of patients receiving palliative care: a randomized controlled trial. *J Pain Symptom Manage*. 2005;30:329–341. doi:10.1016/j.jpainsymman.2005.04.006

33. Hileman JW, Lackey NR, Hassanein RS. Identifying the needs of home caregivers of patients with cancer. *Oncol Nurs Forum*. 1992;19:771–777.

34. Milberg A, Strang P. Met and unmet needs in hospital-based home care: qualitative evaluation through open-ended questions. *Palliat Med*. 2000;14:533–534. doi:10.1191/026921600701536282

35. Goldberg RJ, Wool MS. Psychotherapy for the spouses of lung cancer patients: Assessment of an intervention. *Psychother Psychosom*. 1985;43:141–150. doi:10.1159/000287871

36. Reele B. Effect of counseling on quality of life for individuals with cancer and their families. *Cancer Nurs*. 1994;17:101–112. doi:10.1097/00002820-199404000-00004

37. Kozachik S, Wyatt G, Given C, et al. Patterns of use of complementary therapies among cancer patients and their family caregivers. *Cancer Nurs*. 2006;29:84–94. doi:10.1097/00002820-200603000-00002

38. Walsh K, Jones L, Tookman A, et al. Reducing emotional distress in people caring for patients receiving specialist palliative care: randomised trial. *Br J Psychiatry*. 2007;190:142–147. doi:10.1192/bjp.bp.106.023960

39. Bucher JA, Trostle GB, Moore M. Family reports of cancer pain, pain relief, and prescription access. *Cancer Pract*. 1999;7:71–77. doi:10.1046/j.1523-5394.1999.07207.x

40. Schubart JR, Kinzie MB, Farace E. Caring for the brain tumor patient: family caregiver burden and unmet needs. *Neuro Oncol*. 2008;10(1):61–72.

41. Nijboer C, Tempelaar R, Triemstra M, et al. The role of social and psychologic resources in caregiving of cancer patients. *Cancer*. 2001;91:1029–1039. doi:10.1002/1097-0142(20010301)91:5<1029::AID-CNCR1094>3.0.CO;2-1

42. Sorensen S, Pinquart M, Duberstein P. How effective are interventions with caregivers? An updated meta-analysis. *Gerontologist*. 2002;42:356–372. doi:10.1093/geront/42.3.356

43. Cameron JI, Shin JL, Williams D, et al. A brief problem-solving intervention for family caregivers to individuals with advanced cancer. *J Psychosom Res*. 2004;57:137–143. doi:10.1016/S0022-3999(03)00609-3

44. McMillan S, Small B, Weitzner M, et al. Impact of coping skills intervention with family caregivers of hospice patients with cancer. *Cancer.* 2005;106:214–222. doi:10.1002/cncr.21567

45. Bevans M, Wehrlen L, Castro K, et al. A problem-solving education intervention in caregivers and patients during allogeneic hematopoietic stem cell transplantation. *J Health Psychol.* 2014;19(5):602–617. doi:10.1177/1359105313475902

46. Sahler OJ, Varni JW, Fairclough DL, et al. Problem-solving skills training for mothers of children with newly diagnosed cancer: a randomized trial. *J Dev Behav Pediatr.* 2002;23(2):77–86. doi:10.1097/00004703-200204000-00003

47. Toseland RW, Blanchard CG, McCallion P. A problem solving intervention for caregivers of cancer patients. *Soc Sci Med.* 1995;40:517–528. doi:10.1016/0277-9536(94)E0093-8

48. Blanchard CG, Toseland RW, McCallion P. The effects of a problem-solving intervention with spouses of cancer patients. *J Psychosoc Oncol.* 1996;14:11–21. doi:10.1300/J077v14n02_01

49. Kurtz ME, Kurtz JC, Given CW, et al. Depression and physical health among family caregivers of geriatric patients with cancer — a longitudinal view. *Med Sci Monit.* 2005;10:CR447–CR456.

50. Heinrich RL, Schag CC. Stress and activity management: Group treatment for cancer patients and spouses. *J Consult Clin Psychol.* 1985;53:439–446. doi:10.1037/0022-006X.53.4.439

51. Nezu AM, Nezu CM, Felgoise SH, et al. Project genesis: Assessing the efficacy of problem-solving therapy for distressed adult cancer patients. *J Consult Clin Psychol.* 2003;71:1036–1048. doi:10.1037/0022-006X.71.6.1036

52. Campbell LC, Keefe FJ, Scipio C, et al. Facilitating research participation and improving quality of life for African American prostate cancer survivors and their intimate partners: a pilot study of telephone-based coping skills training. *Cancer.* 2006;109:S414–S424. doi:10.1002/cncr.22355

53. Bevans M, Castro K, Prince P, et al. An individualized dyadic problem-solving education intervention for patients and family caregivers during allogeneic HSCT: a feasibility study. *Cancer Nursing.* 2010;33:E24–E32. doi:10.1097/NCC.0b013e3181be5e6d

54. Dionne-Odom JN, Azuero A, Lyons KD, et al. Benefits of early versus delayed palliative care to informal family caregivers of patients with advanced cancer: outcomes from the ENABLE III Randomized Controlled Trial. *J Clin Oncology.* 2016;33(13):1446–1452. doi:10.1200/JCO.2014.58.7824

55. Robinson KE, Gerhardt CA, Vannatta K, Noll RB. Parent and family factors associated with child adjustment to pediatric cancer. *J Pediatr Psychol.* 2007;32(4):400–410. doi:10.1093/jpepsy/jsl038

56. Askins MA, Sahler OJ, Sherman SA, et al. Report from a multi-institutional randomized clinical trial examining computer-assisted problem-solving skills training for English- and Spanish-speaking mothers of children with newly diagnosed cancer. *J Pediatr Psychol.* 2009;34(5):551–563. doi:10.1093/jpepsy/jsn124

57. Kazak AE. Research priorities for family assessment and intervention in pediatric oncology. *J Pediatr Oncol Nurs.* 2004;21(3):141–144. doi:10.1177/1043454204264394

58. Northouse L, Kershaw T, Mood D, et al. Effects of a family intervention on the quality of life of women with recurrent breast cancer and their family caregivers. *Psycho-Oncology.* 2005;14:478–491. doi:10.1002/pon.871

59. Kissane DW, McKenzie M, Bloch S, et al. Family focused grief therapy: a randomized, controlled trial in palliative care and bereavement. *Am J Psychiatry.* 2006;163:1208–1218. doi:10.1176/ajp.2006.163.7.1208

60. McLean LM, Jones JM, Rydall AC, et al. A couples intervention for patients facing advanced cancer and their spouse caregivers: outcomes of a pilot study. *Psycho-Oncology.* 2008;17(11):1152–1156. doi:10.1002/pon.1319

61. Christensen DN. Postmastectomy couple counseling: an outcome study of a structured treatment protocol. *J Sex Marital Ther.* 1983;9:266–275. doi:10.1080/00926238308410913

62. Stehl ML, Kazak AE, Alderfer MA, et al. Conducting a randomized clinical trial of a psychological intervention for parents/caregivers of children with cancer shortly after diagnosis. *J Pediatr Psychol.* 2009;34(8):803–816. doi:10.1093/jpepsy/jsn130

63. Kuijer RG, Buunk BP, De Jong GM, et al. Effects of a brief intervention program for patients with cancer and their partners on feelings of inequity, relationship quality, and psychological distress. *Psycho-Oncology*. 2004;13:321–334. doi:10.1002/pon.749

64. Scott J, Halford WK, Ward B. United we stand? The effects of a couple-coping intervention on adjustment to early stage breast or gynecological cancer. *J Consult Clin Psychol*. 2004;72:1122–1135. doi:10.1037/0022-006X.72.6.1122

65. Northouse LL, Mood DW, Schafenacker A et al. Randomized clinical trial of a family intervention for prostate cancer patients and their spouses. *Cancer*. 2007;110(12):2809–2818. doi:10.1002/cncr.23114

66. Baucom DH, Porter LS, Kirby JS, et al. A couple-based intervention for female breast cancer. *Psycho-Oncology*. 2009;18:276–283. doi:10.1002/pon.1395

67. Wellisch D, Mosher M, van Scoy C. Management of family emotion stress: family group therapy in a private oncology practice. *Int J Group Psychother*. 1978;28:225–231. doi:10.1080/00207284.1978.11491608

68. Mokuau N, Braun KL, Wong LK, et al. Development of a family intervention for Native Hawaiian women with cancer: a pilot study. 2008. *Soc Work*. 2008;53(1):9–19. doi:10.1093/sw/53.1.9

69. Moore JB, Beckwitt AE. Children with cancer and their parents: self-care and dependent-care practices. *Issues Compr Pediatr Nurs*. 2004;27(1):1–17. doi:10.1080/01460860490279518

70. Lu YF, Wykle M. Relationships between caregiver stress and self-care behaviors in response to symptoms. *Clin Nurs Res*. 2007;16(1):29–43. doi:10.1177/1054773806295238

71. Wiener L, Viola A, Kearney J, et al. Impact of caregiving for a child with cancer on parental health behaviors, relationship quality and spiritual faith: do lone parents fare worse? *J Pediatr Oncol Nurs*. 2016;33(5):378–386. doi:10.1177/1043454215616610

72. Dodd MJ, Miaskowski C. The PRO-SELF Program: a self-care intervention program for patients receiving cancer treatment. *Semin Oncol Nurs*. 2000;16(4):300–308; discussion 308–316. doi:10.1053/sonu.2000.16586

73. Applebaum AJ, Buda KL, Schofield E, et al. Exploring the cancer caregiver's journey through web-based Meaning-Centered Psychotherapy. *Psycho-Oncology*. 2018;27(3):847–856. doi:10.1002/pon.4583

Rebecca Berger and M. Jennifer Cheng

INTRODUCTION

Following the initial therapy for cancer, survivorship can extend for many more years. Survivors experience a myriad of physical, psychosocial, and spiritual effects that can last months, years, or the remainder of their life. This chapter touches on these after-effects of cancer and its treatment, offering healthcare providers advice on how to diagnose and manage these late-term effects in their patients.

SURVIVORSHIP AND PHYSICAL SYMPTOMS

Pain

- Reported prevalence of pain among cancer survivors is varied, reported to be as high as 40% (1).
- Screening for each encounter:
  - "Have you had frequent or persistent pain since the last time you were seen?"
  - "How severe has this pain been, on average, during the past week?"
  - A comprehensive pain assessment should follow, exploring the physical, psychological, social, and spiritual factors contributing to and affected by pain (2).
- Change in quality or severity of pain and new onset pain should prompt consideration for recurrent disease and secondary malignancies.
- Pain shifts from being a short-term issue to chronic concern. Management of pain will need to also shift to chronic pain management strategies and an interdisciplinary approach focusing on rehabilitation, and recognizing the limitations of long-term use of opioids (3).
- For comprehensive assessment of pain and treatment and care options, see Chapter 14.

Fatigue

- Cancer-related chronic fatigue is defined as "a distressing, persistent, subjective sense of physical, emotional, and/or cognitive tiredness or exhaustion that is not proportional to recent activity and interferes with usual functioning"(4) (Figure 20.1).
- Fatigue is one of the most common symptoms among cancer survivors (5), affecting quality of life, and has been underreported, underdiagnosed, and undertreated (4).

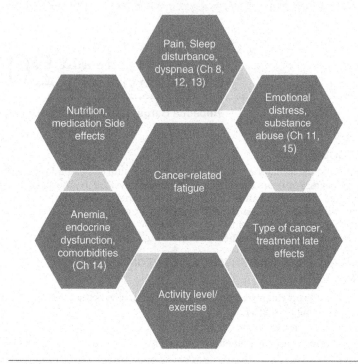

Figure 20.1 Frequent causative elements and/or concurrent symptoms in fatigue that should be assessed and addressed if present.

- The National Comprehensive Cancer Network (NCCN) guidelines recommend screening for fatigue at initial visits, regular intervals as a vital sign, and as clinically indicated. If symptoms are present, use a quantitative (0–10), semi-quantitative (mild, moderate, or severe) assessment, and/or impact on daily function and proceed with a focused history (see Chapter 13) (4).
- If new, assess for recurrence or secondary malignancy.

Neurocognitive Effects

- Cancer-related cognitive impairment (CRCI) commonly described as "chemobrain" or "chemofog" occurs in up to 70% of cancer survivors, with 30% to 40% reporting objective cognitive impairment including changes in memory, impairment in the ability to learn new things, concentrating, planning, and making everyday life decisions (6,7) (Table 20.1).
- CRCI has been associated with a variety of cancer types and treatments (chemotherapy, radiation, hormone therapies) (8).
- CRCI has significant impact on survivors' quality of life, emotional well-being, long-term functioning, and ability to return to work (8).

Table 20.1 Interventions for Cognitive Symptoms Based on Available Evidence

Behavioral approaches	CRCI education Environmental enrichment (regularly undertake mentally stimulating activities such as learning new and complex skills) Compensatory strategies (taking notes, setting alarms for reminders, minimizing distractions at work) Cognitive rehabilitation focusing on cognitive behavioral approaches, retraining of impaired cognitive abilities, and/or teaching compensatory strategies • In-person programs, and/or • Online cognitive rehabilitation programs that are web-based and done from home (e.g., Insight program at brainhq.com)
Exercise	Drawing from general aging and other disease groups: • Aerobic and resistance-based exercise Preliminary evidence in cancer survivors with yoga Balance training
Pharmacological agents	Currently, there is a lack of evidence to recommend any pharmacological interventions outside of a clinical trial

Source: From Vardy JL, Bray VJ, Dhillon HM. Cancer-induced cognitive impairment: practical solutions to reduce and manage the challenge. *Future Oncol.* 2017;13(9):767–771. doi:10.2217/fon-2017-0027

- Screening: A combination of neuropsychological testing by a neuro-psychologist and self-report measures of cognitive functioning is preferred for diagnosis and establishing an intervention plan. (9).

Reproductive Health and Genitourinary Symptoms

Fertility Issues in Females (Table 20.2)

Table 20.2 Fertility Risks for Women

Baseline ovarian reserve before treatment	Older patients typically are more likely to experience signs and symptoms of diminished ovarian reserve during gonadotoxic therapy Resuming menses after treatment is not a direct measure of fertility
Radiotherapy	The severity of depletion depends on: proximity of the ovaries to the irradiated field, the dose of radiation, and single high-dose vs. several fractionated doses

(*continued*)

Table 20.2 Fertility Risks for Women (*continued*)	
Chemotherapy	Mechanism of damage to ovary typically involves impaired follicular maturation and/or primordial follicle depletion • Alkylating agents are most studied for their gonadotoxic effects
Biologicals	Existing studies suggest that gonadotoxcity is agent-specific rather than a class-wide characteristic • Bevacizumab has a higher incidence of acute ovarian failure and a lower incidence of ovarian function recovery in those who received bevacizumab in addition to standard chemotherapy regimen

Source: From Kort JD, Eisenberg ML, Millheiser LS, Westphal LM. Fertility issues in cancer survivorship. *CA Cancer J Clin.* 2014;64(2):118–134. doi:10.3322/caac.21205

Fertility Issues in Males (Table 20.3)

Table 20.3 Fertility Risks for Men	
Cancer	Testicular and hematologic malignancies are often associated with impaired sperm production (oligospermia and some with azoospermia)
Chemotherapy	Impact on spermatogenesis through direct damage to spermatogonia (stem cells) Main classes that impact fertility: alkylating agents and platinum-based agents
Radiotherapy	Cumulative dose is important Can be due to direct exposure or scatter when other organs are targeted (e.g., prostate) Brain irradiation can impair pituitary function resulting in secondary hypogonadism
Surgery	Radical pelvic surgery (for prostate, bladder, or rectal cancer) can impair erections Removal of prostate and seminal vesicles from prostate and bladder surgery interrupts genital tract, leading to loss of ejaculation Retroperitoneal lymph node dissection can interrupt sympathetic nerves, resulting in anejaculation or retrograde ejaculation in some cases Orchiectomy for testicular cancer can impair (unilateral) or eliminates (bilateral) sperm production

Source: From Kort JD, Eisenberg ML, Millheiser LS, Westphal LM. Fertility issues in cancer survivorship. *CA Cancer J Clin.* 2014;64(2):118–134. doi:10.3322/caac.21205

- See Chapter 16 for further information regarding fertility and fertility preservation

Sexual Dysfunction in Men and Women

- Sexual dysfunction due to hormonal, physical, and emotional impact of cancer and cancer treatment can contribute to subfertility through decreased interest in sexual activity, intimacy, or even aversion to intercourse (Figure 20.2).
- Addressing sexual dysfunction requires consideration of the anatomical, psychosocial, and existential impact of cancer and cancer treatment on survivors and their intimate partners. Recommended interventions include: encourage couples to discuss their sexual intimacy, psychotherapy/counseling, pharmacotherapy, and alternative positions or techniques. Consider referrals to a urologist, sexual health specialist, and/or psychotherapist to review treatment options (10,11).

Nutrition and Health

- Recommend a dietary input that is high in vegetables, fruits, whole grains, and legumes, low in saturated fats and limit high-calorie foods and beverages.
- Alcohol consumption limited to no more than one drink per day for women and two drinks per day for men.
- Recommend adults engage in at least 150 minutes of moderate physical activity per week or 75 minutes of vigorous intensity activity each week
- Recommend children and adolescents engage in at least 1 hour of moderate or vigorous intensity activity each day, with vigorous intensity activity occurring at least 3 days each week.
- Avoid excess weight gain at all ages. Losing even a small amount of weight for those who are currently overweight or obese can have health benefits.

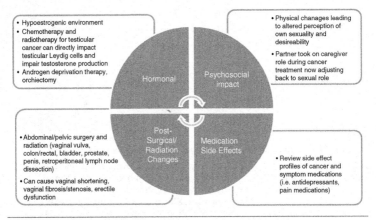

Figure 20.2 Contributors to sexual dysfunction.

- For more information, see the American Cancer Society (ACS) Guidelines on Nutrition and Physical Activity for Cancer Prevention and other ACS cancer specific survivorship guidelines (11–13).

Physical Disfigurement

- Many survivors of cancer report some level of physical disfigurement, which impacts their general well-being. 33% of adult childhood cancer survivors compared to 1.5% to 4.5% of the general population reported treatment related scarring and disfigurement in a small study (14,15). See Figure 20.3.
- Implications for providers
  - Identify patients at high risk of distress and refer to mental health professionals.
  - Promote positive coping skills and emotional adjustment, focusing on other positive aspects of the patient's being.
  - Locate resources for patients including free or reduced-cost wigs, plastic surgeons in cases of severe disfigurement, support groups.

Late-Term Comorbidities

- 80% of survivors of pediatric cancers will have disabling or life-threatening long-term effects by age 45, and 95% will have a chronic health problem (16). Patients require life-long monitoring for long-term health complications. For patients under 30 years of age, refer to

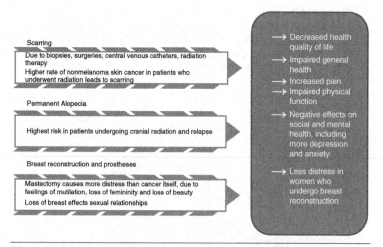

Figure 20.3 Impact of physical disfigurement in survivors of cancer.

Source: From Kinahan KE, Sharp LK, Seidel K, et al. Scarring, disfigurement, and quality of life in long-term survivors of childhood cancer: a report from the Childhood Cancer Survivor study. *J Clin Oncol.* 2012;30(20):2466–2474. doi:10.1200/jco.2011.39.3611; Shaw LK, Sherman KA, Fitness J, Breast Cancer Network A. Women's experiences of dating after breast cancer. *J Psychosoc Oncol.* 2016;34(4):318–335. doi:10.1080/07347332.2016.1193588

Children's Oncology Group Long-Term Follow-Up for Survivors of Childhood, Adolescent, and Young Adult Cancers for further screenings (17). For adult patients, refer to institutional guidelines.

SURVIVORSHIP AND PSYCHOSOCIAL/SPIRITUAL HEALTH
Cancer Recurrence and Secondary Cancers
Recurrence

- Recurrence depends on type of cancer and stage at diagnosis, with surveillance specific to each disease and stage.
- Routine surveillance for metastases often are not beneficial for patients with early stage disease, due to low risk of metastases and no benefit to survival in detecting recurrence early (19).
- The fear of recurrence in patients often causes them to request increased surveillance, which causes increased health costs with no benefit to survival. Healthcare practitioners must educate patients on potential harms of increased screenings and reasons why surveillance is not required (19).

Secondary Malignant Neoplasms (SMNs)

- Refer to Table 20.4 for long-term comorbidities in cancer survivors.
- The death rate from SMNs is higher than for any other cancer-related death, including recurrence. The incidence of developing a SMN at 30 years is 20.5%, with childhood cancer survivors having a greater than four times increased risk than the general public of developing an SMN. Patients with inherited cancer predisposition syndromes are at an even higher risk of developing SMNs. Life-long surveillance is required for all patients at risk (16,20). See Children's Oncology Group (COG) for screening guidelines which can be applied to all at-risk patients (Table 20.5).

Vocational
Issues of Unemployment

- Survivors of cancer are more likely than age-matched peers to be unemployed (18,21).
- Survivors report continued cancer-related symptoms and physical limitations as reasons for unemployment (21).
- Survivors are three times likely as controls to receive disability benefits (21).
- Not only does loss of work result in loss of income, but results in lower quality of life, lower self-esteem, and less sense of normalcy (22).

Return to School and Work

- Those who do return to work have decreased productivity and greater limitations at work than the general population due to job discrimination, hostility in the work place, and lack of support from managers/coworkers (22).
- Survivors often switch jobs or do not go back to school for career of choice in order to maintain health insurance and other benefits, so they are not working to full potential (18).

Table 20.4 Late-Term Comorbidities in Survivors of Cancer

System	Exposures	Other risk factors	Late effects	Screening
Cardiovascular	Chest radiation therapy, anthracyclines, platinums	Hypertension, lipid abnormalities, diabetes, obesity, smoking, illicit drug use, alcohol	Myocardial infarction, stroke, congestive heart failure, valvular disease, cardiomyopathy	Risk-based; periodic echocardiograms and EKG, focused cardiac exam
Pulmonary	Lung radiation therapy, bleomycin, carmustine, thoracotomy	Aging, smoking, illicit drug use	Restrictive lung disease, pulmonary fibrosis, exercise intolerance	Risk-based, serial pulmonary function tests and focused pulmonary exam
Urological/renal	Radiation therapy, platinums, ifosphamide, cyclophosphamide	Alcohol, illicit drug use, diabetes, hypertension, nephrectomy	Renal insufficiency, hemorrhagic cystitis, bladder cancer	Focused history, periodic monitoring of blood pressure, renal function tests, urinalysis
Endocrine	Radiation therapy, alkylating agents, steroids	Smoking, alcohol, carbonated beverages, lack of exercise, younger age at treatment	Obesity, infertility, dyslipidemia, insulin resistance/diabetes, growth hormone deficiency, precocious puberty, thyroid cancer, thyroid abnormalities	Evaluation of height, weight, BMI, Tanner staging in children until mature, lab evaluations (FSH, LH, testosterone, estradiol, T4, TSH, fasting glucose and lipids, HbA1c)

(continued)

Table 20.4 Late-Term Comorbidities in Survivors of Cancer (*continued*)

System	Exposures	Other risk factors	Late Effects	Screening
Central nervous system	Radiation therapy including TBI, intrathecal chemotherapy, corticosteroids	Age younger than 3 years at time of treatment, pre-existing learning disability or family history, sickle cell, higher rates of stroke	Learning disability, cognitive dysfunction, leukoencephalopathy, stroke, Moya-moya	Evaluation of educational or vocational progress, neurologic exam, head CT when concerning findings

All patients should be counseled on healthy living including maintaining healthy weight, avoidance of illicit drugs, smoking, and alcohol, regular exercise, and sun protection measures.

BMI, body mass index; FSH, follicle-stimulating hormone; LH, luteinizing hormone; TBI, traumatic brain injury; TSH, thyroid-stimulating hormone.

Source: From Record EO, Meacham LR. Survivor care for pediatric cancer survivors: a continuously evolving discipline. *Curr Opin Oncol.* 2015;27(4):291–296. doi:10.1097/CCO.0000000000000195; Children's Oncology Group. Long-Term Follow-Up Guidelines for Survivors of Childhood, Adolescent, and Young Adult Cancers 2013. http://www.survivorshipguidelines.org; Nass SJ, Beaupin LK, Demark-Wahnefried W, et al. Identifying and addressing the needs of adolescents and young adults with cancer: summary of an Institute of Medicine workshop. *Oncologist.* 2015;20(2):186–195. doi:10.1634/theoncologist.2014-0265

Table 20.5 Secondary Malignant Neoplasms in Cancer Survivors

Secondary malignant neoplasm	Exposure*	Time period†	Other
Acute myeloid leukemia/ myelodysplastic syndrome	Alkylators Epipodophyllotoxins	3–5 years 6 months–3 years	Usually refractory to treatment
Breast cancer	Chest irradiation: patients with Hodgkin disease at highest risk	10–20 years	Frequently bilateral disease, risk in Hodgkin patients similar to that of patients with BRCA1
Solid tumors: thyroid, sarcomas, brain tumors, basal cell carcinoma	Radiation	10+ years	Sarcomas poor response to treatment, BCC most common SMN

*Risk of radiation induced secondary malignant neoplasms increases with increased dose of radiation.

†Patients at younger age, especially less than 30, at highest risk of secondary malignant neoplasms.

Source: Record EO, Meacham LR. Survivor care for pediatric cancer survivors: a continuously evolving discipline. *Curr Opin Oncol.* 2015;27(4):291–296. doi:10.1097/CCO.0000000000000195; Bhatia S, Francisco L, Carter A, et al. Late mortality after allogeneic hematopoietic cell transplantation and functional status of long-term survivors: report from the Bone Marrow Transplant Survivor Study. *Blood.* 2007;110(10):3784–3792. doi:10.1182/blood-2007-03-082933

- Potential interventions to improve work reentry include better control of pain and fatigue, paid sick leave, preemptive counseling about careers, role playing common difficult situations patients may experience at work, developing a comprehensive work re-entry plan, including issues such as gradual return to work with limited hours and accommodations for disabilities, and assistance in resume writing and organizing a job search (22).

Pediatric Issues: Survivors of Childhood Cancer

- Childhood Cancer Survivor Study (CCSS) demonstrated 23% of childhood cancer survivors require special education services, compared to 8% of siblings. Those at greatest risk are children with brain tumors, children with leukemia, children treated with cranial irradiation, those with treatment-induced hearing loss, and those treated at younger than 5 years of age (23).

- Risk factors for nonemployment in adult survivors of childhood cancer include not finishing high school, cranial radiation, female sex, age less than 4 years at diagnosis, and chronic medical conditions including physical disability after therapy (23).

- As adult survivors of childhood cancer are less likely than healthy siblings to be employed, they are more likely to have difficulty obtaining health insurance, relying on Medicaid or Medicare (23)

- Unemployed survivors and those making less than $20,000 per year are more likely to suffer from depression, somatic distress, and anxiety (23).

Dating and Friendships After Cancer

- Variety of factors, both physical and physiological, make dating harder after the diagnosis of cancer. Those who are single lack the emotional and social support that a partner can provide. Support from partners increases posttraumatic growth, improves physical health, and facilitates sexual adjustment. Cancer survivors report issues such as physical changes, less trust in others, fear of rejection, and issues of disclosure associated with dating (15).

- Physical changes including permanent alopecia and scarring make socializing more difficult for some survivors due to feelings of decreased attractiveness. Survivors report long-term isolation due to friends not maintaining the relationship after the diagnosis (18).

Issues Unique to Survivors of Childhood and Adolescent Cancer

- Survivors of childhood cancer achieve fewer psychosocial milestones than healthy peers. Adolescents with cancer rely on their parents more than they would had they not gotten sick, which may stunt their psychosocial development (24) (Table 20.6).

Marriage and Children

- Surgery, radiation, and chemotherapy can be gonadotoxic. There are high level of distress reported by survivors who have issues with infertility. Discussing the issue prior to treatment and making patients aware tends to decrease distress (10).

- Ideal to refer patients to reproductive endocrinologists at the time of diagnosis; however, when this was not completed, refer after treatment to help survivors build a family (10).

- Fertility preservations options (10):
  - Embryo cryopreservation
  - Oocyte cryopreservation
  - Ovarian tissue cryopreservation and testicular tissue cryopreservation both experimental and not considered standard of care for pre-pubertal children

Table 20.6 Social Outcomes of Long-Term Survivors of Adolescent Cancer

	Impact	Other
Psychosexual development	Decreased for females compared to peers	Most significant for those treated with radiation
Long-term relationships	Overall no differences	Younger age, central nervous system tumors, radiation risk factors for not being in a long-term relationship
Marriage	Less likely to be married than peers and marry later	
Parenthood	Survivors less likely to have children and to have them later than peers	Female survivors especially report a strong desire to have children; however, infertility and fears of bad health outcomes in child affect parenthood
Living situation	Male survivors more likely to live with parents	Highest rate in those with central nervous system tumors

Source: From Dieluweit U, Debatin KM, Grabow D, et al. Social outcomes of long-term survivors of adolescent cancer. *Psychooncology.* 2010;19(12):1277–1284. doi:10.1002/pon.1692

- Sperm cryopreservation
- Surrogacy and adoption
- Health of offspring of cancer survivors are not impacted by diagnosis. Women with prior pelvic or abdominal radiation may have higher risk pregnancies (10).
- Women with breast cancer and melanoma may face a lower prognosis if diagnosed during pregnancy. Women with previous cancer diagnosis may delay pregnancy or choose to not get pregnant due to fear of recurrence and potential for worse prognosis (25,26).

Financial Stressors

- Greater than 30% of cancer survivors in the 2010 National Health Interview Survey report financial difficulties (27).
- Younger age at time of diagnosis, minority status, low socioeconomic status prior to diagnosis, recurrences/multiple cancer associated with higher risk (27).
- Financial difficulties stem from higher insurance premiums and deductibles, periods of lost income during treatment and due to

follow-up appointments, childcare expenses, and transportation costs especially for patients who live far from their healthcare providers (27).

- Patients with financial difficulties more likely to forego or delay needed medical care putting them at higher risk of discovering secondary malignant neoplasms, recurrences, and late-term effects later (27).

- Assess all patients for difficulty with finances, including inability to pay for healthcare -elated expenses, and refer to social work when appropriate.

Emotions

- Survivors can experience a myriad of emotions post cancer treatment. There may be a sense of relief and excitement about reintegrating into pretreatment life. Some experience their life-threatening illness in a life-transforming way and report subjective changes that lead to personal growth.

- There are also confusion and difficult emotions that cancer survivors may experience. While family, friends, and clinicians are ready to celebrate cancer remission, there can be ongoing fear of cancer recurrence or developing a second or secondary cancer, which is one of the areas of greatest unmet need (28).

- Survivors may also experience survivor's guilt, when the question of "Why did I get cancer?" transforms into "Why did I survive cancer, while others did not?"(29). Others may think that they did something to cause the cancer, or feel guilty about the burden placed on their caregivers during and after cancer treatment.

- There can be existential distress stemming from how life has changed from pre-cancer compared to post-cancer. Watching others in their peer group move on and progress steadily through expected life milestones while the survivor's life has taken unexpected turns can raise questions about meaning and purpose.

- What to do with these emotions?
  - Adjusting to emotions takes time
  - Name and acknowledge the emotion
  - Reframing and redefining goals and values and a reassessment of what now gives life meaning.
  - Developing a survivorship care plan with healthcare provider.
  - Reach out, don't isolate; talk with loved one, chaplain, support group and/or counselor about these emotions
  - If these emotions are starting to interfere with everyday life, consider referral to professional counselor and/or psychologist for evaluation

SURVIVORSHIP AND MENTAL HEALTH DISORDERS
Anxiety (30)

- Fifty percent to 60% of individuals with depressive disorder will have a comorbid anxiety disorder, most common of which is generalized anxiety disorder (GAD).

- Other anxiety disorders include: posttraumatic stress disorder (PTSD), specific phobias, panic disorder, agoraphobia, obsessive compulsive disorder, and social anxiety disorder.
- If at risk of harm to self and/or others, refer for emergency evaluation by licensed mental health professional and facilitate safe environment and one-to-one observation.
- GAD is the most prevalent of all anxiety disorders and is often comorbid with other mood disorders, so it is recommended to assess cancer survivors on initial visit and when clinical indicated for GAD.
- For additional information on assessment and treatment of GAD, see Chapter 12.

Depression (30)

- All survivors should be screened for depressive symptoms at initial visit, then routinely during follow-up visits when clinically indicated (i.e., disease recurrence, increase symptom burden).
- If at risk of harm to self and/or others, refer for emergency evaluation by licensed mental health professional and facilitate safe environment and one-to-one observation.
- Screening should be done using a valid and reliable measure with clinically meaningful cut-off scores. Start with the 2-item PHQ-9. If either item occurs for more than half the time or nearly every day during the last 2 weeks, proceed to remaining items in PHQ-9.
- Assess follow-through and compliance with recommendations. If after 8 weeks of treatment, the patient has poor symptom reduction or satisfaction with treatment despite good compliance, consider altering treatment course (e.g., add additional therapies, change medication, refer to specialist if not already).
- For additional information on assessment and treatment of depression, see Chapter 12.

Posttraumatic Stress Syndrome (PTSS) and Disorder (PTSD)

- In the *DSM-IV-TR*, PTSD diagnostic criteria was expanded to include diagnosis and treatment of a life-threatening illness as a stressor (31).
- Incidences of cancer-related PTSD ranges from 4.7% to 21% in childhood cancer survivors and 6.2% to 25% in their parents, with lifetime prevalence from 20.5% to 35% in survivors and 27% to 54% in the parents (32).
- Among adult patients, prevalence of current PTSD is estimated to be 6.4%, lifetime prevalence estimate of 12.6%, and 10% to 20% additional suvivors experience subclinical PTSS associated with distress and imparied quality of life (33).
- See *DSM-5* for diagnostic criteria (34).
- Per the NCCN's guidelines, ongoing and routine screening for distress via the distress thermometer and accompanying problem checklist can identify survivors with increased psychosocial–spiritual concerns, which should prompt formal diagnostic assessment and treatment

for PTSD, other mental health disorders, and need for psychosocial–spiritual support.

Substance Use Disorder

- The prevalence of substance use disorder (SUD) among cancer survivors is less certain. Medicare data found 11% of men with advanced prostate cancer have comorbid SUD. 38% to 43% cancer patients on opioids were screened as medium to high risk for opioid abuse on opioid abuse screening tools (35).

- A chart review of almost 400 patients ages 12 to 35 years documented opioid exposure in 94 cases and 12% was documented to have aberrant opioid-associated behavior (36).

- As cancer is increasingly becoming a chronic disease, clinicians need to be aware of the role of opioids in chronic pain management, risks of opioid misuse and diversion, and importance of an interdisciplinary approach to chronic pain (37).

- It is important to treat both addiction and pain in order to appropriately and successfully manage chronic pain.

CANCER AFTER-CARE

- With recent improvements in cancer therapies, 65% of adults with cancer will be alive more than 5 years after diagnosis, and 75% of children will be alive more than 10 years after diagnosis, necessitating long-term follow-up care (38).

Cancer Survivorship Plans (SCPs)

- The Institute of Medicine (IOM) recommends all patients completing treatment for cancer receive a SCP. SCPs help bridge the gap between patient, oncologist, and primary care provider, and allow patients to be active members in their care. Of note, they are time consuming to prepare with lack of reimbursement and clear delineation of who should prepare it for each patient. The American Society of Clinical Oncology has set guidelines for creating SCPs. All should include a treatment summary and a care plan (38,39).

Treatment Summary

- Patient demographics, disease and stage, therapy received, contact information for providers who administered the therapy, toxicities expected from therapies received (39)

Care Plan (39)

- Schedule of surveillance tests and visits required to detect recurrence and late effects, including who will provide the care

- Interventions to manage long-term toxicities of therapy

- General health promotion and screenings, including age-appropriate cancer screenings; specify if patients require testing at early ages than general population

- Long-term therapy the patient requires (such as adjuvant hormonal therapy for breast cancer) and how long the patient will require it
- General information about long-term psychological effects of cancer treatment

Transition From Pediatric to Adult Care (40)

- Adolescent and young adult (AYA) survivors treated in pediatrics, eventually age out of the pediatric setting, requiring transition to adult focused setting for continued long-term follow-up due to intensive therapies received.
- Studies have shown that AYAs are at high risk for becoming lost to care due to the personal and professional changes occurring in their lives. In addition, as not all institutions are familiar with long-term surveillance guidelines, AYAs frequently get lost in the system.
- Risk-based care proposed by the IOM, with a model chosen for each patient depending on availability of resources, anticipated late effects of treatment, and risk of secondary neoplasms.
  - Cancer center care: care led by oncology team or specialized survivorship clinic; best for high-risk survivors
  - Primary care physician (PCP)-led care: general medical care and survivor care led by PCP; best for low-risk survivors
  - Shared care: care shared by oncology providers and PCP with communication between them

Transition From Oncology to PCP Care (38)

- Patients believe oncologists should be more involved in their follow-up care than they are, while PCPs feel they should be more involved in patients' care than they are.
- Timing of transition depends on specific disease, likelihood of recurrence, and long-term effects of treatment.
- PCPs report uncertainty regarding patients' follow-up care, and patients feel uncertainty and fear. This can be alleviated with SCPs and relationships between PCPs and oncologists.

CONCLUSION

As therapies improve, more patients are surviving cancer longer. However, as patients are surviving oftentimes harsh treatments, they are left with a myriad of physical, psychosocial, and spiritual effects of both the cancer and the treatment that can last for months to years. Survivors face issues that include chronic fatigue, pain, impact on fertility and reproductive health, sexual dysfunction, risk of secondary malignancies and recurrences, neurocognitive effects, long-term disfigurement, and impact on cardiovascular, endocrine, and pulmonary health among others. These long-term effects can impact survivors in school and work, in their dating and marriage, and as they prepare to have children. Survivors often suffer from anxiety, depression, and PTSD. As healthcare providers treat cancer survivors, they need to be aware of how the disease impacts the total patient and offer resources as appropriate. Excellent websites include the NCI survivorship website (41) and The Livestrong Foundation (42). Resources specific to AYAs include First Descents (43), Stupid Cancer (44), Critical Mass: The Young Adult Cancer Alliance (45), and the National Comprehensive Cancer Network Guideline for Patients: Adolescents and Young Adults with Cancer (46). Children's Oncology Group (47) is a resource for children with cancer and their families.

REFERENCES

1. van den Beuken-van Everdingen MH, Hochstenbach LM, Joosten EA, et al. Update on Prevalence of Pain in Patients With Cancer: Systematic Review and Meta-Analysis. *J Pain Symptom Manage*. 2016;51(6):1070–1090 e9. doi:10.1016/j.jpainsymman.2015.12.340

2. Paice JA, Portenoy R, Lacchetti C, et al. Management of Chronic Pain in Survivors of Adult Cancers: American Society of Clinical Oncology Clinical Practice Guideline. *J Clin Oncol*. 2016;34(27):3325–3345. doi:10.1200/JCO.2016.68.5206

3. Glare PA, Davies PS, Finlay E, et al. Pain in Cancer Survivors. *J Clin Oncol*. 2014;32(16):1739–1747. doi:10.1200/JCO.2013.52.4629

4. Berger AM, Mooney K, Alvarez-Perez A, et al. Cancer-Related Fatigue, Version 2.2015. *J Natl Compr Canc Netw*. 2015;13(8):1012–1039. doi:10.6004/jnccn.2015.0122

5. Gosain R, Miller K. Symptoms and symptom management in long-term cancer survivors. *Cancer J*. 2013;19(5):405–409. doi:10.1097/01.PPO.0000434391.11187.c3

6. Treanor CJ, McMenamin UC, O'Neill RF, et al. Non-pharmacological interventions for cognitive impairment due to systemic cancer treatment. *Cochrane Database Syst Rev*. 2016;(8):CD011325. doi:10.1002/14651858.CD011325.pub2

7. Vardy JL, Bray VJ, Dhillon HM. Cancer-induced cognitive impairment: practical solutions to reduce and manage the challenge. *Future Oncol*. 2017;13(9):767–771. doi:10.2217/fon-2017-0027

8. Isenberg-Grzeda E, Ellis J. Cancer-related cognitive impairment. *Curr Opin Support Palliat Care*. 2017;11(1):17–18. doi:10.1097/SPC.0000000000000256

9. Duijts SF, van der Beek AJ, Boelhouwer IG, Schagen SB. Cancer-related cognitive impairment and patients' ability to work: a current perspective. *Curr Opin Support Palliat Care*. 2017;11(1):19–23. doi:10.1097/SPC.0000000000000248

10. Kort JD, Eisenberg ML, Millheiser LS, Westphal LM. Fertility issues in cancer survivorship. *CA Cancer J Clin*. 2014;64(2):118–134. doi:10.3322/caac.21205

11. Resnick MJ, Lacchetti C, Bergman J, Hauke RJ, et al. Prostate Cancer Survivorship Care Guideline: American Society of Clinical Oncology Clinical Practice Guideline Endorsement. *J Clin Oncol*. 2015;33(9):1078–1085. doi:10.1200/JCO.2014.60.2557

12. Kushi LH, Doyle C, McCullough M, et al. American Cancer Society Guidelines on nutrition and physical activity for cancer prevention: reducing the risk of cancer with healthy food choices and physical activity. *CA Cancer J Clin*. 2012;62(1):30–67. doi:10.3322/caac.20140

13. Runowicz CD, Leach CR, Henry NL, et al. American Cancer Society/American Society of Clinical Oncology Breast Cancer Survivorship Care Guideline. *J Clin Oncol*. 2016;34(6):611–635. doi:10.1200/JCO.2015.64.3809

14. Kinahan KE, Sharp LK, Seidel K, et al. Scarring, disfigurement, and quality of life in long-term survivors of childhood cancer: a report from the Childhood Cancer Survivor study. *J Clin Oncol*. 2012;30(20):2466–2474. doi:10.1200/jco.2011.39.3611

15. Shaw LK, Sherman KA, Fitness J, Breast Cancer Network A. Women's experiences of dating after breast cancer. *J Psychosoc Oncol*. 2016;34(4):318–335. doi:10.1080/07347332.2016.1193588

16. Record EO, Meacham LR. Survivor care for pediatric cancer survivors: a continuously evolving discipline. *Curr Opin Oncol*. 2015;27(4):291–296. doi:10.1097/CCO.0000000000000195

17. Children's Oncology Group. Long-Term Follow-Up Guidelines for Survivors of Childhood, Adolescent, and Young Adult Cancers 2013. http://www.survivorship-guidelines.org

18. Nass SJ, Beaupin LK, Demark-Wahnefried W, et al. Identifying and addressing the needs of adolescents and young adults with cancer: summary of an Institute of Medicine workshop. *Oncologist*. 2015;20(2):186–195. doi:10.1634/theoncologist.2014-0265

19. Shapiro CL, Jacobsen PB, Henderson T, et al. ReCAP: ASCO Core Curriculum for Cancer Survivorship Education. *J Oncol Pract*. 2016;12(2):145, e08–e17. doi:10.1200/jop.2015.009449

20. Bhatia S, Francisco L, Carter A, et al. Late mortality after allogeneic hematopoietic cell transplantation and functional status of long-term survivors: report from the Bone Marrow Transplant Survivor Study. *Blood*. 2007;110(10):3784–3792. doi:10.1182/blood-2007-03-082933

21. de Boer AG, Taskila T, Ojajarvi A, et al. Cancer survivors and unemployment: a meta-analysis and meta-regression. *JAMA*. 2009;301(7):753–762. doi:10.1001/jama.2009.187

22. Tamminga SJ, de Boer AG, Verbeek JH, Frings-Dresen MH. Return-to-work interventions integrated into cancer care: a systematic review. *Occup Environ Med*. 2010;67(9):639–648. doi:10.1136/oem.2009.050070

23. Gurney JG, Krull KR, Kadan-Lottick N, et al. Social outcomes in the Childhood Cancer Survivor Study cohort. *J Clin Oncol*. 2009;27(14):2390–2395. doi:10.1200/JCO.2008.21.1458

24. Dieluweit U, Debatin KM, Grabow D, et al. Social outcomes of long-term survivors of adolescent cancer. *Psychooncology*. 2010;19(12):1277–1284. doi:10.1002/pon.1692

25. Rodriguez AO, Chew H, Cress R, et al. Evidence of poorer survival in pregnancy-associated breast cancer. *Obstet Gynecol*. 2008; 112(1):71–78. doi:10.1097/AOG.0b013e31817c4ebc

26. Byrom L, Olsen C, Knight L, et al. Increased mortality for pregnancy -associated melanoma: systematic review and meta-analysis. *J Eur Acad Dermatol Venereol*. 2015;29(8):1457–1466. doi:10.1111/jdv.12972

27. Kent EE, Forsythe LP, Yabroff KR, et al. Are survivors who report cancer-related financial problems more likely to forgo or delay medical care? *Cancer*. 2013;119(20):3710–3717. doi:10.1002/cncr.28262

28. Simard S, Thewes B, Humphris G, et al. Fear of cancer recurrence in adult cancer survivors: a systematic review of quantitative studies. *J Cancer Surviv*. 2013;7(3):300–322. doi:10.1007/s11764-013-0272-z

29. Verano M. Surviving sruvivor's guilt after cancer Cure2016. 2016. http://www.curetoday.com/community/mike-verano/2016/01/surviving-survivors-guilt-after-cancer

30. Andersen BL, DeRubeis RJ, Berman BS, et al. Screening, Assessment, and Care of Anxiety and Depressive Symptoms in Adults With Cancer: An American Society of Clinical Oncology Guideline Adaptation. *J Clin Oncol*. 2014;32(15):1605–1619. doi:10.1200/JCO.2013.52.4611

31. American Psychiatric Association. *Diagnostic and Statistical Manual of Mental Disorders*. 4th ed. Washington, DC: Author; 2000.

32. Bruce M. A systematic and conceptual review of posttraumatic stress in childhood cancer survivors and their parents. *Clin Psychol Rev*. 2006;26(3):233–256. doi:10.1016/j.cpr.2005.10.002

33. Cordova MJ, Riba MB, Spiegel D. Post-traumatic stress disorder and cancer. *Lancet Psychiatry*. 2017;4(4):330–338. doi:10.1016/S2215-0366(17)30014-7

34. American Psychiatric Association. *Diagnostic and Statistical Manual of Mental Disorders*. 5th ed. Washington, DC: Author; 2013.

35. Chang YP. Substance abuse and addiction: implications for pain management in patients with cancer. *Clin J Oncol Nurs*. 2017;21(2):203–209. doi:10.1188/17.CJON.203-209

36. Ehrentraut JH, Kern KD, Long SA, et al. Opioid misuse behaviors in adolescents and young adults in a hematology/oncology setting. *J Pediatr Psychol*. 2014;39(10):1149–1160. doi:10.1093/jpepsy/jsu072

37. Pinkerton R, Hardy JR. Opioid addiction and misuse in adult and adolescent patients with cancer. *Intern Med J*. 2017;47(6):632–636. doi:10.1111/imj.13449

38. Jackson JM, Scheid K, Rolnick SJ. Development of the cancer survivorship care plan: what's next? Life after cancer treatment. *Clin J Oncol Nurs*. 2013;17(3):280–284. doi:10.1188/13.CJON.280-284

39. Mayer DK, Nekhlyudov L, Snyder CF, et al. American Society of Clinical Oncology clinical expert statement on cancer survivorship care planning. *J Oncol Pract.* 2014;10(6):345–351. doi:10.1200/JOP.2014.001321
40. Kinahan KE, Sanford S, Sadak KT, et al. Models of Cancer Survivorship Care for Adolescents and Young Adults. *Semin Oncol Nurs.* 2015;31(3):251–259. doi:10.1016/j.soncn.2015.05.005
41. Children's Oncology Group Patients and Families. n.d. https://www.childrensoncologygroup.org/index.php/patients-and-families
42. Critical Mass: The Young Adult Cancer Alliance–Medium. n.d. https://medium.com/critical-mass-the-young-adult-cancer-alliance
43. Outdoor Adventure for Cancer Survivors and Fighters. n.d. https://firstdescents.org
44. Shead D, Hanisch L, Corrigan A, et al. Adolescents and Young Adults with Cancer. n.d. https://www.nccn.org/patients/guidelines/aya/files/assets/common/downloads/files/aya.pdf
45. Simple Healthy Living. n.d. https://www.livestrong.com
46. Stupid Cancer. n.d. http://www.stupidcancer.org
47. Survivorship. 2016, September 16. https://www.cancer.gov/about-cancer/coping/survivorship

Palliative and End-of-Life Care for Adult and Pediatric Cancer Patients 21

Victoria D. Powell and Anne Watson

INTRODUCTION

This chapter covers issues related to end of life for children and adults with cancer. There currently still exists a minimal level of high quality research in this area; the majority of work, and the contents outlined in this chapter, especially symptom management, are based on consensus and expert opinion (1–7).

- Cancer is the leading cause of death by disease in children and the second leading cause of death in adults, worldwide, with large variability in death rates by country income level.
- Most common causes of cancer deaths in children are acute myelogenous leukemia, bone and joint cancers, cancer of the brain and central nervous system (CNS), and soft tissue cancers.
- Most common causes of cancer deaths in adults are lung, liver, colorectal, stomach, and breast cancer.

CARE AT THE END OF LIFE

End-of-life (EOL) care is a special subset of palliative medicine that focuses on care in the last hours to days before death. These domains include, but are not limited to (8,9):

- Physical symptoms
- Psychological, cognitive, and emotional symptoms
- Spirituality
- Family/caregiver needs and well-being, including bereavement care
- Quality of life
- Advance care planning

RIGHTS OF DYING CHILDREN AND THE DUTIES OF THEIR CAREGIVERS INCLUDE (10)

- Effective management of pain and other symptoms causing suffering
- Being allowed to participate and express wishes
- Being listened to and properly informed in an age-appropriate way
- Being surrounded by loved ones
- Having cultural, religious, spiritual, and social needs respected

- Being cared for in an age-appropriate setting
- Having access to pediatric palliative care services

Based on the recognition that dying patients do not receive adequate attention and care from acute hospital staff, some health systems have developed integrated care pathways—systematic approaches to improving the quality of EOL care (8) across a wide variety of settings. These have met with mixed success, and research is ongoing.

LOCATION OF DEATH

People facing imminent death often report a need for privacy and a desire to die in a place of their choice, with up to 70% of adults identifying home as their preferred place (11,12). For parents of dying children, evidence of preference is less clear; families ideally should be involved in a discussion of options (13). Despite increasing utilization of palliative medicine consult services and do-not-resuscitate orders, the proportion of pediatric cases utilizing hospice services and dying at home has remained essentially stable in recent years (14,15). Recently, there has been increasing interest in providing critical care transport at EOL in order to provide the option of withdrawal of life-sustaining treatment in the home (16,17).

HOSPICE

The hospice is a model of excellence in the provision of EOL care involving (18):

- Acceptance of death as the final stage of life
- Focus on quality of life (i.e., pain and other symptom management) rather than treatment with curative intent
- Dignified, compassionate, and family-centered care with a focus on the person, not the disease
- Multidisciplinary team-based approach: supervising physician, nurses, social workers, chaplains, nursing aides, volunteers, and other disciplines

The hospice is also an insurance benefit, initially established by the Medicare Hospice Benefit (MHB) and followed by many private insurance companies (19–24).

- Two physicians (one of whom includes the hospice medical director) must certify that the patient is terminally ill, defined as less than 6 months life expectancy if the disease follows its typical course. Criteria vary depending on the disease process.
- For patients with Medicare, Medicare Part A (acute hospital coverage) is replaced with the Medicare Hospice Benefit, a per-diem capitated reimbursement system to hospice agencies.
- The services covered include (notably, only covered if related to the qualifying diagnosis):
  - Durable medical equipment and medical supplies
  - Prescription medications

- Nursing provides assessment and skilled treatments through routine visits (generally once or twice weekly depending on need) with 24-hour coverage available by phone
- Social work services
- Spiritual care/chaplaincy
- Ancillary services as needed (e.g., nursing aide support, speech language pathology, respiratory therapy)
- Bereavement/grief support for families up to 12 months after patient's death
- A hospice does *not* generally cover blood transfusions, chemotherapy, and total parenteral nutrition, though some hospices and private insurance companies have begun to experiment with an "open-access" model where certain life-sustaining treatments are allowed.

Patients vary in the intensity of care needed at EOL. Medicare requires that certified hospices provide the following levels of care according to need (19,22,25):

- Routine home care: The majority of patients receive care at their existing residence (long-term care facility, private residence, or group home)
- General inpatient: Indicated for patients with severe symptoms in need of acute management requiring round-the-clock supervision and management
- Continuous home care: Indicated for patients primarily with 8 to 24 hour nursing needs due to symptom management. Goal is to keep patient at home while stabilizing crisis/severe symptoms
- Respite care: Families who need a respite from routine home care may utilize this service provided in a facility with 24-hour supervision for up to 5 consecutive days

Pediatric palliative and hospice care differs from adult palliative and hospice care in that it can be provided concurrently with curative care. The difference was mandated by The Patient Protection and Affordable Care Act (ACA) which requires that all state Medicaid programs to pay for both curative and hospice services for children under age 21 who qualify. The new provision, Section 2302, termed the "Concurrent Care for Children" Requirement (CCCR), was signed into law in 2010 (70).

DECISION MAKING AND COMMUNICATION

For children and adults, there is a need to normalize the conversation surrounding the EOL decision making as part of institutional wisdom and lived experience for both families and care providers. Discussions and planning are ideally not to be conducted in acute, crisis situations. If decision making and communication are not done well, complicated grief and regret can be expected. Informational materials provided should be language specific, culturally sensitive, and appropriate for education and development.

Pediatrics:

- EOL decision making is exceptionally challenging often because of overwhelming feelings of parental and professional responsibilities, prognostic uncertainty, and denial (the possibility of death of a child is unexpected and "unnatural") (26).
- There are no long-term negative consequences for parental participation, and to varying extents, most parents want to participate (27).
- A variety of support materials in the form of age-appropriate games, documents, and other tools have been developed to assist with serious illness conversation and EOL decision making. These can empower children and adolescents as well as their families by giving words and clarity, conversation starters, and psychosocial support (28,29):
  - Caring Decisions Handbook (30)
  - Voicing My CHOiCES™ for adolescents and young adults (31)
  - ShopTalk: A board game designed to help youth living with cancer talk about their illness (32)

Adults (4):

- Assess expectations and understanding of the patient as they near EOL, including wishes for loved ones to be present when making decisions, presence of an advance directive or previously stated wishes, and how much information is desired.
- Emphasize open and honest communication, but respect wishes of patient.
- Ask specifically about religious or spiritual practices and preferences.
- Ensure information is communicated to all members of interdisciplinary team and remains easily available (i.e., at top of note, in front of paper chart).
- Legacy: Ask how patient would like to be remembered and if help is needed (e.g., video to grandchildren on future birthday).
- EOL decision-making tools, games, and other initiatives have been used successfully:
  - The Conversation Game™ (33)
  - Five Wishes™ (34)
  - My Gift of Grace™ (35)
  - The Go Wish Game™ (36)

SPIRITUALITY, DIGNITY, AND EXISTENTIAL SUFFERING

Spirituality and the need to preserve dignity and meaning as illness progresses are integral aspects of EOL care. Terminal diagnoses and physical and emotional suffering can threaten or complicate the sense of meaning and purpose for a patient and the family. As EOL draws near, some patients and families experience existential/spiritual distress or death anxiety. While addressing spiritual and existential needs has long been recognized as a central goal of palliative medicine, little is known about what approaches are most effective overall, or whether certain groups may benefit from targeted interventions. Several researchers have sought to relieve existential suffering through interventions that aim to help the dying person identify meaning and legacy (37–39). A sizeable body of research has identified certain aspects of spirituality and religiosity that are associated with positive coping (40). To date, targeted interventions with spiritual or religious components to improve quality of life have shown inconclusive benefit (41). Providers should be aware that spiritual suffering can manifest as physical symptoms (e.g., intractable pain) and should always be addressed.

- Five things that both a dying patient and family member can benefit from hearing and saying (42):
  - I forgive you
  - Please forgive me
  - Thank you
  - I love you
  - Goodbye
- Visions/deathbed experiences (43,44):
  - It is common for patients to report transcendent experiences (e.g., visions of dead relatives, going on a journey).
  - Generally these experiences are comforting and separate from hallucinations which are distressing (43). If experiences are not distressing, they do not need to be treated simply because they are unusual.

ANTICIPATORY GUIDANCE

Observational studies have identified several discrete trajectories of functional decline in the last months of life based on the underlying disease process (see Table 21.1) (45,46). For most adult patients with cancer, functional status is relatively preserved until the last few months of life. Functional status declines more rapidly in the last month of life (45).

As the disease course progresses and EOL is nearer, it is helpful to assess patients' and families' understanding of the illness and their preferences about receiving information. Anticipatory guidance includes an explanation of symptoms that are natural, normal, and expected as EOL nears (see Table 21.2). Families of dying patients with a wide variety of disease processes indicate that accurate information and adequate communication are extremely important; not having these needs met can be highly distressing (11,47–49).

Professionals can help family members and patients recognize that EOL is approaching (see Tables 21.3 and 21.4). For loved ones, this can help mitigate future guilt or fear on the part of the family member that important treatments were withheld at EOL. It can also prevent the presence of normal symptoms/signs (i.e., death rattle) from causing excess distress that the dying patient is suffering. Skilled communication with families may help avoid futile interventions that will not produce a better outcome or result in unwanted side effects.

Table 21.1 At Least Four Distinct Patterns of Functional Decline in the Year Prior to Death in a Representative Sample of Individuals ≥65 Years Old

	Group characteristics	Percentage of sample	Description of functional decline in last year of life
Cancer	Cancer as cause of death on death certificate	21%	• Mostly independent/fully functional 12 months before death • Experienced accelerating decline in the 3 months prior to death • Fastest decline in independence occurred in the last month of life
Organ failure	Congestive heart failure or chronic lung disease on death certificate	20%	• Some disability 12 months before death • Varying functional disability consistent with exacerbations of disease in the following months • Somewhat accelerating decline in last 3 months of life, but not as quickly as group with cancer
Frailty	Those with a nursing home stay	20%	• High baseline disability 12 months before death • Experienced gradual, slow decline in last year of life • Markedly dependent in last month of life
Sudden death	No known history of cancer, organ failure, diabetes, hip fracture, or stroke	15%	• Low levels of dependence in the 12 months before death that persisted throughout last years of life
Other	Unclassified, but 40% had ischemic heart disease as underlying cause of death	24%	• Generally, a gradual decline over 12 months

Source: From Lunney JR, Lynn J, Foley DJ, et al. Patterns of Functional Decline at the End of Life. *JAMA.* 2003;289(18):2387. doi:10.1001/jama.289.18.2387

Table 21.2 Physical Signs/Symptoms in the Last Hours of Life (50)

Frequency	Vital signs and bedside measurements	Sign/symptom
Almost all (~75%–100%)	• Palliative Performance Scale ≤20%	
More than half (50%—~75%)	• Heart rate >100 • RASS of –2 or lower	• Urinary incontinence • Dysphagia
Many (~25%–50%)	• Oxygen saturation ≤90% on measurement • Respiratory rate >20 • Systolic blood pressure <100 mmHg • Urine output <100 mL/12 hr	• Drooping of nasolabial fold • Decreased response to visual and verbal stimuli • Inability to palpate radial artery pulse • Fecal incontinence • Cheyne-Stokes respiration • Death rattle • Periods of apnea • Respirations with mandibular movement • Cyanosis
Less common (<25%), but still potentially normal depending on disease process and patient history	• Fever (>38.5°C) • Systolic blood pressure >140	• Myoclonus

Source: From Hui D, dos Santos R, Chisholm G, et al. Bedside clinical signs associated with impending death in patients with advanced cancer: preliminary findings of a prospective longitudinal cohort study. *Cancer*. 2015;121(6):960–967. doi:10.1002/cncr.29048

ASSESSING AND REDUCING BOTHERSOME SYMPTOMS AT EOL

In general, the most important factor when deciding whether to treat a symptom is the level of distress the symptom is causing (see Table 21.5). Assessing level of distress of the patient is complicated by limitations in communication as the patient nears EOL; nonverbal indicators of discomfort are extremely important to assess at regular intervals, preferably via the use of an instrument validated in the relevant population.

The following behaviors in nonverbal patients should alert providers to presence of pain/discomfort and a search for a source, if unknown (see Table 21.6):

• Facial grimace

Table 21.3 Physical Signs/Symptoms Seen in the Last 2 Weeks of Life Based on Weighted Prevalence From a Systematic Review (51)

Frequency	Sign/symptom
Almost all (~75%–100%)	• Cyanosis • Respirations with mandibular movement
More than half (50%–~75%)	• Bed bound • Dry mouth • Dyspnea • Respiratory secretions • Weakness
Many (~25%–50%)	• Anorexia/reduced appetite • Bowel problems other than constipation and diarrhea • Constipation • Cough • Dysphagia/trouble swallowing • Edema • Fatigue • Fever • Incontinence • Increased sleeping • Pain • Paralysis • Sedation
Less common (<25%), but still potentially normal depending on disease process and patient history	• Abdominal swelling • Cachexia • Candidiasis • Dehydration • Diarrhea and other bowel problems not including constipation • Falls • Hemoptysis • Hemorrhage • Mouth sores • Myoclonus • Nausea/vomiting • Oral problems • Pruritus • Seizures • Skin integrity problems • Sleep problems • Urinary problems

Source: From Kehl KA, Kowalkowski JA. A Systematic Review of the Prevalence of Signs of Impending Death and Symptoms in the Last 2 Weeks of Life. *Am J Hosp Palliat Med.* 2013;30:601–616. doi:10.1177/1049909112468222

Table 21.4 Cognitive and Psychological Signs/Symptoms Seen in the Last 2 Weeks of Life (51)

Frequency	Sign/symptom
Almost all (~75%–100%)	None
More than half (50%–~75%)	None
Many (~25%–50%)	• Confusion
Less common (<25%), but still potentially normal depending on disease process and patient history	• Agitation • Anxiety • Depression • Hallucinations

Source: From Kehl KA, Kowalkowski JA. A Systematic Review of the Prevalence of Signs of Impending Death and Symptoms in the Last 2 Weeks of Life. *Am J Hosp Palliat Med.* 2013;30:601–616. doi:10.1177/1049909112468222

- Withdrawal from stimulus (e.g., moving hand away when it is touched)
- Rubbing or touching painful area
- Moaning
- Restlessness or agitation

For many common symptoms, there is very little high-quality evidence in the form of randomized, placebo-controlled trials available when

Table 21.5 Validated Tools for Assessing Pain/Discomfort in Nonverbal Patients (52)

Instrument	Population for which tool was developed
Behavioral Pain Scale (BPS)	Critically ill adults
Checklist of NonVerbal Pain Indicators (CNPI)	Adults with cognitive impairment
Critical Care Pain Observation Tool (CPOT)	Critically ill adults
Face, Legs, Activity, Cry, and Consolability (FLACC) Pain Tool	Pediatrics
Multidimensional Observational Pain Assessment Tool (MOPAT)	Noncommunicative palliative care populations, except those with dementia
Nociceptive Coma Scale (NCS)	Adults in vegetative or minimally conscious state
Nonverbal Pain Scale (NVPS)	Critically ill adults

Source: From McGuire DB, Kaiser KS, Haisfield-Wolfe ME, Iyamu F. Pain Assessment in Noncommunicative Adult Palliative Care Patients. *Nurs Clin N Am.* 2016;51:397–431. doi:10.1016/j.cnur.2016.05.009

Table 21.6 Commonly Used Interventions to Alleviate Non-Pain EOL Symptoms (4,11,41,53-61)

Symptom	Cause	Commonly used intervention/treatment
System		
Respiratory/pulmonary		
Noisy breathing (aka "death rattle")	• Pooling of oropharyngeal secretions • Ineffective pulmonary toilet	• Reassurance of normalcy to family • Repositioning patient • Gentle oropharyngeal mechanical suction • Anticholinergics such as glycopyrrolate and atropine commonly used, but these can contribute to delirium and have never been demonstrated to be better than placebo
Mandibular or "guppy" breathing	• Poorly understood, likely related to reflexive mechanisms • Death imminent	• Alert family to death within minutes to hours • Reassurance of normalcy, no specific treatment indicated
Cheyne-Stokes respirations (deep breaths followed by periods of apnea and shallow respirations)	• Failure of normal homeostatic mechanisms that control breathing in response to fluctuating oxygen and CO_2 levels (Rudrappa et al., 2017) most commonly due to heart failure or stroke, but occurs also at EOL	• Reassurance of normalcy to family • Diuresis • Position more upright in bed

(continued)

Table 21.6 Commonly Used Interventions to Alleviate Non-Pain EOL Symptoms (4,11,41,53–61) *(continued)*

Symptom		Cause	Commonly used intervention/treatment
Respiratory/pulmonary	Dyspnea	• Pulmonary edema • Hypercarbia • Acidosis • Pulmonary infiltrates/pneumonia • Aspiration • Pleural or pericardial effusion	• Opioids are preferred therapy, with morphine the best studied • Fan blowing cool air or oxygen by nasal cannula • Less evidence exists for benzodiazepines, diuretics, buspirone, SSRIs, but may be considered depending on disease process • Indwelling thoracentesis catheter in patient with recurrent malignant pleural effusions to control dyspnea without need for repeated painful thoracentesis
Gastrointestinal	Dysphagia	• Weakness • Possible obstruction	• Parenteral route of medication administration (i.e., buccal, rectal, subcutaneous, transdermal)
	Thirst, dehydration, dry mouth	• Poor PO intake • Volume depletion • Medication side effect	• Increasing recognition that dehydration may cause discomfort from thirst or contribute to/cause delirium, but giving artificial hydration may not be in line with patient's stated wishes, and may cause problems such as third spacing • Assess aspiration risk and allow PO intake for comfort • Mouth care and lip care reduce discomfort from dry mucous membranes

(continued)

Table 21.6 Commonly Used Interventions to Alleviate Non-Pain EOL Symptoms (4,11,41,53-61) *(continued)*

Symptom	Cause	Commonly used intervention/treatment
Anorexia or reduced appetite	• Exact cause unknown, suspected to be related to decreased ability to digest nutrients	• Recognize that food is often used to provide comfort and care and can be highly distressing to families when patients stop eating • Provide anticipatory guidance that body is changing and no longer requires energy input • Reassure families that loved ones' disinterest in food is not a rejection of their attempts to show care
Neurologic/ psychiatric	• Exact cause unknown • May be exacerbated by medication side effects	• Behavioral and environmental modification should be cornerstone of treatment through minimizing excess noise, promoting normal sleep–wake cycle, reorienting the patient, avoiding restraints if possible, involving family to talk to and calm patient • Antipsychotics/neuroleptics are commonly used, but limited high quality evidence exists regarding efficacy exists in terminally ill patient populations, and a very recent RCT demonstrated placebo was superior to haloperidol or risperidone in patients receiving palliative care • Benzodiazepines should not be used to treat delirium; if used for another indication, their need should be reassessed as they can contribute to delirium and agitation paradoxically
Restlessness and delirium		

deciding which treatments, if any, to employ (53). In such instances and in absence of evidence of patient discomfort, informing caregivers and family that such symptoms are natural, normal, and expected may ease concerns. If symptoms are accompanied by verbal or nonverbal indications of discomfort, attempting treatment is then indicated. When adding a new medication, a common effective approach is to "start low and go slow," that is, starting at the lowest possible effective dose and increasing dose slowly, over 24 to 48 hours typically with frequent reassessment for efficacy and unwanted side effects.

SPECIAL SITUATIONS RELEVANT TO EOL MEDICATION MANAGEMENT

- De-escalation of nonessential medications that are not directly treating symptoms can help avoid excessive pill-burden. Medications that are not controlling active symptoms but could cause discomfort or complications if discontinued (e.g., long-term steroids, antiarrhythmics) should typically be continued.
- Ensure caregivers are trained in non-oral routes of administration for medications for patients with dysphagia and have medications available.
- Pain medications can pre-emptively be given prior to situations that are known to cause discomfort, such as turning or moving patient.
- Anticipatory prescribing is the process of ensuring that essential medications for control of symptoms are available in a 24- to 72-hour supply such as opioids and benzodiazepines, especially if the patient is dying outside of an acute care hospital (62).

END-OF-LIFE EMERGENCIES

Certain situations that occur at EOL are so distressing, uncomfortable, or traumatizing for the patient or family that they warrant addressing even if they are part of the normal progression of the disease process. These situations may necessitate escalation of treatment to a higher level of care for the purpose of symptom control, such as an inpatient hospice unit or palliative medicine unit. For patients in especially high-risk groups for certain emergencies, advance planning and discussion of contingency plans may mitigate distress (see Table 21.7) (63).

PALLIATIVE SEDATION

For some patients with refractory symptoms, including pain and agitation, palliative sedation with the intent to relieve symptoms by suppressing consciousness (but not hasten death) is used. The efficacy of this technique to relieve symptoms, improve well-being, and quality of life has not been rigorously demonstrated. However, it does not appear to decrease survival time (67). It may be considered as an option for patients with truly refractory and highly distressing symptoms. Practitioners considering palliative sedation should document prior treatments and outcomes, need for sedation, and obtain informed consent in the presence of patient and family.

Table 21.7 End-of-Life Emergencies (64,65,66)

	Cause/pathophysiology	At-risk population	Recommended approach
Hemorrhage	• Disseminated intravascular coagulation most commonly from infection or malignancy • Liver failure • Anticoagulant side effect	• Intra-abdominal tumors • Hematologic malignancies	• Epinephrine-soaked tamponades • Tranexamic acid • Desmopressin • Keep dark towels/sheets easily available • Have line in place if patient is high-risk for administration of rapid palliative sedation in case of uncontrollable hemorrhage
Airway obstruction	• Mass effect (i.e., tumor compressing trachea)	• Intrathoracic malignancy	• Palliative sedation
Opioid-induced neurotoxicity: myoclonus, hyperalgesia, seizures	• Buildup of opioid metabolites, especially in renal failure • Idiosyncratic	• Those on high doses of opioids, especially morphine with renal failure • Those receiving meperidine	• Avoid morphine in ESRD • Avoid meperidine for pain control at EOL • Rotate opioid • Benzodiazepines

(continued)

Table 21.7 End-of-Life Emergencies (64,65,66) *(continued)*

	Cause/pathophysiology	At-risk population	Recommended approach
Seizures	• CNS metastases or primary tumors • Metabolic derangements • Withdrawal of medications in patient with pre-existing epilepsy • CNS hemorrhage	• Those with known CNS metastases or primary tumors • Those with prior CVA and suspected hemorrhagic conversion • Those with pre-existing epilepsy	• IV or SC lorazepam 2 to 4 mg, repeated in several minutes if seizure continues • Diazepam or midazolam also likely effective • Phenytoin or phenobarbital second line for status epilepticus
Acute bowel obstruction	• Mass effect (compression or invasion of bowel by tumor) • Intestinal adhesions	• Intra-abdominal or pelvic malignancy	• Nasogastric tube placement to suction if available • Corticosteroids • Somatostatin analogues

CNS, central nervous system; CVA, cerebrovascular accident; ESRD, end-stage renal disease.

Source: From Schrijvers D. Emergencies in palliative care. *Eur J Cancer.* 2011;47:S359–S361. doi:10.1016/S0959-8049(11)70203-9; Smith LN, Jackson VA. How do symptoms change for patients in the last days and hours of life? In: Goldstein N, Morrison R, eds. *Evidence-based practice of palliative medicine.* Philadelphia, PA: Elsevier Saunders; 2013:218–226; Tradounsky G. Seizures in palliative care. *Can Fam Physician.* 2013;59(9):951–955. http://www.pubmedcentral.nih.gov/articlerender.fcgi?artid=3771721&tool=pmcentrez&rendertype=abstract

- Medications used for palliative sedation, either alone or in combination (68):
  - Benzodiazepines: Primarily midazolam, but also lorazepam and diazepam
  - Phenobarbital
  - Propofol
  - Dexmedetomidine

OTHER ASPECTS OF EOL CARE IMPORTANT TO PATIENTS AND FAMILIES

In addition to treatment of physical, cognitive, psychological, and spiritual needs, patients and families have indicated other concerns for EOL care.

Patients at the end of life report the following aspects as extremely important (11,48,49):

- Reassurance they will receive expert care from interdisciplinary staff who know the patient as an individual
- Good communication with providers regarding prognosis and expectations
- Avoidance of being perceived as a burden to others and the maintenance of dignity

Families of patients who are at EOL additionally reported the following aspects as important (48,49):

- Valuing the family's role in care, such as their knowledge of their loved one's preferences and history, and including family in conversations and decision making
- Receiving information about financial affairs, funeral planning, and support (varies by health system and country)

Family members should be informed of their options for funeral/memorial services as well as arrangements for their loved one's body (cremation, burial). If a patient wishes, he or she may express preferences for the family to consider. Choosing a funeral home can assist with arrangements and can be done prior to the patient's death. These vary by locality.

Healthcare providers should inform families that the funeral home will be contacted after a patient dies to transport the patient's body.

CARE AFTER DEATH

Care after death is very important to families and should not be overlooked or minimized (see Table 21.8) (69). Attention to the following aspects helps provide closure to family members and assists with the burden of detail planning.

- Immediately after death, ask family permission to clean and prepare the body and dress in clean clothes or gown.
- Allow family to spend time with patient's body if desired, including time for additional family members to arrive.

Table 21.8 Examples of Post-Mortem Body Care and Rituals by Non-Christian Religions

Religion	Body care	Rituals
Islam	Autopsies avoided as body is seen as sacred Care should be provided by member of religion and same sex Body may be positioned to face the East Burial to occur as soon as possible because embalming is uncommon Body is bathed and wrapped in a plain cloth Body is given a ground burial	The Muslim call to prayer at time of death Iman not required to be present at time of death
Judaism	Euthanasia forbidden Withdrawal of care controversial Limited use of autopsies The body should not be left alone	Any personal belongings with the patient's blood must be buried with body Cremation is forbidden Death is followed by an intense mourning period called "shiva" with multiple requirements for dress and household arrangements
Buddhism	Autopsies or embalming should not happen until 3 days after death Western routine postmortem body care accepted Body is cremated	Death seen as a "rebirth" so a clear calm mind and serene surroundings important Mourning is lengthy so that loved ones can help the deceased through the death transformation
Hinduism	Cremation is preferred and done soon after death, as some loved ones desire to fast until completed Body is laid in a coffin decorated with sandalwood paste and garlands	Remains are usually scattered in a body of water Anniversaries of the death are commemorated with sacred rites Extensive, lengthy mourning is discouraged

Source: Adapted from Wolfe J. (2011). Easing distress when death is near. In: Wolfe J, Hinds PS, ed. *Textbook of interdisciplinary pediatric palliative care*. Philadephia, PA: Elsevier Saunders; 2011:368–384.

- Assess whether family would like presence of chaplain or other spiritual support.
- Engage interdisciplinary team to offer assistance with identifying a funeral home or document choice of funeral home, and assess family's plan for patient's body (i.e., cremation or burial).
- Assess whether family is planning memorial service or funeral; if so, encourage family to consider gathering music, photos, or other special memories in anticipation of the service.

ETHICS

Ethical factors related to death and dying are central to many cultural and legal aspects of societies. Thus, variability in perceptions and practices with respect to death and dying is to be expected and appreciated.

- Controversy continues regarding withdrawal or withholding of life-sustaining care that is not in the patient's best interest.
- Brain death
  - Usually caused by neurological injuries such as from traumatic brain injury from abuse, motor vehicle accidents, or asphyxia/anoxia
  - Defined by essentially universal neurological criteria, including a series of tests, and irreversibility
  - May require agreement of multiple practitioners to diagnose
  - Not recognized by all religions, although once cardiorespiratory support is withdrawn, death is imminent
- Many steps in EOL process have come to have legal manifestations
  - Pronouncement, medical record documentation, and death certificate completion
  - Notification to the medical examiner if any circumstances surrounding the death are unusual or unclear
- Organ donation is becoming increasingly necessary given wider access to transplant surgeries worldwide, but is still a difficult topic to raise for care providers in many situations

REFERENCES

1. Childhood Cancer Statistics. (n.d.). https://curesearch.org/Childhood-Cancer-Statistics
2. *Comprehensive Cancer Care for Children and Their Families: Summary of a Joint Workshop by the Institute of Medicine and the American Cancer Society.* (2015). *The National Academies Collection: Reports funded by National Institutes of Health.* Washington; DC: National Academic Press. http://eutils.ncbi.nlm.nih.gov/entrez/eutils/elink.fcgi?dbfrom=pubmed&id=26203485&retmode=ref&cmd=prlinks%5Cnpapers3://publication/uuid/0C6027CD-D9EC-4089-816D-4B48D24AFA41
3. WHO Cancer Fact Sheet. *WHO.* 2017. http://www.who.int/mediacentre/factsheets/fs297/en
4. National Institute for Health and Care Excellence. *Care of Dying Adults in the Last Days of Life.* 2015. nice.org.uk/guidance/ng31
5. Ranallo L. Improving the Quality of End-of-Life Care in Pediatric Oncology Patients Through the Early Implementation of Palliative Care. *J Pediatr Oncol Nurs.* 2017;34:374–380. doi:10.1177/1043454217713451
6. Villanueva G, Murphy MS, Vickers D, et al. End of life care for infants, children and young people with life limiting conditions: summary of NICE guidance. *BMJ.* 2016;355:i6385. doi:10.1136/BMJ.I6385

7. Wolfe J, Orellana L, Ullrich C, et al. Symptoms and distress in children with advanced cancer: prospective patient-reported outcomes from the PediQUEST study. *J Clin Oncol*. 2015;33:1928–1935. doi:10.1200/JCO.2014.59.1222

8. Chan RJ, Webster J, Bowers A. End-of-life care pathways for improving outcomes in caring for the dying. *Cochrane Database Syst Rev*. 2016. doi:10.1002/14651858. CD008006.pub4

9. Mularski RA, Dy SM, Shugarman LR, et al. A systematic review of measures of end-of-life care and its outcomes. *Health Serv Res*. 2007;42:1848–1870. doi:10.1111/j.1475-6773.2007.00721.x

10. Benini F, Vecchi R, Lazzarin P, et al. The rights of the dying child and the dutes of healthcare providers: the "Trieste Charter." *Tumori*. 2017;103:33–39. doi:10.5301/tj.5000566

11. Clark K. Care at the very end-of-life: dying cancer patients and their chosen family's needs. *Cancers*. 2017;9:11. doi:10.3390/cancers9020011

12. Teno JM. Family Perspectives on End-of-Life Care at the Last Place of Care. *JAMA*. 2004;291:88. doi:10.1001/jama.291.1.88

13. Bluebond-Langner M, Beecham E, Langner R, Jones L. Preferred place of death for children and young people with life-limiting and life-threatening conditions: a systematic review of the literature and recommendations for future inquiry and policy. *Palliat Med*. 2013;27(278):705–713. doi:10.1177/0269216313483186

14. Brock KE, Steineck A, Twist CJ. Trends in End-of-Life Care in Pediatric Hematology, Oncology, and Stem Cell Transplant Patients. *Pediatric Blood & Cancer*. 2016;63(3):516–522. doi:10.1002/pbc.25822

15. Centers of Disease Control and Prevention, Multiple causes of death data. http://wonder.cdc.gov/mcd.html

16. Noje C, Bernier ML, Costabile PM, et al. Pediatric critical care transport as a conduit to terminal extubation at home: a case series. *Pediatric Crit Care Med*. 2017;18(1):e4–e8. doi:10.1097/PCC.0000000000000997

17. Sanderson A, Burns JP. Withdrawal of Life-Sustaining Therapy at Home. *Pediatr Crit Care Med*. 2017;18(1):92–93. doi:10.1097/PCC.0000000000001005

18. McConnell T, Porter S. The experience of providing end of life care at a children's hospice: a qualitative study. *BMC Palliat Care*. 2017;16(1):15. doi:10.1186/s12904-017-0189-9

19. Centers for Medicare and Medicaid Services Hospice Center. (n.d.). https://www.cms.gov/Center/Provider-Type/Hospice-Center.html

20. Medicare Hospice Benefits. *Center for Medicaid and Medicare Services*. Baltimore, MD: U.S. Department of Health and Human Services; 2017. https://www.medicare.gov/Pubs/pdf/02154-Medicare-Hospice-Benefits.pdf

21. Gazelle G. Understanding Hospice — An Underutilized Option for Life's Final Chapter. *N Engl J Med*. 2007;357(4):321–324. doi:10.1056/NEJMp078067

22. Turner R, Rosielle D. Medicare Hospice Benefit Part I: Eligibility and Treatment Plan. 2015. https://www.mypcnow.org/blank-jvz8r

23. Turner R, Rosielle DA. Medicare Hospice Benefit Part III: Special Interventions. 2015. https://www.mypcnow.org/blank-mj26x

24. Turner R, Rosielle DA. Medicare Hospice Benefit Part II: Places of Care and Funding. 2016. https://www.mypcnow.org/blank-ipt3p

25. National Hospice and Palliative Care Organization (NHPCO). *The Medicare Hospice Benefit*. 2015; https://www.nhpco.org/sites/default/files/public/communications/Outreach/The_Medicare_Hospice_Benefit.pdf

26. Henderson A, Young J, Herbert A, et al. Preparing pediatric healthcare professionals for end-of-life care discussions: an exploratory study. *J Palliat Med*. 2017;20(6):662–666. doi:10.1089/jpm.2016.0367

27. Sullivan J, Monagle P, Gillam L. What parents want from doctors in end-of-life decision-making for children. *Arch Dis Child*. 2014;99:216–220. doi:10.1136/archdischild-2013-304249

28. Psychosocial Support and Research Program- Educational Materials. (n.d.). https://ccr.cancer.gov/Pediatric-Oncology-Branch/psychosocial/education

29. Wiener L, Zadeh S, Battles H, et al. Allowing adolescents and young adults to plan their end-of-life care. *Pediatrics*. 2012;130(5):897–905. doi:10.1542/peds.2012-0663

30. Delany C, Xafis V, Gillam L, et al. A good resource for parents, but will clinicians use it?: Evaluation of a resource for paediatric end-of-life decision making. *BMC Palliat Care*. 2017;16(1):12. doi:10.1186/s12904-016-0177-5

31. Zadeh S, Pao M, Wiener L. Opening end-of-life discussions: how to introduce Voicing My CHOiCES™, an advance care planning guide for adolescents and young adults. *Palliat Support Care*. 2015;13(3):591–599. doi:10.1017/S1478951514000054

32. Wiener L, Battles H, Mamalian C, Zadeh S. ShopTalk: a pilot study of the feasibility and utility of a therapeutic board game for youth living with cancer. *Support Care Cancer*. 2011;19(7):1049–1054. doi:10.1007/s00520-011-1130-z

33. End of Life Games. (n.d.). https://www.dyingmatters.org/page/end-life-games

34. Five Wishes. Tallahassee, Florida: Aging with Dignity. 2011. https://agingwithdignity.org/docs/default-source/default-document-library/product-samples/fwsample.pdf?sfvrsn=2

35. My Gift of Grace: A Conversation Game for Living and Dying Well. (n.d.). https://www.mygiftofgrace.com

36. The GoWish (TM) Game. (n.d.). http://www.gowish.org

37. Ando M, Morita T, Akechi T, et al. Efficacy of short-term life-review interviews on the spiritual well-being of terminally ill cancer patients. *J Pain Symptom Manage*. 2010;39(6):993–1002. doi:10.1016/j.jpainsymman.2009.11.320

38. Chochinov HM, Hack T, Hassard T, et al. Dignity therapy: A novel psychotherapeutic intervention for patients near the end of life. *J Clin Oncol*. 2005;23:5520–5525. doi:10.1200/JCO.2005.08.391

39. Chochinov HM, Kristjanson LJ, Breitbart W, et al. Effect of dignity therapy on distress and end-of-life experience in terminally ill patients: a randomised controlled trial. *Lancet Oncol*. 2011;12(8):753–762. doi:10.1016/S1470-2045(11)70153-X

40. Puchalski C. Spirituality. In: Berger A, Shuster JL, Von Roenn JH, eds. *Principles and Practice of Palliative Care and Supportive Oncology*. Philadelphia, PA: Lippincott Williams and Wilkins; 2013:702–718.

41. Candy B, Jones L, Varagunam M, et al. Spiritual and religious interventions for well-being of adults in the terminal phase of disease. *Cochrane Database Syst Rev*. 2012;(5):CD007544. doi:10.1002/14651858.CD007544.pub2

42. Byock I. *Dying Well-Peace and Possibilities at the End of Life*. New York, NY: Berkley Publishing Group; 1997.

43. Broadhurst K, Harrington A. A thematic literature review: the importance of providing spiritual care for end-of-life patients who have experienced transcendence phenomena. *Am J Hosp Palliat Med*. 2016;33(9):881–893. doi:10.1177/1049909115595217

44. Fenwick P, Brayne S. End-of-life experiences: reaching out for compassion, communication, and connection-meaning of deathbed visions and coincidences. *Am J Hosp Palliat Care*. 2011;28(1):7–15. doi:10.1177/1049909110374301

45. Lunney JR, Lynn J, Foley DJ, et al. Patterns of functional decline at the end of life. *JAMA*. 2003;289(18):2387–2392. doi:10.1001/jama.289.18.2387

46. Seow H, Barbera L, Sutradhar R, et al. Trajectory of performance status and symptom scores for patients with cancer approaching the last six months of life. *J Clin Oncol*. 2011;29:1151–1158. doi:10.1200/JCO.2010.30.7173

47. Dikkers MF, Dunning T, Savage S. Information needs of family carers of people with diabetes at the end of life: a literature review. *J Palliat Med*. 2013;16:1617–1623. doi:10.1089/jpm.2013.0265

48. Virdun C, Luckett T, Davidson PM, Phillips J. Dying in the hospital setting: a systematic review of quantitative studies identifying the elements of end-of-life care that patients and their families rank as being most important. *Palliat Med*. 2015;29:774–796. doi:10.1177/0269216315583032

49. Virdun C, Luckett T, Lorenz K, et al. Dying in the hospital setting: a meta-synthesis identifying the elements of end-of-life care that patients and their families describe as being important. *Palliat Med*. 2017;31(7):587–601. doi:10.1177/0269216316673547

50. Hui D, dos Santos R, Chisholm G, et al. Bedside clinical signs associated with impending death in patients with advanced cancer: Preliminary findings of a prospective longitudinal cohort study. *Cancer*. 2015;121(6):960–967. doi:10.1002/cncr.29048

51. Kehl KA, Kowalkowski JA. A Systematic Review of the Prevalence of Signs of Impending Death and Symptoms in the Last 2 Weeks of Life. *Am J Hosp Palliat Med.* 2013;30:601–616. doi:10.1177/1049909112468222

52. McGuire DB, Kaiser KS, Haisfield-Wolfe ME, Iyamu F. Pain Assessment in Noncommunicative Adult Palliative Care Patients. *Nurs Clin N Am.* 2016;51:397–431. doi:10.1016/j.cnur.2016.05.009

53. Jansen K, Haugen DF, Pont L, Ruths S. Safety and effectiveness of palliative drug treatment in the last days of life - a systematic literature review. *J Pain Symptom Manage.* 2017;55:508–521.e3. doi:10.1016/j.jpainsymman.2017.06.010

54. Agar MR, Lawlor PG, Quinn S, et al. Efficacy of Oral Risperidone, Haloperidol, or Placebo for Symptoms of Delirium Among Patients in Palliative Care. *JAMA Intern Med.* 2017;177:334. doi:10.1001/jamainternmed.2016.7491

55. Awan S, Wilcock A. Nonopioid medication for the relief of refractory breathlessness. *Curr Opin Support Palliat Care.* 2015;9:227–231. doi:10.1097/SPC.0000000000000149

56. Barbetta C, Currow DC, Johnson MJ. Non-opioid medications for the relief of chronic breathlessness: current evidence. *Exp Rev Respir Med.* 2017;11(4):333–341. doi:10.108 0/17476348.2017.1305896

57. Barnes H, McDonald J, Smallwood N, Manser R. Opioids for the palliation of refractory breathlessness in adults with advanced disease and terminal illness. In: Barnes H, ed. *Cochrane Database of Systematic Reviews.* Chichester, UK: John Wiley & Sons, Ltd; 2016, vol. 3:CD011008

58. Grassi L, Caraceni A, Mitchell AJ, et al. Management of Delirium in Palliative Care: a Review. *Curr Psychiatry Rep.* 2015;17. doi:10.1007/s11920-015-0550-8

59. Mccann RM, Hall WJ, Groth-Juncker A. Comfort Care for Terminally Ill Patients The Appropriate Use of Nutrition and Hydration. *JAMA.* 1994;272:1263–1266. doi:10.1001/jama.1994.03520160047041

60. Rosseau P, Vaughan L. Management of Symptoms in the Actively Dying Patient. In: Berger AM, Shuster JL, Von Roenn JH, eds. *Principles and Practice of Palliative Care and Supportive Oncology.* Philadelphia, PA: Lippincott Williams and Wilkins; 2013:688–701.

61. Wee B, Hillier R. Interventions for noisy breathing in patients near to death. In: Wee B, ed. *Cochrane Database of Systematic Reviews.* Chichester, UK: John Wiley & Sons, Ltd; 2008.

62. Finucane AM, Stevenson B, Gardner H, et al. Anticipatory prescribing at the end of life in Lothian care homes. *Br J Commun Nurs.* 2014;19(11):544–547. doi:10.12968/bjcn.2014.19.11.544

63. Nauck F, Alt-Epping B. Crises in palliative care-a comprehensive approach. *Lancet Oncol.* 2008;9:1086–1091. doi:10.1016/S1470-2045(08)70278-X

64. Schrijvers D. Emergencies in palliative care. *Eur J Cancer.* 2011;47:S359–S361. doi:10.1016/S0959-8049(11)70203-9

65. Smith LN, Jackson VA. How do symptoms change for patients in the last days and hours of life? In: Goldstein N, Morrison R, eds. *Evidence-based practice of palliative medicine.* Philadephia, PA: Elsevier Saunders; 2013:218–226

66. Tradounsky G. Seizures in palliative care. *Can Fam Physician.* 2013;59(9):951–955. http://www.pubmedcentral.nih.gov/articlerender.fcgi?artid=3771721&tool=pmcentrez&rendertype=abstract

67. Beller EM, van Driel ML, McGregor L, et al. Palliative pharmacological sedation for terminally ill adults. In: Beller EM, ed. *Cochrane Database of Systematic Reviews.* Chichester, UK: John Wiley & Sons, Ltd; 2015. doi:10.1002/14651858.CD010206.pub2

68. Bodnar J. A review of agents for palliative sedation/continuous deep sedation: pharmacology and practical applications. *J Pain Palliat Care Pharmacother.* 2017;31:16–37. doi:10.1080/15360288.2017.1279502

69. Steinhauser KE, Voils CI, Bosworth H, Tulsky JA. What constitutes quality of family experience at the end of life? Perspectives from family members of patients who died in the hospital. *Palliat Support Care.* 2015;13(4):945–952. doi:10.1017/S1478951514000807

70. National Hospice and Palliative Care Organization (NHPCO). Pediatric concurrent care. 2016; https://www.nhpco.org/sites/default/files/public/ChiPPS/Continuum_Briefing.pdf

Advance Care Planning for Adult and Pediatric Cancer Patients 22

Katalin Eve Roth and Maureen E. Lyon

INTRODUCTION

Advance care planning (ACP) is a process that provides patients and their families guided time to communicate about their treatment goals and preferences, and to convey these preferences to their physicians. In pediatrics ACP has afforded children, parents and families the precious space and the language to navigate the disease trajectory and to enhance their autonomy even as their illness might advance. For adults it affords the opportunity for patients to participate in their medical decision making and provides a forum for the expression of goals and values as well as a means to control their illness journey.

Modern medicine has helped thousands of seriously ill infants and children live longer lives. Pediatric advance care planning (pACP) is essential to bring attention to the quality of these longer lives—for both the affected children and their families and to prepare them for future medical decision making. Barriers to pACP include legal issues unique to advance care planning (ACP) with children and adolescents. Legally they have no voice in decisions about their own end-of-life (EOL) care. The legal guardian is the decision maker and presumed to act in the best interest of the child. It is assumed that children and adolescents lack the maturity or capacity to discuss these issues. There is fear of distressing already vulnerable children and adolescents. Furthermore, there is the dread of the powerful emotions that are stirred up in ourselves when facing a death that is "out of season." Finally, some providers and researchers believe initiating end-of-life discussions with children is inappropriate, potentially harmful, ineffective or will cause the patient and family to lose hope. But hope has many constellations. To quote one mother, Victoria Sardi-Brown, Mattie's Mother of Mattie Miracle Cancer Foundation, "Once I found out we were dealing with EOL care, I did have hope. Hope changes along the continuum. When hope for a cure went out the window, then we hoped for a more sound, humane, and less painful death. Empowerment and communication go hand in hand." As we illustrate, there is now an evidence base to support high quality and effective pACP, which minimizes suffering, while increasing the family's understanding of their child's wishes through facilitated communication in a developmentally sensitive and culturally informed way about EOL treatment preferences, if the worst were to happen.

WHAT IS ACP?

ACP is a process that provides patients and their families guided time to communicate about their treatment goals and preferences, and to convey these preferences to their physicians.

ACP may include documentation of wishes, such as completion of an Advance Directive or a Living Will document, and designation of surrogate decision makers, but it may also take the form of extended conversations between patients and their treating physicians, and patients and their loved ones or their trusted healthcare proxies. Documentation of ACP may be used to guide physicians and family members on choices regarding interventions, surgeries, and initiation of life support. Conversations regarding ACP may be in written format, in a Living Will or Advance Directive, or in another document format such as "Five Wishes" (fivewishes.org) or in an online module like the "Letter to My Doctor" in the Stanford Letter Project (med.Stanford.edu/letter/advancedirective.html). Some ACP takes place in conversations in the doctor's office, and office notes that describe patient preferences may constitute evidence of ACP. Legal requirements for ACP may vary among jurisdictions, and some jurisdictions may require witnessed or notarized documentation of wishes, particularly preferences to refuse life-saving interventions or treatment.

ACP provides designation of a healthcare proxy or surrogate decision maker, who can step in and honor the patient's preferences if and when the patient becomes unable to speak for himself or herself. Such a surrogate decision maker, also known as a Durable Power of Attorney, or DPOA, should ideally speak from the perspective of the patient, articulating the known values and aspirations of the patient who becomes incapacitated. While decision making may default by law or custom to the nearest kin, nearest relatives may not agree with or know the treatment and outcome preferences of the patient, and ACP provides a mechanism to designate a surrogate who is respectful of the patient's values. When there are a number of adult children who may disagree among themselves about treatment goals and acceptable quality of outcome, the designated surrogate speaks for the patient.

WHAT ARE THE ADVANTAGES OF ACP?

Research has demonstrated that:

- **ACP improves patient participation in healthcare decision making and improves autonomy and patient dignity.**
- **ACP can improve communication between patients and their healthcare providers.**
- **ACP may increase the use of palliative care and hospice, and most importantly, may increase patient satisfaction and quality of life.**
- **ACP has been shown to decrease readmission to hospitals.**

DEFINITIONS

While definitions vary, recent working groups in America and Europe have achieved consensus regarding what ACP for adults should include (1,2). ACP is seen as a *process* rather than a discrete moment in time, which acknowledges that patient choices and preferences may change as their circumstances change and patients adapt to serious health limitations. A document such as a Living Will or Advance Directive or a Physician Orders for Life-Sustaining Treatment (POLST) form (polst.org) may embody ACP at a specific time and may be relied upon to guide treatment decisions. However, it is well understood that patient preferences may change over the course of a treatment journey.

Traditionally ACP has not been undertaken except when persons faced severe or life- threatening illness, but it is increasingly viewed as an important process for persons facing the infirmities of aging as well. As illness may strike suddenly and unpredictably and is no respecter of age, it may be important for persons to share their life goals and preferences for treatment with their physicians and their family members whenever challenges might be anticipated.

Many cancer centers now include recommendations for a palliative consultation, including ACP, at the beginning of embarking on a course of treatment, particularly when the diagnosis is severe. The American Society of Clinical Oncology (ASCO) now recommends an initial palliative care consultation for all new stage 3 and stage 4 solid tumors and for all newly diagnosed hematologic malignancies. When facing serious disease and treatments, which themselves carry risks of serious side effects, it is an excellent time for persons to reflect upon their goals.

Doctors are not always comfortable discussing potential bad outcomes and most physicians feel that projecting confidence gives patients courage. Furthermore, given the paternalism and power differential inherent in the doctor–patient relationship, it may be difficult for patients to assert limitations on treatment plans or to disagree with physician choices for aggressive care. Other members of the healthcare team, such as social workers, nurses or patient navigators, may be more neutral initiators of ACP conversations. Patients and surrogates can also undertake ACP alone, utilizing some of the excellent online resources now readily available (e.g., theconversationproject.org; med.Stanford.edu/letter/advance-directive.html).

Many states now require that there be some discussion between physicians and their patients prior to hospital discharge and that patients have available to them formal implementation of their wishes through POLST legislation. POLST is an approach to improving end-of-life care in the United States, encouraging providers to speak with patients and create specific medical orders to be honored by healthcare workers during a medical crisis. POLST includes order sets that can follow the patient from clinic to hospital to discharge to nursing home to hospice, stipulating the kinds of interventions the patient does or does not want. Typical treatments addressed in POLST forms are resuscitation, comfort care, intubation, blood transfusions, kidney dialysis, and artificial nutrition. POLST forms also serve as directives to ambulance and emergency personnel so that patient wishes are respected at all times.

Historical, Ethical, and Legal Considerations

In the United States, the principles of autonomy and informed consent have long established that individuals may refuse medical treatments and may make choices regarding different therapies. Dramatic legal cases such as those involving Karen Ann Quinlan, Nancy Cruzan, and Terry Schiavo have established that patients and families may choose to terminate or withhold medical treatment that does not accord with patient or surrogate wishes. In 1990, in response to patients' concerns, the Patient Self-Determination Act (PSDA) was passed, establishing firmly that medical providers must respect the wishes of patients to continue, choose, or discontinue treatment, and recognize that different individuals may place different weights on the benefits, burdens, and risks of treatment.

Bioethical principles of autonomy, beneficence, and respect for persons requires:

- Patient participation in medical decision making
- Informed consent for treatments
- An understanding of the person's life history, values, and goals
- Consideration of the patient as an individual in a social and psychological context

ACP supports palliative medicine and the ethical provision of medical care through:

- Respect for individual treatment choices
- Reflection about treatment goals
- Reflection about how to live one's life in the face of serious illness
- Communication between patient and physician
- Communication between patient and family and loved ones
- Consideration and designation of a trusted individual to act as surrogate decision maker
- Conversation between patient and surrogate regarding goals

Severe illness raises the possibility of mortality, and thorough ACP requires persons to consider the possibility that they may not get better. Although doctors traditionally avoid financial discussions, at times it is imperative to raise the issue of financial disposition, wills, and guardians with patients. Patients who have minor children and those who are caregivers for dependent adults may be especially concerned about how their illness and treatment choices might impact their responsibilities. Elderlaw specialists are attorneys who help patients plan for aging, disease, and infirmity; with the skill sets of traditional trusts and estate lawyers, they also have special sensitivity for health-related decision making. Elderlaw attorneys may help foresee complicated situations and help patients feel confident that they and their loved ones will be properly cared for. These lawyers also understand that illness may require one or more visits to the hospital or bedside to complete necessary paperwork.

Palliative specialists may also wish to become familiar with the concept of "ethical wills," in which people consider important life concerns. Repayment of debts, financial or emotional, reconciliation with old friends or relatives from whom the person may have become estranged, and charitable gifts to beloved religious, educational, or other institutions may give the person peace of mind before undergoing arduous treatment.

ACP IS A PROCESS AND A PROCEDURE

The palliative specialist understands that ACP is not something that can be done quickly, or be accomplished merely by leaving some forms at a bedside. Conversations may take place over a long period of time, and need to elicit patient concerns and values. Use of interactive tools may help clarify the patient's values, but these are adjuncts, not substitutes for conversation.

Respect for process is very important. The Center to Advance Palliative Care (CAPC; www.capc.org) and other sites are helpful to provide practical tools for the palliative specialist undertaking ACP. It is impossible to clarify goals and values without knowing something about a person's life—these are not "magic" questions but they require a true curiosity for a patient's biography and life journey. The first step is to find out where the patient has been and hoped to go before illness interrupted this life journey—the patient grew up, went to school, and worked, and the status of relationships with parents, family, and others, as well as avocations, hobbies, and passions. Often, what the patient's experience of severe illness and loss may have been in the past will also have a bearing on future choices and concerns. When the patient feels understood by the palliative team, future discussions about care preferences and goals are eased.

The palliative specialist should have the names and phone numbers of a few trusted elderlaw specialists, so that referrals can be made. Relatedly, in the case of individuals who have young children or who have dependents such as older parents or a disabled sibling, ACP gives them an opportunity to plan for substitutes to help shoulder their responsibilities. ACP may involve consideration of writing letters to one's children or grandchildren, or videotaping messages.

ACP With Children and Adolescents

ACP is the gold standard in the care of patients with life-limiting illnesses, but its practice is limited in pediatrics (3). To date, there is no national or international consensus regarding the definition of pACP. The ultimate goal of pACP is to relieve suffering (physical, psychological, spiritual) through timely conversations, and thereby maximize quality of life for seriously ill children and their families. In multiple studies, adolescents and young adults with cancer and HIV have reported that ACP was useful and worthwhile (11,12), and that having an ACP document that addressed end-of-life issues was useful as well (4). Every child and family should be invited to decide on an end-of-life plan to the degree each finds it comfortable and be provided with care and support during this process (5). The Initiative for Pediatric Palliative Care (IPPC; www.ipfcc.org/best-practices/ipe/ippc.html) was a national project that supported informing children with life-threatening illnesses and involving them in decisions regarding their care as fully as possible, given their developmental abilities and desires; the American Academy of Pediatrics (6) and the World Health Organization (7) also support this.

For the purposes of this chapter, pACP is operationally defined as a process that has three key elements for effective achievement of these aims:

- Supporting communication with children/adolescents at any stage of a serious illness in understanding and sharing their understanding of their illness, complications, fears, worries, and hopes/life goals, as well as treatment preferences regarding future medical care with their family.

- Communication of these goals of care and treatment preferences to the treating physician.
- Documentation of these goals of care and end-of-life treatment preferences in the electronic health record.

The best timing of these conversations from the adolescent's point of view should be before death is imminent, as adolescents living with HIV and cancer have expressed the thought that waiting too long would be too stressful and expressed concern that their families might think they were "giving up" (4). This timing preference is illustrated in Figure 22.1 where adolescents living with HIV were surveyed (8), replicating an earlier survey of adolescents with cancer (9).

The field of pediatric palliative care is still determining if trained/certified facilitators are an essential component of the pACP communication process with seriously ill adolescents. If this is a key component, who should these trained certified facilitators be? Should the conversation between the adolescent and family be facilitated by the treating physician, or certified/trained healthcare professionals, paraprofessionals, or volunteer peers? In surveys adolescents with HIV have reported a preference to have these conversations with their physician (8).

There is a consensus that conversations matter and that advance directives alone are insufficient. How critical is the inclusion of the family to this process? Is it the family who will speak for the child or adolescent

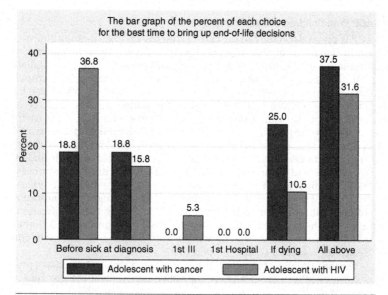

Figure 22.1 Adolescents' preference for timing of discussions about end-of-life care.

if the child or adolescent cannot communicate? Or is it sufficient to have a conversation between a healthcare professional and the adolescent? Currently there are three pediatric hospital-based models available. Adolescent and family responses to participating in the FACE-pACP model are presented in Box 22.1.

- *FOOTPRINTS*[SM] is a model developed for adolescents living with a life-limiting illness and includes ACP facilitated by staff and care coordination and treatment plans directed by the "continuity physician" regardless of site of care. More than 90% of families and healthcare providers reported satisfaction with this model (10).

- *FAmily CEntered (FACE™ pACP) pACP* is a recognized, theoretical and evidence-based model, which engages seriously ill adolescents (cancer, HIV) and their families in conversations facilitated by trained/certified staff. FACE is a structured weekly 3-session intervention (Lyon Advance Care Planning Survey©; Next Steps: Respecting Choices Interview®; advance directive the Five Wishes®). Documented outcomes of the FACE model include (a) high ratings of satisfaction by both adolescents and their families (11); (b) increased family understanding of adolescents' goals of care and end-of-life treatment preferences (12,13); (c) improved quality of life (14,15); (d) decreased physical symptoms (16); (e) increased antiretroviral medication adherence (17,18); and (f) increased feelings of peace (15,18). Additionally documented is the significant influence of religious practices and spiritual beliefs on quality of life outcomes of FACE adolescents (16,19), as well as end-of-life treatment preferences (20), making it important

---

Box 22.1 Adolescent Responses to FACE pACP

Adolescent Responses to Participating in FACE pACP

- "I felt that it helped a lot and it helps my family and healthcare provider with more insight if I have a life-threatening illness."
- "I liked the situation questions because they made me think."
- "It was a good session. I learned a lot about what to think about—good thought process."

Family Responses to Participating in FACE pACP

- "This was a relief. This session got me to think about a family member's death and it was nice to know what that person would like. I always want to know what my son thinks."
- "I think it was outstanding, essential. I pray that after the research is done, it will become standard for the hospital."
- "It was productive in that it went to a place I hadn't gone to before in a subtle way."

FACE pACP, FAmily CEntered pediatric Advance Care.

for healthcare professionals to inquire about both when working with these adolescents and their families. Finally, FACE was documented as being included in the medical chart and easy to locate there by healthcare professionals (15,21)

- *Voicing My CHOICES*™ is a model currently being tested with young adults by Wiener and colleagues. This model was originally developed with adolescents diagnosed with HIV and cancer (4,22). Wiener and colleagues are now exploring whether having an ACP document completed with a healthcare professional fosters future discussions with family and friends and the primary healthcare provider regarding the adolescent's personal goals, values, or beliefs.

In conclusion, comparative effectiveness trials of these different models of ACP and pACP are needed, as well as a consensus on culturally sensitive outcomes of interest to seriously ill adolescents and their families. ACP requires effective communication to clarify the goals of care and establish agreement on what treatments may or may not be appropriate to achieve these goals, including resuscitative and palliative measures (23).

Pediatric Resources

- The National Institute of Nursing Research (NINR), Palliative Care: Conversations Matter® campaign to increase the use of palliative care for children and teens living with serious illnesses. Web site contains information for children, teens and families. www.ninr.nih.gov/newsandinformation/conversationsmatter/conversations-matter-newportal

- National Cancer Institute, Research-tested Intervention Programs (RTIPS). FAmily-CEntered Advance Care Planning for Teens with Cancer (FACE-TC) is designed to enhance the quality of life for teens with cancer or HIV and their caregivers. (2013). The program focus is psychosocial–coping and was developed for adolescents (11–18 years) and young adults (19–21 years). rtips.cancer.gov/rtips/programDetails.do?programId=17054015

- My Wishes,® *Voicing My CHOICES*™ and Five Wishes® can be viewed and obtained at www.agingwithdignity.org

- PEDIATRIC CONVERSATION STARTER KIT. A new resource created by The Conversation Project for parents of critically ill children, Pediatric Starter Kit: Having the Conversation with Your Seriously Ill Child, is available for free download. The kit offers advice and provides stories from parents and palliative care specialists who have been there, and offers questions that can help parents navigate the approach to the conversation based on the personality and cognitive level of the child. theconversationproject.org/starter-kits

- ChiPPS E-Journal Pediatric Palliative and Hospice Care Issue #39; May, 2015 Issue Topic: Advance Planning in Pediatric Hospice/Palliative Care, Part Two Produced by the ChiPPS E-Journal Work Group. www.nhpco.org/sites/default/files/public/ChiPPS/ChiPPS_ejournal_Issue-39.pdf

- Speak Up Ontario has many resources for pACP, including videos. www.advancecareplanning.ca/national-community-of-practice-for-advance-care-planning-educators/document-library/pediatric-advance-care-planning
- Center to Advance Palliative Care (CAPC)–Courageous Parents Network has training available in pACP media.capc.org/filer_public/0b/61/0b616f5d-84db-4730-b131-474a11951806/courageous_parents_network_peds_cme_course_flyer.pdf
- CAPC Pediatric Care Field Guide: A Catalogue of Resources, Tools and Training to Promote Innovation, Development and Growth media.capc.org/filer_public/58/70/587067d2-ba65-4263-a29e-25dca6b2e0df/peds_pc_field_guide_111116.pdf

REFERENCES

1. Sudore RL, Lum HD, You JJ, et al. Defining advance care planning for adults: a consensus definition from a multidisciplinary delphi panel. *J Pain Symptom Manage.* 2017;53(5):821–832. doi:10.1016/j.jpainsymman.2016.12.331
2. Rietjens JAC, Sudore RL, Connolly M, et al. Definition and recommendations for advance care planning:an intrnational consensus supported by the European Association for Palliative Care. *Lancet Oncol.* 2017;18:e543–e550. doi:10.1016/S1470-2045(17)30582-X
3. Lotz JD, Jox RJ, Borasio GD, Fuhrer M. Pediatric advance care planning: a systematic review. *Pediatrics.* 2013;131(3):e873–e880. doi:10.1542/peds.2012-2394
4. Wiener L, Ballard E, Brennan T, et al. How I wish to be remembered: the use of an advance care planning document in adolescent and young adult populations. *J Palliat Med.* 2008;11(10):1309–1313. doi:10.1089/jpm.2008.0126
5. Wolff T, Browne J. Organizing end of life care: parallel planning. *Pediatr Child Health.* 2011;21:378–384. doi:10.1016/j.paed.2011.04.007
6. Feudtner C, Friebert S, Jewell J, from the American Academy of Pediatrics. Pediatric palliative care and hospice care commitments, guidelines, and recommendations: Section on hospice and palliative medicine and committee on hospital care. *Pediatrics.* 2013;132:966–972. doi:10.1542/peds.2013-2731
7. World Health Organization. WHO Definition of Pediatric Palliative Care. 2014. http://www.who.int/cancer/palliative/definition/en
8. Lyon ME, Dallas RH, Garvie PA, et al. A pediatric advance care planning survey: Congruence and discordance between adolescents with HIV/AIDS and their families. *BMJ Support Palliat Care.* (In Press).
9. Jacobs S, Perez J, Cheng YI, et al. Teen end of life preferences and congruence with their parents' wishes: results of a survey of teens with cancer. *Pediatr Blood Cancer.* 2015;62:710–714. doi:10.1002/pbc.25358
10. Toce S, Collins MA. The FOOTPRINTS^SM model of pediatric palliative care. *J Palliat Med.* 2003;6:989–1000. doi:10.1089/109662103322654910
11. Dallas RH, Kimmel A, Wilkins ML, et al. A randomized controlled trial of FAmily-CEntered (FACE) advanced care planning for adolescents with HIV/AIDS: Emotions, acceptability, feasibility. *Pediatrics.* 2016;138(6):e20161854. doi:10.1542/peds.2016-1854
12. Lyon ME, Jacobs S, Briggs L, et al. Family Centered Advance Care Planning for Teens with Cancer. *JAMA Pediatr.* 2013;167:460–467. doi:10.1001/jamapediatrics.2013.943
13. Lyon ME, D'Angelo LJ, Dallas, R, et al. A randomized controlled clinical trial of adolescents with HIV/AIDS: pediatric advance care planning. *AIDS Care.* 2017;29(10):1287–1296. doi:10.1080/09540121.2017.1308463
14. Lyon ME, Garvie PA, Briggs L, et al. Is it safe? Talking to teens with HIV/AIDS about death and dying: A 3-month evaluation of family centered (FACE) advance care planning – anxiety, depression, quality of life. *HIV/AIDS Res Palliat Care.* 2010;2:27–37. doi:10.2147/hiv.s7507

15. Lyon ME, Jacobs J, Briggs L, et al. Longitudinal Randomized Controlled Trial of Advance Care Planning for Teens with Cancer: Anxiety, Depression, Quality of Life, Advance Directives, Spirituality. *J Adolesc Health*. 2014;54:701–717. doi:10.1016/j.jadohealth.2013.10.206

16. Lyon ME, Garvie PA, D'Angelo LJ, et al. Advance Care Planning and HIV Symptoms in Adolescence. *Pediatrics*. 2018;142(5):e20173869. doi:10.1542/peds.2017-3869

17. Lyon ME, Dallas, R, Wilkins, M, et al. Does advance care planning increase medication adherence in HIV+ teens? (ind143432). 122nd Annual convention of the American Psychological Association: Washington, DC; August 2014.

18. Lyon ME, Garvie PA, Kao E, et al. Spirituality in HIV-infected adolescents and their families: FAmily CEntered (FACE) advance care planning and medication adherence. *J Adolesc Health*. 2011;48:633–636. doi:10.1016/j.jadohealth.2010.09.006

19. Lyon ME, Kimmel AL, Cheng YI, Wang J. The role of religiousness/spirituality in health-related quality of life among adolescents with HIV: a latent profile analysis. *J Relig Health*. 2016;55(5):1688–1699. doi:10.1007/s10943-016-0238-3

20. Lyon ME, Cheng YI, Wang J, for the Adolescent Palliative Care Consortium. Longitudinal randomized controlled trial of advance care planning for teens: religiousness and end of life treatment preferences. *J Adolesc Health*. 2016;58:S84. doi:10.1016/j.jadohealth.2015.10.180

21. Lyon ME, Garvie PA, McCarter R, et al. Who Will Speak for Me? Improving end-of-life decision-making for adolescents with HIV and their families. *Pediatrics*. 2009;123:e199–e206. doi:10.1542/peds.2008-2379

22. Wiener L, Zadeh S, Battles H, et al. Allowing adolescents and young adults to plan their end-of-life care. *Pediatrics*. 2012;130:891–905. doi:10.1542/peds.2012-0663

23. Tsai E; Canadian Paediatric Society (CPS), Bioethics Committee. Advance care planning for paediatric patients. *Paediatr Child Health*. 2008;13(9):791–796. doi:10.1093/pch/13.9.791

Index